Travel Medicine for Health Professionals

Calderdale and Huddersfield NHS
NHS Trust

Travel Medicine for Health Professionals

Larry I Goodyer

BPharm MPharm PhD MRPharmS
Head of Leicester School of Pharmacy
Faculty of Health and Life Sciences
De Montfort University
Leicester
UK

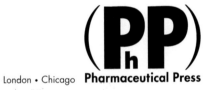

London • Chicago **Pharmaceutical Press**

Published by the Pharmaceutical Press
Publications division of the Royal Pharmaceutical Society of Great Britain

1 Lambeth High Street, London SE1 7JN, UK
100 South Atkinson Road, Suite 206, Grayslake, IL 60030-7820, USA

© Pharmaceutical Press 2004

(**PP**) is a trade mark of Pharmaceutical Press

First published 2004

Text design by Barker/Hilsdon, Lyme Regis, Dorset
Typeset by Photoprint, Torquay, Devon
Printed in Great Britain by TJ International, Padstow, Cornwall

ISBN 0 85369 511 3

A catalogue record for this book is available from the British Library

I would like to dedicate this book to my wife Sandy who has enabled me to complete this project in so many ways, from that first trip to India to the final proofreading.

I would also like to give special thanks to my brother Paul and the staff at Nomad who gave so much inspiration towards my attempt at making this a practical text for those working in diverse areas of travel medicine.

Contents

The colour plate section is between pages 144 and 145

Preface

My interest in travel medicine probably dates to a backpacking trip to India with my wife in 1988. At the time I was working as a hospital pharmacist in London so was well equipped with medicines and first-aid supplies, and had a reasonable knowledge of how to minimise the risk of gastrointestinal disease and other travel-related health problems. While we were travelling around Northern India we met two broad categories of fellow backpackers: those whose only medical supplies consisted of a box of plasters and those who carried a veritable field hospital in their rucksacks, the latter often being sons and daughters of doctors. Fortunately we remained fit and well throughout our trip; however we gave away much of our supplies to various travellers. Also both my wife and I, who is a nurse, were frequently asked for advice about managing the usual range of problems that such travellers encounter. This convinced me of the need for better preparing these types of traveller for their trips overseas. At this time travel medicine was not a recognised speciality, and the International Society of Travel Medicine (ISTM) was only founded in the early 1990s.

The spur for a direct involvement in travel medicine came when I helped to set up Nomad Medical in 1989. This company caters for a range of travellers, from young backpackers on their gap year through to expatriates and those planning large expeditions far from medical facilities. The Nomad stores consist of areas for specialist travel equipment and clothing, vaccination clinics and, uniquely, a dedicated travel pharmacy. The experience gained through Nomad has contributed greatly to the contents of this book.

There are now some excellent texts on travel medicine available to the health professional. The focus of this book fills a gap in having a product-oriented approach, in that it delves more deeply and broadly than other texts into the often-asked question by the traveller: 'What medicines and other health-related supplies do I need for my trip overseas?' The book is therefore aimed at the health professional who needs to give evidence-based advice addressing this important question. Medical products are the special province of the pharmacist and this book is particularly aimed at those working in community pharmacies. In addition the practice nurse and general practitioner with any involvement in travel medicine will find this text of practical use.

Inevitably one cannot separate a consideration of the supplies and prophylactic vaccinations from the general health promotion issues and the verbal advice given to travellers pre-departure. In order to highlight the most important points a section of frequently asked questions has been included in each chapter. The inspiration for some of these was derived from the TravelMed e-mail discussion group, run through the ISTM. This international group discusses a range of topical and varied questions raised by experts and practitioners. It has to be stressed that the answers quoted in response to these questions do not necessarily reflect the opinions of any members of this group and are based largely upon my own understanding of the available evidence.

Much, but by no means all travel medicine concerns avoiding and managing infections, whether contracted through insect bites, food and water or direct contact. The first few chapters are therefore devoted to this general subject area with an emphasis on medication, vaccination, water purification and bite avoidance. Adventure holidays are becoming more popular and a chapter is devoted to considering health problems associated with extreme environmental condition. There has been much media attention recently on the problems associated with air travel, particularly the risk of deep-vein thrombosis or exposure to contagious diseases such as severe acute respiratory syndrome (SARS). A chapter considers these areas together with the perennial problem of motion sickness. Another very well recognised area of health promotion associated with travel is overexposure to the sun and the chapter dealing with the potential dangers of sunburn and suntanning focuses particularly on the use of sunscreens. The final chapter presents an overview of medical and first-aid supplies that could be considered for different types of travellers and also discusses the management of bites and stings.

The role of the health professional is to consider the risks likely to be encountered by different travellers, and to help with preparation in terms of vaccination, malaria prophylaxis, health promotion, medical/first-aid supplies and other equipment. Nurses, general practitioners and pharmacists all have a role to play and I hope this book will provide a useful reference and educational tool for any health professional involved in preparing travellers for their trips overseas.

Larry Goodyer
September 2003

About the author

Professor Goodyer is currently Head of the Leicester School of Pharmacy at De Montfort University, Leicester. In 1989 he helped to set up and became a Director of the Nomad Travel Pharmacy, which specialises in the medical provision for those travelling overseas, from large sponsored expeditions to private individuals. As superintendent pharmacist of this company, Professor Goodyer is called upon to give advice to both members of the public and the medical profession. He lectures on many topics related to travel medicine and regularly contributes to a variety of books, journals and magazines. He has appeared on a number of live television and radio broadcasts concerning travel medicine.

Apart from travel medicine, his research interests include medicines management, non-medical prescribing and multimedia computer presentation systems in the pharmacy.

1

The role of the health professional and sources of information

Introduction

The discipline of travel medicine has grown in recent years, in parallel with the general rise in tourist travel, to the extent that in the USA it has been given its own name of 'emporiatrics', derived from the Greek for seafarer. The history of travel-related disease is a long one and can even be traced back to ancient times. For instance, it is recorded that the Athenian plague of 430 BC was probably spread via the trade routes. The first public health attempts to contain travel-related epidemics date to the plagues of the Middle Ages, where the practice was to detain ships and crews for 40 days, the word 'quarantine' being derived from the Latin for 40. The roots of the study of travel medicine date back to the late nineteenth century where morbidity and mortality amongst explorers and missionaries were extremely high. In one study at the time it was revealed that over a quarter of workers had to return due to their own or their family's ill health.[1] The subject of travel medicine is now a very broad term, referring to any travel-related hazard that can affect the individual's health, and the terms 'travel medicine' and 'travel health' are often used synonymously.

The risk to an individual's health may have two sources: the presence or increased incidence of diseases at the country of destination (e.g. tropical disease) or the hazards of travel and travel-related pursuits (e.g. travel sickness, environmental problems and accidents). In some cases it is the absence or poor quality of local medical facilities that also presents a hazard to health. Not to be underestimated is the likely impact of tourists on an overstretched health system. For the longer-term traveller there are additional psychological problems of adapting to a new culture and environment. More recently travel medicine has tended to include a study of health implications due to movement of displaced peoples, i.e. refugees, into host nations. The general range of travel health-related problems is shown in Box 1.1.

Box 1.1   Travel health hazards

- Infections: spread by insects, food- and water-borne, contact/inhalation
- Accidents
- Altitude/climate
- Travel sickness
- Dermatological, including sun hazards
- Iatrogenic
- Chronic illness

Much in the field of travel health involves preventive medicine, that is education of the travelling public in how to minimise the various hazards. For instance, appreciation that insect vectors transmit many tropical diseases encourages the use of methods for bite prevention. Similarly, knowing the ways in which diarrhoeal diseases are contracted will help define the various steps to be taken regarding food and water hygiene.

Pharmaceutical and related supplies also tend to be 'preventive' in nature – these include vaccines, antimalarial tablets, sunblocks and kits containing sterile equipment and chemicals for water purification. The management of medical problems once they occur should also be considered. Certain medicines may be in short supply or of poor quality and so should usually be purchased before travel.

For many people, the first consideration given to travel health is the planning of any recommended vaccinations, although, as will be discussed later, this does not necessarily represent the group of diseases posing the greatest risk. However, it does bring the traveller into contact with a health professional, usually the practice nurse or general practitioner (GP). The nurse or GP may only have a limited time for screening and advice, and, as in other general areas of health promotion, the community pharmacist also has an important role to play.

International travel, morbidity and mortality

International travel has undoubtedly increased over recent years. For instance, total visits abroad by UK residents rose from 11.8 million per year in 1970 to 31 million by 1989. Also there is a trend for increased travel to the tropics, with a 7% average annual growth rate to South-East Asia and a 5–10% growth in journeys to Africa. This compares with a growth of travel to Europe and the USA of just 5%, although these destinations still have by far the largest market share. These figures are based on predicted growth rates 1995–2020.[2]

The size and extent of the problem of travel-related illnesses have been quite well defined by a number of studies, the largest being carried out in Scotland,[3] Finland[4] and Switzerland.[5] The results are summarised in Table 1.1. A number of factors have been shown to increase risk, including area to be visited, age and length of time away. The Swiss study found that 75% of travellers to the tropics had at least one health-related problem, although only 5% of these were serious enough to warrant medical attention. The Finnish and Scottish studies mainly consisted of travellers to Spain or North America and reported health-related complaints in 48% and 43% of individuals respectively. Generally, the further south – and in Europe the further east – you go, the greater the chances of health-related problems. Both the Scottish and Swiss studies confirmed the highest number of problems in the 20–29-year age group.

Diseases for which vaccinations are available by no means account for the most likely source of morbidity and mortality. A number of studies[6–9] have established that the largest cause of death amongst travellers is related to cardiovascular disease, usually myocardial infarction, and this has been placed at between 35% and 70% of reported deaths. This trend may be partly due to an increase in travel by elderly people, although these deaths are not necessarily related to travel *per se*. Injury, mostly from motor accidents or drowning, is next on the list, at around 20% of deaths. This may be a reflection of the tendency for individuals to undertake activities that are more adventurous and dangerous than they would consider doing at home. It is interesting to note that death from infectious disease accounts for just 1–3% of cases.

Table 1.1 Incidence of illness as a percentage of holiday-makers

Condition	Incidence as percentage of holiday-makers		
	Swiss[5] (n = 10 555)	Scottish[3] (n = 2211)	Finnish[4] (n = 2665)
Diarrhoea	34	34	18
Respiratory	13	6	8
Sunburn/skin	6	4	10
Other	32 (14% constipation)	N/A	6

Potential problems associated with travel

The requirements and potential problems will vary depending on the profile of the traveller, as classified in Table 1.2.

Holiday-makers on short trips to westernised destinations, e.g. southern Europe, form the greatest proportion of travellers overseas and are not likely to visit a GP for pre-travel health advice, although many will visit pharmacies. In this group, advice regarding sun awareness and gastrointestinal infections might be the main areas of concern. Some individuals may also need help with problems connected to air travel or travel sickness. Reactions to bites or stings may also cause problems. High altitude may represent a hazard in a variety of destinations.

Holiday-makers to developing countries, in particular the tropics, e.g. sub-Saharan African or South-East Asia, will need additional advice relating to disease contracted from biting insects, particularly malaria. Also, for these destinations a vaccination schedule would need to be planned, ideally 2 or 3 months before travel.

Travellers and backpackers on longer-term trips tend to be of a younger age group and may be travelling independently or with one of the 'overland' companies. An example of the latter would consist of a group of 10–20 individuals in trucks on a 6-month trans-African tour.

Table 1.2 Levels of advice and support

Type of traveller	Requirements
Holiday-makers and travellers to westernised countries	Sun care Gastrointestinal Travel sickness Air travel Bites and stings
Holiday-makers and travellers on short trips to the tropics and developing nations	As above plus: Bite avoidance and malaria Vaccination (Altitude)
Travellers/backpackers on longer trips to the tropics	As above plus: Comprehensive medical kit
Expeditions	As above plus: Specialised medical kit Altitude and climate problems Envenomation

This type of traveller would be well advised to carry a fairly comprehensive medical kit, perhaps including antibiotics. The overland truck may well have an extensive kit, but individuals are always recommended to have their own supplies.

Providing a service to an expedition, whether scientific or exploratory, lies somewhat outside the scope of this book. Special considerations relating to medical supplies and climatic conditions will need to be taken.

Areas of involvement for health professionals

The health professional will be involved with four broad types of activity:

1. pre-travel advice (health promotion)
2. prescription and recommendation of medicines and medically related goods
3. vaccinations
4. problems of the returned traveller

The GP or practice nurse activity would tend to focus on the administration of vaccines, whereas the community pharmacist is also in a position to supply and advise on the use of medication and any other supplies for a medical kit.

There is the potential for travellers to receive conflicting advice. This may result, for instance, from a traveller inquiring after malaria prophylaxis from the GP and then using the internet, telephone advice lines or the local pharmacy as further sources of information. A further dimension is that the travel agent may offer different advice, with the tendency to underplay any particular requirements. A number of studies have identified that travel agents offer a generally poor level of service in this respect,[10,11] giving inconsistent and often incorrect advice. One study identified that few would offer advice spontaneously.[12] Also noted in a number of studies is that GPs themselves do not always offer the best support for travellers.[13] Unacceptable variability in advice of GPs has been noted, particularly regarding malaria prophylaxis. This may be due to the relatively small proportion of people seen by GPs for travel health advice. A further study has confirmed that practice nurses offer more pre-travel health advice and vaccinations than do GPs in the UK.[14] A reasonable level of knowledge concerning a variety of travel health-related issues was found in a study of Swiss pharmacists.[15] For interviews conducted over the phone pharmacists often gave incorrect advice concerning malaria prophylaxis, although half said that they would have

Table 1.3 Pre-travel interviews

Areas to be covered	Specific questions
Destination and itinerary	Reason for travel, e.g. business/pleasure Type of travel, e.g. hotel/backpack Special activities, e.g. trekking
Health status	Chronic conditions Current medication Recurrent conditions Allergies Psychological status Special needs
Pregnancy	
Previous history	Vaccinations given Reaction to malaria prophylaxis Altitude problems

referred to official documentation in reality. In a further interview scenario when such documents were used, correct advice was usually given.

This book considers a broad range of topics to help health professionals prepare the public for travel overseas. A particular emphasis is placed on the pharmaceutical and supply aspects of travel and in this area pharmacists in particular have an important role to play.

In order to determine what type of advice or range of supplies would be required, it is important to gather some basic information from the traveller, as outlined in Table 1.3. Of course, it may be unrealistic to cover all the points described in this table and health professionals would do well to identify the higher-risk groups referred to earlier for more in-depth discussion. Certain of these points should be covered by anyone asking for general support with a more adventurous holiday.

Most of the areas briefly discussed below will be considered in some detail in the specific chapters (see also Table 1.4).

Gastrointestinal disease

Clear advice on the management of diarrhoeal illness is important, as it is one of the most common problems and can be debilitating. The government publications listed in the section on sources of information, below, offer general advice to the public.

Table 1.4 Role of the health professional

Problem	Advice	Supplies and prophylaxis
Gastrointestinal	Food and water hygiene	Electrolyte replacement Antidiarrhoeal Antibiotics[a] Water purification
Sun	Sun protection	Sunscreens
Motion sickness	Measures to minimise	Anti-motion-sickness medication
Altitude problems	Measures to avoid	Drug treatments[a]
Sexual activity	Safe sex	Condoms Oral contraceptives[a]
Diseases spread by biting insects	Bite avoidance measures and prophylaxis	Repellents, insecticides, mosquito nets, malaria prophylaxis[b]
Vaccinations	General advice on schedules	Vaccines[a]
Wounds, bites and stings	Wound care	Dressings and antiseptic Sting relief
General hygiene and precautions	Specific advice	
Travellers with special needs	Ensuring necessary medical advice given	Medication for chronic conditions[a] Medication for exacerbation of acute problems[b]

[a] Prescribed.
[b] May need to be prescribed.

Sun care

There is a range of leaflets produced in response to a number of sun hazard awareness campaigns that can be used in conjunction with verbal advice. The supply and choice of sun screens are an important area for the pharmacist.

Air and sea travel

Although there are a number of medications available to prevent motion sickness particularly associated with sea travel, it is important to remember that practical advice can be given to help minimise the problem. The particular danger associated with developing deep-vein thrombosis during long-haul air flights has received much attention in recent years.

Altitude problems

Altitude sickness is potentially fatal, and simple useful advice can be offered to those intending a trip where this may be a risk. In certain circumstances drug treatment may be necessary, and health professionals should be aware of the various protocols that could be used.

Sexual activity

All health professionals have the general responsibility of promoting safe sexual practices. The advice offered will be the same, whether at home or abroad. It is also worth considering contraceptive advice, as some women of child-bearing age may wish to carry hormonal emergency contraception that may be difficult to obtain in certain countries.

Diseases spread by biting insects

All health professionals have an important part to play regarding malaria prophylaxis and recommendations for bite avoidance. The recommendation of the appropriate antimalarial prophylaxis is perhaps one of the most important, and sometimes contentious, areas in travel medicine. Access to the relevant sources of information, an understanding of the basic principles and the recognition of cases that should be referred for expert opinion is the responsibility of all offering advice in this area. Pharmacists in particular can supply most of the products employed in bite avoidance, as well as certain antimalarial tablets.

Vaccinations

One of the major motivations for travellers to seek advice is to obtain vaccination prior to travel. The usual point of contact in this case is the practice nurse, who must have a knowledge of the appropriate protocols to be followed in terms of selection and administration of vaccines.

Wound care

In the tropics, particularly if travelling in rough conditions, even a minor wound can develop into a chronic sore. Good wound care and the availability of a basic first-aid kit can avoid this.

General measures

There are a number of areas where specific advice may be needed. For instance, swimming in fresh water in Africa should be avoided owing to the risk of bilharzia. Dehydration or heat stroke is a potential hazard in hot climates if sensible measures are not taken.

Medication for chronic conditions

Of particular concern to the pharmacist would be the need to travel with medicines for chronic conditions. Any legal requirements, packaging, stability or general supply problems in the country of destination must be considered. In addition, even an occasional recurrent condition such as mild asthma or cystitis may be difficult to treat when overseas and it may be appropriate to carry a supply of any medication required. The general screening of individuals for fitness to travel and work overseas, which is determined by the mental and physical health of the individual, is beyond the scope of this book. Some consideration will be given to fitness for air travel.

The returned traveller

It would be virtually impossible for a primary care health worker to diagnose a tropical disease as in the first instance the symptoms can be non-specific. Inquiry after travel may be important if there are flu-like symptoms or general tiredness and lethargy. Current advice is to test for malaria if anyone describes flu-like symptoms after visiting a malaria-endemic area. Ideally, anyone presenting with such symptoms should be asked about travel over the previous year. Unusual eruptions or skin sores can sometimes be related to tropical diseases and may also need referral to specialists. Finally, a history of diarrhoea of a longer duration than a week may be related to a dysentery contracted overseas. General screening for tropical diseases in the returned traveller is not usually performed unless specific problems have been identified.

Sources of information

One of the most important aspects of travel medicine is ascertaining the potential health hazards for a particular destination and keeping abreast of current advice. This section aims to outline some of the resources that are available (Table 1.5).

Table 1.5 Sources of information

Organisation	Contact
Aventis Pasteur helpline	(44) 1628 773737
British Travel Health Association	(44) 141 300 1132 www.btha.org
Centers for Disease Control (US) Travelers' Health	www.cdc.gov/travel
Department of Health	PO Box 410, Wetherby LS23, UK (also Ceefax pp. 460–464)
Fit for Travel	www.fitfortravel.scot.nhs.uk
Foreign and Commonwealth Office	www.fco.gov.uk/travel
Health advice for travellers, Department of Health	www.doh.gov.uk/traveladvice/index.htm
Health Protection Agency, UK	www.hpa.org.uk
Hospital of Tropical Diseases, London	(44) 906 133 7733 www.uclh.org/services/htd/departments.shtml
International Society of Travel Medicine	www.istm.org/news.html
International Travel and Health, World Health Organization	www.who.int/ith/english/index.htm
Medical Advisory Service for Travellers Abroad (MASTA)	(44) 906 822 4100 www.masta.org/index.html
National Travel Health Network and Centre	(44) 207 380 9234 (9 a.m.–4.30 p.m.)
NHS Direct	www.nhsdirect.nhs.uk/
ProMed	www.promedmail.org
Royal Free, London	(44) 207 830 2885
Travax	www.travax.scot.nhs.uk/
Travelhealth, UK	www.travelhealth.co.uk
World Health Organization disease outbreaks	www.who.int/disease-outbreak-news/

Books, texts and charts

There are two major specialist texts on travel medicine. Richard Dawood's *Travellers' Health*[1] is written principally for the layperson but is of immense value to the health professional. Each chapter is written by an expert in the field and covers just about every aspect of the subject. The *Textbook of Travel Medicine and Health*[2] is written more for the health professional and, while not quite as broad as Dawood's book, covers some subjects in greater depth. A further similar text is *Principles and Practice of Travel Medicine*,[16] which gives further in depth insight and information regarding travel medicine.

The World Health Organization guide[17] gives a detailed description of the risks related to various destinations, and there are a number of charts and lists available that outline the current UK recommendations for vaccination and antimalarial prophylaxis. The main drawback is that they may not contain the most up-to-date information. Both the National Pharmaceutical Association and *British National Formulary* (BNF) guides on malaria prophylaxis are updated every 6 months. The GP magazine *Pulse* and *Medical Index of Monthly Specialities* (MIMS) produce regular updates on malaria and vaccine requirements. A useful regularly updated wall chart can also be obtained from Glaxo-SmithKline. Texts on specific subjects are referenced in each chapter in this book.

Leaflets

Leaflets on general travel health matters are produced from time to time by companies marketing vaccines or antimalarials. They may also produce more specialist information leaflets related to their field. General practices and pharmacies should stock supplies of the Department of Health booklet *Health Advice for Travellers* as well as leaflets relating to sun care as supplied by the health promotion units.

Advice lines

There are a number of advice lines, some of which are open to the general public, others taking calls from health professionals only. Those relating specifically to malaria prophylaxis are listed in the BNF. Contact details are summarised in Table 1.5.

Hospital of Tropical Diseases in London

This automatic phone line is open to the general public. By identifying the destination through a menu system, appropriate advice is given regarding malaria prophylaxis and vaccinations.

National Travel Health Network and Centre (NaTHNaC)

This network was set up in April 2003 in the UK as a collaboration between the PHLS, London School of Hygiene and Tropical Medicine and the HTD in order to consolidate and improve the various travel health resources available to health professionals within the UK. The centre is based in the HTD and has three initial priorities: operating a telephone advice service for health professionals, surveillance of travel-associated illness and administration of yellow fever vaccination centres.

Nomad Medical

Advice can be obtained from a travel health nurse or pharmacist and is open to the public. They specialise in advising and equipping longer-term travellers and expeditions.

Medical Advisory Service for Travellers Abroad (MASTA)

This was one of the first commercial organisations offering tailor-made advice to travellers on health issues. Members of the public can telephone MASTA and an automatic menu system will allow identification of a particular itinerary. A full briefing is then sent by post.

Royal Free Travel Health Centre

Specialist nurses offer a health line.

Communicable Disease Surveillance Centre

The services previously offered by this centre regarding travel health advice have been transferred to NaTHNaC.

Aventis Pasteur

This company runs a special health line as part of its product information service.

Electronic databases and internet sites

A large number of sites on the internet are based in the USA and do not reflect current UK guidelines. However, numerous sites contain information on general issues in travel medicine as well as searchable databases that identify malaria prophylaxis and vaccination requirements. Below is a selection of those available at time of print. Unfortunately, uniform resource locators (URLs) are liable to change or sites close down completely. As these sites tend to provide hyperlinks to others, mentioned below, it is worth persisting to find one that is running and then using that to access others whose web address may have changed.

Travax

This is an online database available from the Scottish Centre for Infection and Environmental Health. It provides accurate up-to-date information on vaccination schedules, malaria prophylaxis and other health hazards to specified destinations. Registration is available free for general practices. Also available to the general public is a shortened version, Fit for Travel, which lists vaccination schedules and malaria prophylaxis advice. Also included are useful maps showing the distribution of malaria in various countries.

World Health Organization (WHO)

For those keen on the latest news regarding disease outbreaks, the WHO website gives a listing of confirmed problems in its Communicable Disease Surveillance and Response (CSR) network. Also go to the International Travel and Health Section for general advice and detailed vaccination and malaria information. Be aware that advice on prophylaxis and vaccinations may not represent UK practice. Much of the country information found in the handbook described above can also be found at this site.

ProMed

This is an e-mail discussion group which acts as an early-warning system for unconfirmed reports of disease outbreaks from around the world. It is also possible for health professionals to sign up for postings from ProMed, although you will have to wade through a deluge of communications from health experts around the world discussing the latest outbreaks.

MASTA

This website contains a very useful search engine and database that allows you to enter an entire itinerary of many countries for a trip and then produces a list of recommendations for malaria prophylaxis and vaccinations. In addition, any country-specific problems are outlined as well as more general advice on staying healthy whilst away. Another interesting section is a jet lag calculator in which you enter the details of the flight and then a recommendation regarding alteration of sleeping patterns and sun exposure is produced. MASTA has an e-commerce section for its own products.

Foreign and Commonwealth Office

Misadventure due to crime or political instability in a country is also an important component of safe and healthy travel. This site provides country-by-country information regarding any potential threats to British nationals as well as tips of a general nature to avoid or resolve potential problems.

University College London Hospital of Tropical Diseases (HTD), Department of Travel Medicine

This website lists the contact numbers for their help lines and details regarding certain health-related products.

Travelhealth.co.uk

This is a nurse-led site, offering general travel health promotion to the travelling public.

Public Health Laboratory Service (PHLS) (now part of the Health Protection Agency)

On this site can be found the most recent guidelines concerning malaria prophylaxis from the malaria reference laboratory (see Chapter 4). Reviews also offer insights into trends for imported diseases amongst travellers.

Department of Health

The Department of Health has made available an electronic version of the *Health Advice to Travellers* booklet, described above.

Centers for Disease Control

This is a US government-run organisation and has a large section on travellers' health. Country-specific recommendations are given reflecting US policy.

Nomad

The Nomad website contains travel health information. You can also order general and more difficult to obtain travel health products.

Organisations

The International Society of Travel Medicine (ISTM) runs a biannual conference and is associated with the *International Journal of Travel Medicine*. It also runs a worthwhile website and members can join the informal but very informative e-mail discussion group. The British Travel Health Association (BTHA) is very active and all health workers with any involvement in travel medicine in the UK should join. All members are given free access to Travax as well as receiving their educational/news bulletin *Travelwise* and the BTHA research journal.

References

1. Dawood R, ed. *Travellers' Health: How to Stay Healthy Abroard*, 3rd edn. Oxford: Oxford University Press, 2002.
2. DuPont H L, Steffen R, eds. *Textbook of Travel Medicine and Health*, 2nd edn. Hamilton, Canada: BC Decker, 2001.
3. Reid D, Dewar R D, Fallon R J *et al*. Infection and travel: the experience of package tourists and other travellers. *J Infect* 1980; 2: 356–370.
4. Peltola H, Kyronseppa H, Holsa P. Trips to the south – a health hazard. *Scand J Infect Dis* 1983; 15: 375–381.
5. Steffen R, Rickenbach M, Willhelm U *et al*. Health problems after travel to developing countries. *J Infect Dis* 1987; 156: 84–91.
6. Hargarten S W, Baker T D, Guptill K. Overseas fatalities of United States citizen travellers: an analysis of deaths related to international travellers. *Ann Emerg Med* 1991; 20: 622–626.
7. Sniezek J E, Smith S M. Injury mortality among non-US residents in the United States 1979–1984. *Int J Epidemiol* 1991; 19: 225–229.

8. Pociv P. Deaths of Australian travellers overseas. *Med J Aust* 1995; 163: 27–30.

9. Piaxao M L T, Dear R D, Cossar J H *et al.* What do Scots die of when abroad? *Scot Med J* 1991; 36: 114–116.

10. Lawler D A, Burke J, Bouskill E *et al.* Do British travel agents provide adequate health advice for travellers? *Br J Gen Pract* 2000; 50: 567–568.

11. Harris C B, Welshy P D. Health advice and the traveller. *Scot Med J* 2000; 45: 14–16.

12. Grabowski P, Behrens R H. Provision of health information by British travel agents. *Trop Med Int Health* 1997; 4: 102–103.

13. Leggat P. Sources of health advice given to travelers. *Int J Travel Med* 2000; 7: 85–88.

14. Carroll B, Behrens R H, Crichton D. Primary health care needs for travel medicine training in Britain. *J Travel Med* 1998; 5: 3–6.

15. Kodkani N, Jenkins J M, Hatz C F. Travel advice given by pharmacists. *J Travel Med* 1999; 6: 87–93.

16. Zuckerman J, ed. *Principles and Practice of Travel Medicine.* Chichester, UK: Wiley, 2001.

17. International Travel and Health. Geneva, World Health Organization. Available online at: www.who.int/ith/index.html.

2

Travellers' diarrhoea

Montezuma's revenge, Aden gut, Basra belly . . . there is an almost endless list of names used to describe the syndrome referred to as travellers' diarrhoea (TD). Of all the travel health hazards, a bout of diarrhoea is the most likely. It has been estimated that 30–50% of travellers from industrialised nations who visit developing countries will suffer from an episode of TD, representing around seven million individuals a year[1] (Fig. 2.1). Although it is usually a self-limiting problem resolving within 3–5 days, there are some important considerations:

- 3–5 days out of a 2-week holiday could still represent a ruined itinerary, which could be particularly distressing if the trip was expensive. This becomes even more important if the holiday was only of a week's duration.
- For important business or political meetings, a bout of TD could inhibit performance to the extent that the trip would be regarded as a failure.
- Some travellers are at a potentially greater risk from the effects of TD, e.g. the young, old or immunosuppressed.
- A developing country gaining a reputation for a high incidence of TD can suffer a loss of vital revenue from tourism.
- Persistent diarrhoea, continuing on return from abroad, can result in days lost from work and reduced performance.

The high incidence of TD in developing countries is believed to be linked to problems concerning sanitation and food handling which, due to economic and other constraints, are not as well regulated as in industrialised nations. This has resulted in the concept that travellers should be educated in hygiene measures, about both food and water, in an attempt to reduce the incidence of TD. This will be dealt with in greater depth in Chapter 3.

For the health professional, the most important issues are an understanding of both the potential role of prophylactic measures and the management of TD using oral rehydration, antimotility agents and antimicrobials. These aspects will be discussed in this chapter, together with other important considerations linked to the epidemiology, aetiology and symptoms of TD.

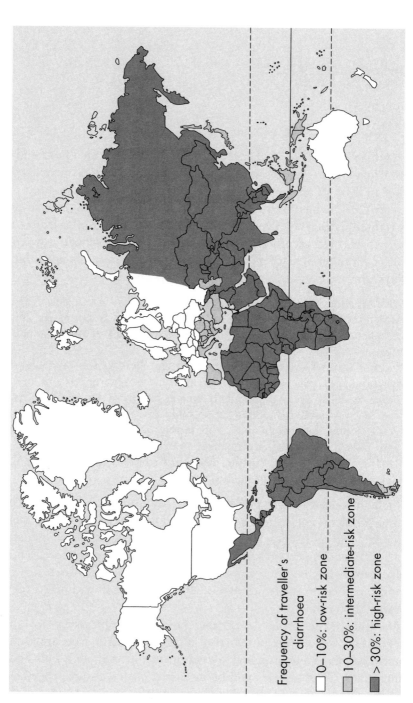

Figure 2.1 Distribution of travellers' diarrhoea. Courtesy of Eric Caumes.

Definition and symptoms of travellers' diarrhoea

A recognised working definition of the syndrome of TD[2] is accepted as: three to four unformed stools in 24 hours and at least one of the following symptoms:

- abdominal pain
- nausea
- vomiting
- fever
- cramps
- blood or mucus in the stools
- faecal urgency

Some of the enteric symptoms, such as cramps, abdominal pain and urgency, will occur quite frequently. Vomiting and blood in the stools occur in fewer than 10% and fever in up to 30% of cases.

Typically, TD is considered an acute problem and diarrhoea lasting longer than 14 days might be classified as a chronic or persistent diarrhoea, considered by some as a separate entity.[3] It has been suggested that the term 'persistent TD' is used to describe symptoms for more than 14 days and chronic TD for symptoms of greater than 30 days.[4] Whether or not the TD is classified as acute, persistent or chronic will largely depend upon the causative agent; *Giardia* is listed as a potential cause of TD and symptoms of infection with this organism can persist for many weeks or months if untreated.

There is also some difficulty in classifying the relative severity of a bout of TD. The following system has been proposed:[1]

- mild – one to two unformed stools in 24 hours with tolerable symptoms
- moderate – more than three unformed stools in 24 hours with distressing symptoms
- severe – fever and/or blood in the stools, plus more than three unformed stools in 24 hours with incapacitating symptoms

There is a fine line between the symptoms individuals would consider tolerable or those they might find distressing. For instance, in which category would you place a woman suffering just one or two massive bouts of diarrhoea that she finds particularly distressing? The definition of severe diarrhoea is perhaps more helpful, implying a dysentery which would need further investigation with a view to specific antimicrobial therapy.

TD tends to be seen within the first week of travel and peaks 3 days after arrival; over 90% of cases have occurred within the first 2 weeks.[5] A study in travellers to Mexico staying longer than 2 weeks found a wider spread in reports, with nearly half of the subjects experiencing diarrhoea in the second 2 weeks of their stay.[6]

Around 30% of patients may be bed-ridden and 40% are forced to change their itinerary. Fewer than 1% will require hospitalisation. Only 3% are reported to develop persistent diarrhoea lasting longer than 2 weeks and 1–2% have diarrhoea lasting longer than a month. The severity of symptoms does vary to some extent with the pathogen involved and there is a weak association between severity and the likelihood of identifying a responsible pathogen. In around 50% of cases the diarrhoea will resolve spontaneously after 48 hours, the average duration being 4 days.

Epidemiology

The risk of contracting diarrhoea in some areas is remarkably similar to that observed amongst children in the local population,[7] leading to the assumption that adaptation and developing immunity to certain pathogens play an important part. There are a number of factors that must be taken into account.

Destination

The relative risk of TD for various destinations is summarised in Table 2.1. Underreporting tends to occur in many of the studies which attempt to assess the scale of the problem and the figures in the higher range are probably more representative. Generally, TD is more likely if visiting countries in the summer months, perhaps reflecting an increase in the local fly population. This variation in incidence due to destination has been well illustrated in a study[8] which examined 322 patients returning to Austria who presented to their GP with persistent diarrhoea, from

Table 2.1 Incidence of travellers' diarrhoea: percentage of travellers affected for each country visited[2]

<7%	10–20%	20–50%
USA	Southern Europe	Africa
Canada	Israel	Latin America
Middle Europe	Japan	Middle East
Australia	South Africa	Asia
New Zealand		

which 97 were found to have one or more pathogens in their faeces. A much higher incidence of diarrhoea was reported for Asia than any other destination. A large study of over 60 000 people returning from visits to Kenya, India, Jamaica and Brazil found that Kenya and India represented the highest risk with around 50% of visitors reporting TD.[9] Surprisingly the rate was significantly higher amongst those from the UK who also appeared to suffer more severe symptoms than those originating from other countries. The authors could find no obvious explanation for this observation.

Length of stay and prior travel

There is a relationship between length of stay and a tendency to develop immunity to subsequent bouts of TD. This is supported by the observation that those travelling from one developing nation to another are at less risk than those travelling from industrialised countries.[10]

In a study involving a large number of American travellers away for less than 90 days[11] the risk of diarrhoea appeared to rise by 2% for each day of travel despite the destination. This increase in risk with duration appeared to rise across the whole length of stay and over half of those who had more than one bout of diarrhoea travelled for longer than 1 month.

The risk to expatriates does fall over time but there is still a substantial occurrence of diarrhoeal illness, as was evident from a study conducted in Nepal.[12] Furthermore, the expatriates in this study showed a high level of pathogens present in normal stool samples. It is likely that tolerance can develop to enterotoxigenic *Escherichia coli* (ETEC), but individuals remain susceptible to the other organisms responsible for TD.

Other work by Shlim *et al.*[7] has indicated that those living overseas might be at risk for up to the first 2 years of residence. Forty-two per cent of cases of diarrhoea amongst those living in Nepal were still identified as being due to ETEC within the first 3 months of residence, although this incidence of infection due to ETEC diminished significantly after that time. This may explain the observation by Hill[11] that multiple episodes of TD were still observed in travellers after a month. Other organisms observed within this time period included: *Cyclospora* (32%), *Giardia* (16%) and *Entamoeba* (6%). They did note a reduction in TD in those who had been away for longer than 2 years.

It is also likely that inexperienced travellers are at a greater risk of TD (possibly due to inadequate food and water hygiene measures), as are those travelling independently.[13] Reinthaler *et al.*[8] observed that those who were away for longer than 2 months were more likely to develop a parasitic infection. In their study *Giardia lamblia* was the most important parasite, reflecting the large proportion visiting India, an area known to have a high association with this disease. For bacterial infections they found an association with trips of 1–2 weeks.

Overall it appears that the risk of TD does fall over time and it has been suggested that this reduced risk will be apparent after 12 months of stay in a tropical area.[4] In view of the above evidence this may well be due to resistance to ETEC. The risk of TD from other causes, particularly parasitic infections, would tend to diminish only over a much greater period of time.

The important message is that longer-term travellers, e.g. expatriates staying in a developing country for longer than a year, should not treat mild to moderate TD with antibiotics because some immunity should be allowed to develop. The immunity will be lost on returning home and frequent travellers from industrialised countries show the same incidence of TD as infrequent travellers. The evidence that immunity can develop to ETEC does encourage research into the development of a vaccine against this organism, although none is currently available.

Host factors

Age appears to be a risk factor,[2,8] with young adults (20–30 years) being at greater risk than older people. Possible explanations for this age difference might be more adventurous eating habits and less previous immunological exposure to certain pathogens. Children under 3 years old seem to be at the highest risk. Surprisingly, children of 3–6 years may have the lowest incidence of all.

Dietary habits

This will be dealt with in the next chapter, but one of the most important risk factors appears to be associated with eating out in restaurants. In a study on Austrian tourists[8] it was found that TD due to bacteria was more likely in those staying in hotels and parasitic infection more common in those on trekking holidays.

It seems to make little difference whether staying and eating in a five-star hotel or in budget accommodation.

Other illness and medication

It has recently been found that those with reduced stomach acid are much more prone to TD.[14] This is because many pathogens are removed by stomach acid to levels unlikely to cause TD. Therefore, travellers taking proton pump inhibitors (PPIs) and, to a lesser extent, longer-acting H_2-antagonists, may be at risk of TD.

In patients in whom acid suppression is essential, an H_2-antagonist should be given in preference to a PPI and they should be warned about the risks. Possible consideration could be given to antimicrobial prophylaxis if visiting very-high-risk areas.

The effect of TD on drug absorption has not been widely studied, but a decrease in gastrointestinal tract transit time is theoretically possible. Many travellers to the tropics will be taking malaria prophylaxis and one study has shown that blood levels of proguanil (but not chloroquine) are reduced by TD.[15] Travellers should therefore be aware of paying particular attention to precautions against biting insects if this is likely to be a problem. They should not take extra medication except on medical advice.

People who are immunocompromised, e.g. those receiving chemotherapy or patients with acquired immune deficiency syndrome (AIDS) who have a low CD4 count, would be at an increased risk of TD. In the young and elderly there may be a greater potential for dehydration as a result of TD. Patients with inflammatory bowel disease (IBD) may experience a worsening of the condition following TD.

Aetiology

A number of non-infectious causes of TD have been proposed. The most important might include:[2]

- changes in diet compared to that usually followed at home, e.g. additives/food intolerance, high fat intake
- changes in gut flora due to a different profile of organisms present in the country being visited.
- increased alcohol consumption, resulting in gastrointestinal irritation
- menstruation

These non-infectious causes appear to be supported by the observation that over 50% of stool samples from TD patients prove negative for a pathological organism. However, in many studies, a response rate of over 95% is observed with antimicrobial treatment. Therefore, the current view is that the majority of cases of TD are infective in origin, even though a pathogen may fail to be detected by stool culture.

It is convenient to classify diarrhoea due to infective organisms in one of three ways:

1. Organisms causing a non-inflammatory diarrhoea. The diarrhoea produced is usually watery with nausea and vomiting and there is little or no inflammation of the bowel. The usual causes of this type of diarrhoea amongst travellers are viruses or bacteria producing enterotoxin (e.g. ETEC, discussed later).
2. Organisms causing an inflammatory diarrhoea. As a result of inflammation of the colon, pus and blood will be seen in the diarrhoea. There may be fever associated with bacterial infections together with abdominal cramps. Generally the presence of pus and blood in diarrhoea is referred to as a dysentery; this may be either a bacterial or an amoebic dysentery.
3. Organisms causing systemic infections. In this case the organisms are able to penetrate the bowel, causing systemic symptoms and infection of other tissues. The prime organism of relevance is *Salmonella typhi*.

The role of *E. coli* in travellers' diarrhoea

The most common and widely quoted causative agent is ETEC.[16] This bacteria produces a toxin similar to that of *Vibrio cholerae*, which disrupts sodium pump function in the bowel, resulting in a watery diarrhoea. The incidence of ETEC as the causative agent of TD varies in different parts of the world. It is highest in Latin America, with a mean isolation rate of around 40%, in comparison with 30% in parts of Africa and just 16% in Asia.[17] However, those figures are mean values and there are large variations: for example, in Latin America studies show results of between 17 and 70%. The study by Sonnenburg *et al.*[9] found that ETEC was responsible for around 30% of cases in India and Kenya, with a somewhat higher incidence due to viruses than in some other studies. There are other forms of *E. coli* implicated in TD: enteroinvasive *E. coli*, enterohaemorrhagic *E. coli*, enteropathogenic *E. coli* and enteroaggregative *E. coli*.

The causative agent may also be influenced by the season. For instance, in Mexico, ETEC is more commonly implicated in the summer and rainy season but *Campylobacter* is more common in the winter.[18,19]

A large range of organisms other than ETEC are known to be responsible for TD. Table 2.1 gives a crude comparison of the risk of acquiring pathogens in different regions. Unfortunately, it is not always possible to ascertain the likely causative agents from clinical symptoms alone. For instance, although *Shigella* is more commonly associated with fever and blood in the stools, such symptoms can also occasionally be observed for ETEC. However, in general, ETEC is associated with a milder disease. Some of the important strains of organisms listed in Table 2.2 are described below.

Other bacteria

In total, bacterial infections may account for up to 85% of cases of TD. There are a number of other important bacteria that are implicated other than *E. coli*.[4] *Campylobacter* tends to cause a longer-lasting disease than ETEC and may be preceded by fever. Blood and mucus may be present in the stools, and symptoms of malaise and colic continue after the diarrhoea has resolved. It has been implicated as a relatively common cause of TD in some areas of the world, in particular Thailand.[20] *Campylobacter* has been observed to be responsible for a higher proportion of cases of TD than ETEC in the winter months in both Mexico and Morocco.[19] In the study of Reinthaler *et al.*[8] it was the most frequent bacterial cause of TD, being identified in 37% of stool samples, compared to just 24% for ETEC and other forms of *E. coli*. However, stool samples were taken from tourists who had visited their general practitioner on return due to a persistent diarrhoea. As ETEC is known mainly to affect travellers soon after arriving at their destination, and then rarely for longer than 5 days, it is expected that incidence

Table 2.2 Organisms other than *Escherichia coli* which are responsible for travellers' diarrhoea

	Asia	Latin America	Africa
Campylobacter jejuni	+++	+	++
Salmonella spp.	+++	++	++
Shigella spp.	++	+++	+
Aeromonas spp.	+++	+	+
Rotavirus	+	+	+++
Entamoeba histolytica	++	−	−
Giardia lamblia	++	−	−
Cryptosporidium	+	−	+
Cyclospora	+	−	−
Vibrio cholerae (non-01)	−	−	−

The quantity of reported isolates in studies by percentage:
−, rarely reported (< 5%); +, 5–10%; ++, 10–30%; +++, some studies reporting > 30%.

would be relatively low. It was not specifically reported what countries the individuals had visited, but it was noted that three patients from southern Europe were carrying quinolone-resistant strains. One can conclude that *Campylobacter* is an important agent for persistent diarrhoea on returning home.

Aeromonas spp. are a potential cause of TD, particularly in Asia. It has not been widely studied but can be associated with a persistent diarrhoea.

Food poisoning by *Salmonella* spp. is a possibility in any situation where hygiene is poor. It is therefore not surprising that this is a regular cause of TD, often associated with reported outbreaks in hotels. The symptoms can vary greatly in severity and duration, lasting from just 1–2 days to up to 3 weeks. Septicaemia and systemic invasion are potential complications.

Shigella spp. are responsible for the condition often described as bacillary dysentery. The diarrhoea is usually of abrupt onset, accompanied by fever and vomiting. Mucus and blood may be observed in the stools and other enteric symptoms can be present. Symptoms may persist for 2 or 3 weeks.

Parasites

These organisms may be more of a concern to longer-term travellers. In total, around 5% of cases of TD are caused by parasites.[2]

Entamoeba histolytica is an unlikely cause of TD, resulting in amoebic dysentery. It has a somewhat slower onset than bacillary dysentery and there is a more formed stool, which has an offensive smell and contains blood and mucus. Fever will be absent. Although symptoms may resolve after a few weeks, there is a danger of relapse and complications such as perforation and haemorrhage of the gastrointestinal tract (Plate 1). In addition, organisms can travel from the gastrointestinal tract, resulting in abscess formation in the lung, liver or brain. A typical presentation in travellers, sometimes referred to as non-dysenteric amoebiasis, is a day of crampy diarrhoea followed by a few days of no symptoms or even constipation. Such fluctuations in symptoms may delay presentation for treatment.[21] At the other end of the spectrum, a severe amoebic colitis is rare in travellers and potentially life-threatening due to a danger of colon perforation.

Giardia infection has been found more commonly among travellers to Nepal and some parts of Russia and Eastern Europe. It is a potential risk to trekkers and campers using a natural water supply. Recently, it has been identified as a cause of 'bushwalkers' diarrhoea' in Tasmania.[22] Infection is usually water-borne and it is believed that wild animals may be an important vector. Initially the diarrhoea may be watery before the other symptoms, mostly related to malabsorption, become apparent. In particular a reduced fat absorption will lead to the production of a frothy, foul-smelling type of diarrhoea known as steatorrhoea. In addition there may be nausea, abdominal discomfort, flatulence and bloating. As symptoms can persist for more than 7 weeks, weight loss may also occur in 25% of people. A study in German travellers[23] identified the Indian subcontinent and West Africa as areas of highest risk, with 4–5% of travellers contracting *Giardia*. It was not stated whether travellers spent longer at these destinations than others, as this would increase the risk. A further observation was that in 11% of patients cure was not achieved on the first course of metronidazole, and some required albendazole to achieve a cure. They also found that asymptomatic parasitaemia was only present in 10% of individuals.

Cyclospora is not a common cause of TD,[24] but incidence can vary in particular circumstances. *Cyclospora* is a reported cause in Nepal[25] and may be responsible for up to 30% of cases of diarrhoea in expatriates in this country during the months of April–June.[7] The symptoms of severe watery diarrhoea can appear abruptly and are associated with gas and bloating, although symptoms do tend to become less severe after a few days. Anorexia and fatigue are common, resulting in weight loss if symptoms persist.

Cryptosporidium has caused problems in contamination of water supplies in recent years in the UK. It is self-limiting but very dangerous in those who are immunocompromised, in particular in patients with AIDS. Diarrhoea caused by this organism can be quite severe, but in otherwise healthy individuals it will resolve in 1–3 weeks.

Others

Viral disease may account for around 10% of all TD, but cholera is extremely rare in travellers. However, news of cholera outbreaks are frequent enough to deter tourists from visiting particular destinations.[26] This is largely unfounded as the massive fluid loss and sudden dehydration associated with classic cholera are now rarely seen in healthy individuals when due to the El Tor 01 strain of cholera, which is responsible for the current pandemic. A more virulent strain, known as the 0139 serotype, was identified in Bangladesh in 1992[26] but so far has not posed a danger to travellers. Cholera is a far more serious problem in a malnourished population, where it is more likely to claim the lives of the young or elderly. In the healthy traveller, cholera can have quite a mild course, with some sufferers perhaps remaining undiagnosed in the belief that they have had no more than a bout of TD.

Helminth (worm) infestation of the gastrointestinal tract is not considered as a cause of TD *per se*, although those with chronic *Strongyloides* (round worm) infestations may present with diarrhoea. These infestations are contracted by eating contaminated food and are considered in more detail in Chapter 5. Schistosomiasis (bilharzia) is another important helminth infection discussed in Chapter 5.

Prophylaxis

As the majority of cases of TD respond to an antimicrobial, it might seem reasonable to use such agents prophylactically. The use of Streptotriad by the UK team during the 1960 Olympics in Rome won general admiration for the achievement of fewest cases of diarrhoea.

Agents that can be used for prophylaxis

Antimicrobials have been employed in the prophylaxis of TD for many years. Until the 1980s, sulphonamides were generally used. Owing to the development of worldwide resistance to these agents, co-trimoxazole can only offer 60–70% protection. In addition, the adverse drug reactions of the sulphonamides would make them largely redundant for this indication.

The quinolones are now considered the first choice, providing over 90% protection.[3] The recommended dose for ciprofloxacin is 500 mg once a day. It must be emphasised that this is a non-licensed indication in the UK and physicians should be aware of this fact before prescribing. As will be discussed later, the regimens described for the self-treatment of TD using ciprofloxacin are also not covered by the product licence.

Doxycycline may also shorten the duration of TD,[27] but this has not been as widely investigated as the quinolones. Concerns have also been expressed regarding the generally high level of resistance to the tetracycline group of antibiotics by enteropathogens.[28] The question also arises as to whether doxycycline used for malaria prophylaxis (see Chapter 4) would also offer some protection against TD. Again, there is little evidence for or against this assumption. One trial indicated that doxycycline[29] conferred 85% protection if used on a regular basis twice a week. In another study on travellers to Mexico, 40% of isolates of potentially enteropathogenic *E. coli* were found to be resistant to doxycycline, whereas none were observed to be resistant to ciprofloxacin.[30]

The only other products marketed in the UK that have the potential for the prevention of TD are the *Lactobacillus* preparations. Some trials have shown *Lactobacillus acidophilus* to be ineffective in the prevention of TD.[31] One preparation containing *L. casei* GG has been examined in a few small-scale trials and appears to provide a maximum 40% protection.[32] At this low level of protection it is important to address the potential for a false sense of security leading to complacency regarding dietary advice, which would still need to be followed. The good side-effect profile of *Lactobacillus* may be an attraction for some travellers who are willing to pay for a product which may only provide partial protection. For the future, genetically modified *Lactobacillus* may hold a potential for use as a probiotic in the prevention of TD.

In the USA, bismuth salicylate (Pepto-Bismol) has been recommended for the prophylaxis of TD.[3] It must be taken four times a day to provide around 60% protection. However, it would not be practical to carry sufficient liquid to cover a 2-week trip and tablets are not available in the UK. In any case, in the UK, TD is not a licensed indication for Pepto-Bismol. Apart from having to remember to take medication four times a day, other minor side-effects, such as the tendency to cause a blackening of the tongue and stools, may reduce compliance.

In the near future, a vaccine against ETEC should be available, to offer at least partial protection against TD. Similarly, a new oral cholera vaccine seems to offer some cross-protection against ETEC.

Indications for antimicrobial prophylaxis

Perhaps the strongest argument against chemoprophylaxis is that TD is invariably a self-limiting condition, which would hardly warrant the continuous use of expensive antimicrobial agents. A consensus development conference in the USA ruled that prophylaxis against TD is not warranted.[33] Generally, the arguments against such use are:

- adverse reactions – there is the added complication of developing a reaction without access to medical help. Also, there may be overgrowth of other organisms such as *Candida* and *Clostridium*
- cost
- complacency – ciprofloxacin would not protect against parasites or viruses and therefore food and water hygiene must still be observed

- resistance – the use of these agents by travellers would probably have little impact on the overall level of resistance in the area visited if they were already being used by the local population. However, there is still the potential for travellers to develop and harbour ciprofloxacin-resistant organisms
- treatment is more effective – as antimicrobials can potentially relieve symptoms within 24 hours, it is more realistic to use treatment courses if indicated

There may be a few indications for prophylaxis in high-risk individuals, e.g. those who are immunosuppressed, achlorhydric (as a result of taking PPIs) or who have IBD. A case could also be made for those at particular risk from dehydration or electrolyte disturbance, for instance those receiving digoxin therapy. The importance of a trip could be a consideration, although, as discussed below, if antimicrobials are to be used at all, self-treatment with short courses is the preferred option.

Those with human immunodeficiency virus (HIV) would not normally be provided with a prophylactic agent and should instead carry antimicrobials for self-treatment and be warned to take extra precautions regarding food and water hygiene. It has been suggested that CD4+ counts should guide whether prophylaxis is given; those with a count less than 200 would be offered antimicrobial prohylaxis and those with less than 500 would be given bismuth salicylate.[34]

Management of travellers' diarrhoea

There are three approaches to the management of TD – antimotility agents, oral rehydration and antimicrobial therapy.[35] In the majority of cases travellers will self-treat their TD, as was illustrated in a study by Hill.[11] This study examined retrospectively 784 travellers from the USA, of whom 46% reported diarrhoea, this being more likely when travelling to the higher risk destinations. Thirty-four per cent had diarrhoea according to the classification system described above, in the section Definition and symptoms of travellers' diarrhoea, and a further 11% simply had 'loose motions'. Despite many episodes of diarrhoea being reported as severe, nearly all the travellers self-treated. For those with TD, 47% took antibiotics and the rest antimotility agents, whereas for those with loose motions 74% took antimotility agents and 27% antibiotics. This highlights the two approaches available to travellers for the self-treatment of TD: antibiotics and/or loperamide. However, antibiotics are not as widely prescribed in many countries as they appear to be in the USA for the self-treatment of TD. The other important consideration concerning management of TD is the place of rehydration therapy, and specifically the use of oral rehydration solutions (ORS). All these aspects of self-management will be discussed below.

Antimotility agents

The most useful agent in this class is loperamide, because of its specific effects on the gastrointestinal tract. Others, such as codeine and diphenoxylate/atropine, are no more effective than loperamide and carry a far higher risk of systemic side-effects. Loperamide decreases large-bowel motility and therefore, to some extent, promotes an increased reabsorption of fluid.[36] However, it is always prudent to maintain fluid intake when using loperamide.

For mild to moderate TD, loperamide will improve symptoms such as faecal frequency and cramping,[37] allowing the traveller some freedom to carry on with the planned agenda. It should not be used in children where rehydration is the primary goal.

There are a few perceived drawbacks to using loperamide, which need to be addressed. Taking loperamide at the maximum dosage for more than a day or so could well lead to a bout of constipation as the TD resolves. No studies have indicated that this is a particular problem associated with loperamide, although due to changes in diet and inadequate fluid intake, constipation can be as much a problem for travellers as TD. Another theoretical drawback is that antimotility agents have been shown to prolong infection caused by *Shigella* spp.,[38] presumably because of retention of the organism. This may be related to the observation that only a relatively few organisms need to be present to cause the symptoms of shigellosis. Therefore, the retention of even a small number of organisms could have an adverse effect.

Recently manufacturers of loperamide[39] have claimed that the product is perhaps under-utilised, with an overemphasis being placed on rehydration alone. In a survey of general practitioners, nurses and pharmacists[40] only one-quarter would have recommended an antimotility agent for treating TD. Over a half strongly agreed with statements that described the use of antimotility agents as prolonging the illness and further damaging the gastrointestinal tract. There was widespread belief that such agents delayed the excretion of pathogens and toxins. The authors commented that the *British National Formulary* inappropriately discourages the use of loperamide for TD.

Certainly, in the case of TD, where the inconvenience of bouts of diarrhoea is an important consideration, loperamide does therefore have a useful role. In the absence of any good evidence that antimotility agents have a detrimental effect on the course of TD, many are of the opinion that, in the absence of any dysenteric symptoms, they are safe to use. Even in the presence of dysentery they could still be used, providing appropriate antibiotic therapy has been initiated.

An approach to using loperamide in TD might be to use it for mild to moderate TD where there is no fever or blood in the stools. Loperamide should preferably be reserved for use in situations where TD may affect travel plans and for not longer than 24 hours. It should be used in addition to maintaining good hydration.

Oral rehydration

The use of ORS in the management of diarrhoeal illness has saved millions of lives in developing countries. The balance of salt and glucose (or other carbohydrate) allows the most efficient absorption of fluid. The addition of potassium and bicarbonate also helps to correct electrolyte imbalance. The use of ORS in diarrhoeal illness in the very young and elderly is well established. However, in otherwise healthy adults it has been suggested that they are unnecessary when managing TD, which is not usually a dehydrating disease in this age group. Simply maintaining fluid intake using sugary drinks and eating, for instance, salt crackers, should suffice in healthy adults. Some direct evidence that such therapy is not required for adults is provided by a study carried out on visitors to Mexico.[41] Subjects were randomised either to receive loperamide or ORS plus loperamide to self-treat their TD. No difference was found between the two groups in terms of symptoms or duration of diarrhoea.

A case may still be made for some travellers to carry electrolyte sachets for emergency use as the more intrepid traveller may not have suitable soft drinks or foods readily to hand. It may also be necessary for such travellers to make up their own solution using salt and sugar; a suitable formula is half a teaspoon of salt and eight level-teaspoons of sugar in 1 litre of clean water. Honey could be substituted if sugar is not available.

Children and the elderly should use commercial rehydration sachets (e.g. Dioralyte, Rehidrat). Although these are readily available overseas, they usually contain the higher-sodium-content World Health Organization (WHO) formulation, which can be less palatable although the recommended WHO formulation was changed in 2003. Table 2.3 compares the formulation of some of the available ORS solutions. The

Table 2.3 Some oral rehydration solutions (ORS)

Solutes (mmol/L)	WHO ORS 2003	WHO ORS (Pre-2003)	UK ORS (Dioralyte)	Dioralyte Relief (UK)
Sodium	75	90	60	60
Potassium	20	20	20	20
Chloride	65	30	60	50
Bicarbonate		30		
Citrate	10		10	10
Glucose	75	111	90	
Rice/starch				(6g sachet)
Osmolarity	245	331	240	

WHO, World Health Organization.

older WHO formulation is hypertonic due to the high sodium concentration. The formulations used in the UK contain less sodium and are therefore hypotonic. There is good evidence that water absorption is actually greater if a hypotonic solution is used.[42] At one time it was queried whether they would reverse hyponatraemia associated with very-high-output diarrhoea as might be associated with cholera.[43] It is believed that a sodium concentration between 50 and 75 mmol/L is sufficient for children who contract cholera.[44] In any case this would be an extremely rare event for children travelling from developed countries.

Maintaining fluid intake can also help to improve general symptoms and well-being, although faecal fluid output can actually increase with aggressive rehydration therapy.[5] Whether or not electrolyte solutions offer any benefit to adults over simply increasing fluid intake has not been studied.

There is some evidence that formulations based on complex carbohydrates such as rice are more efficient in promoting absorption and retention of fluid than glucose formulations.[43,44] A starch-based product (Dioralyte Relief) is now available in the UK and an additional advantage is that it would form a more solid stool. Whether this product offers any specific advantages to sufferers of TD needs further study.

Antimicrobial therapy

Self-treatment of TD with antimicrobials can be very successful. Whether or not travellers should be supplied with such agents is a contentious issue. At one time, co-trimoxazole was considered the antimicrobial of choice for the empirical treatment of TD. This has now been replaced by the quinolones which have been shown to be highly effective in a number of trials.[1]

When a quinolone is supplied to travellers for self-treatment at the first sign of diarrhoea, both the severity and duration of the illness are reduced.[20,45] In one widely quoted study carried out using British troops in Belize, it was reported that a single 500 mg dose of ciprofloxacin reduced the mean duration of TD from around 50 hours to under 24 hours.[46] Furthermore, over 90% of the participants in the trial experienced no further episodes of unformed stools by 72 hours, compared to 79% in the placebo group. The study involved only 84 volunteers and the population may not be representative of the majority of travellers. Almost identical results were obtained when a 3-day course of ciprofloxacin was taken by travellers to Mexico, where time to cure was reduced from 60 to 20 hours.[30] Other trials using single doses of ciprofloxacin have shown considerable improvements in the duration and severity of diarrhoea.[20,45]

There appears to be reasonable evidence, although further studies are required, that single doses of ciprofloxacin, taken as soon as possible after the first sign of diarrhoea, are a useful approach in reducing the duration of TD. If symptoms persist on the second day, after single-dose therapy, a 3–5-day course (500 mg twice a day) might be advisable.

A systematic review of the efficacy of antibiotics in TD has recently been carried out by the Cochrane Collaboration.[47] They identified 20 trials that were suitable for inclusion, but there were insufficient data to perform a full meta-analysis. Ten trials examined the primary outcome measure of time to last unformed stool, demonstrating that this was significantly reduced in those receiving antibiotics. However, the analysis of this outcome was criticised as not using or properly reporting a time to event analysis. The secondary endpoint of number of unformed stools passed in 24 hours was reduced in those taking antibiotics, and there was a greater proportion of people cured in 72 hours. The conclusion was therefore that antibiotics shorten the duration and reduce the severity of TD. As expected, the incidence of side-effects was greater in those receiving antibiotics, but none were serious and resolved on discontinuing antibiotic treatment. The review did not comment on the effectiveness of one regimen over another, e.g. between long or short courses.

There are some important considerations when supplying such therapy to travellers. As has been mentioned, TD is not a licensed indication for ciprofloxacin. Also, the regimens usually employed are not those covered by the product licence for infective diarrhoea, the usual length of therapy being 5–7 days.

As shown in Table 2.4 (below), ciprofloxacin is effective against many, but not all, of the responsible bacterial pathogens. *Campylobacter* infections may respond to a quinolone,[48] but treatment failures and recurrence have been reported[20] and erythromycin is the usual drug of choice. There is some promising work indicating that azithromycin may be the agent of choice against *Campylobacter* and it would be effective against a number of other pathogens responsible for TD.[49] *Cyclospora* is only sensitive to co-trimoxazole and *Cryptosporidium* infection responds to no available agents. For *Giardia* or amoebic dysentery, metronidazole or tinidazole is required.

Therapy should probably be avoided for the first bout of diarrhoea in long-term travellers in order to allow some immunity to develop.

A promising new agent, rifaximin,[50] is being assessed for use against bacterial forms of TD. It is structurally similar to rifampicin, but the addition of a pyridoimidazole ring results in oral bioavailability being reduced to less than 1%. As it is not absorbed, high concentrations of the antibiotic will remain in the gastrointestinal tract. Although the minimum inhibitory concentration of rifaximin against bacteria associated with TD is quite high, this is greatly exceeded by the concentration attainable within the gastrointestinal tract at therapeutic doses. The efficacy studies so far conducted do indicate that rifaximin is at least as effective as ciprofloxacin in treating TD, and superior to placebo, with a low incidence of adverse effects. Although its usefulness in patients with dysentery was not specifically examined, rifaximin does have activity against causative bacterial agents such as *Shigella* spp. One concern is that use of the agent may induce a cross-resistance to *Mycobacterium tuberculosis*. In practice, studies have shown that such resistance does not appear to occur and that bacterial resistance is not carried by plasmid transfer.

General approach to management of travellers' diarrhoea

There is no internationally accepted consensus on the place of antimicrobials in treating TD. If an antimicrobial is to be used, then travellers may be supplied with a course of ciprofloxacin and instructed to use them as described in the bottom half of Table 2.5 (below). In the USA, bismuth salicylate would also be considered as an option for mild TD, as around 60% of cases may improve with such treatment. This approach is generally not followed in the UK, where the regimen described in the top half of Table 2.5 would be considered more appropriate for most travellers. The instructions given are therefore to seek

Table 2.4 Antimicrobial treatment of travellers' diarrhoea

Organism	Clinical syndrome	Incubation/ duration	Principal symptoms	Antimicrobial of choice
Viruses e.g. rotavirus	Non-inflammatory	Incubation 3 days Duration 1 week	Watery diarrhoea Nausea and vomiting	N/A
Enterotoxigenic *Escherichia coli* (ETEC)	Non-inflammatory	Incubation 16–72 hours Duration 3–5 days	Watery diarrhoea Abdominal cramps	Quinolone
Campylobacter jejuni	Inflammatory	Incubation: sudden onset	Fever Diarrhoea with pus, mucus and blood	Macrolide
Salmonella spp.	Inflammatory	Incubation: sudden onset	Fever Diarrhoea with pus, mucus and blood	Quinolone
Shigella spp.	Inflammatory	Incubation: sudden onset	Fever Diarrhoea with pus, mucus and blood	Quinolone
Entamoeba histolytica	Inflammatory	Symptoms of gradual onset	Diarrhoea with pus, mucus and blood. Flatulence, discomfort and moderate weight loss.	Metronidazole
Giardia lamblia	Non-inflammatory	Incubation: 2 weeks. Gradual onset, can persist for months untreated	2–5 semi-formed stools per day. Gas/bloating. Mild weight loss	Metronidazole Tinidazole
Cyclospora	Non-inflammatory	May be sudden onset. Duration up to 6 weeks	Watery diarrhoea with gas/bloating. Weight loss, fatigue and anorexia	Co-trimoxazole

Table 2.4 continued

Organism	Clinical syndrome	Incubation/ duration	Principal symptoms	Antimicrobial of choice
Cryptosporidium	Non-inflammatory	Sudden onset. Incubation 1 week. Duration 1–3 weeks	Watery diarrhoea. Mild gas/bloating and weight loss	None

Table 2.5 Management of travellers' diarrhoea

	Severity of diarrhoea		
	Mild	Moderate	Severe
Travellers not carrying antimicrobials	Fluid replacement (loperamide if required)	Fluid replacement and a short course of loperamide	Seek medical help
Travellers carrying an antibiotic	Fluid replacement (loperamide if required)	Loperamide and quinolone (single dose/short course)	Quinolone 3–5 days and metronidazole if longer than 14 days

medical attention if there is blood in the stools, if fever is present and/or the diarrhoea persists for more than 5 days. This assumes that such help is available and that the appropriate antimicrobials can be easily obtained. For the minority of travellers on longer trips to developing countries, this may not be the case and, in my opinion, antimicrobials should be carried; both ciprofloxacin and metronidazole may be needed. The advice should always be to use such medication under medical supervision. In comparatively rare circumstances, i.e. when travelling to very remote regions, individuals might need to be instructed on self-medication, particularly if a more severe or persistent diarrhoea develops.

For young children, the recommended approach to treating acute diarrhoea of any cause should be followed, with an emphasis on oral rehydration.

Dietary restriction is not necessary in adults or children, but given a tendency for certain foods to increase gastrointestinal motility, eating more bland foods (e.g. bread, potatoes, bananas) may help with symptoms. Some advocate avoiding dairy products due to a potential for lactose intolerance.

A more difficult question relates to the demands of a business executive or politician on an important trip, where time is critical. There is evidence that combining a single 500 mg dose of ciprofloxacin with loperamide after the first loose stool will improve symptoms within the first 24 hours, particularly if caused by ETEC.[20,45] The advantages of adding the loperamide do not appear to be great, but some consider it worthwhile.[49] Although ciprofloxacin is not licensed for this regimen, there may occasionally be circumstances when it is prescribed. This has also been demonstrated with the combination of another fluoroquinolone, ofloxacin, with loperamide.[51]

The argument for antimicrobial treatment can be justified on pharmacoeconomic terms, where cost of therapy would be less than the cost of the time lost on the trip.[28] It is also of interest to note that it may well be the treatment of choice for those in the medical profession; 25% of microbiologists attending a conference overseas were found to be carrying antimicrobials for TD.[52]

In summary, the following course of action might be recommended for the self management of TD in healthy adults, using the definitions described previously:

- A mild TD with only one or two loose stools in 24 hours requires no particular treatment.
- For mild to moderate diarrhoea, loperamide could be used, perhaps adding an antimicrobial if the symptoms worsen or are distressing. A single dose is sufficient, but if symptoms persist longer than 24 hours or there are dysenteric symptoms, a full 3-day course may be required, e.g. ciprofloxacin 500 mg b.d. However, it must be remembered that many studies have been conducted when the antibiotic is taken at the first sign of diarrhoea, so there is limited evidence of benefit when treatment is delayed in order to assess the severity of the diarrhoea. Some experts recommend taking antimicrobials if less than two bouts of distressing diarrhoea are experienced within 24 hours;[34] others state that they should be taken at the first sign of diarrhoea.[35]
- For severe dysenteric symptoms a full course of antimicrobials should be taken.

Persistent diarrhoea

In about 3% of cases, symptoms persist for longer than 14 days and inevitably the returning traveller will seek medical help.[53]

There are a number of reasons for persistent diarrhoea; giardiasis is one of the most important, although the other parasites listed in Table 2.2 may also be responsible. Bacterial infections can also cause a persistent diarrhoea, especially *Shigella* and *Aeromonas* spp. Occasionally, *E. coli*, particularly the enteropathogenic forms, can cause a longer-lasting diarrhoea. There are cases of outbreaks of very severe diarrhoea with chronic sequelae and where no causative agent can be identified, possibly due to the disappearance of the agent soon after the acute phase, such that stool sample fails to detect any pathogens. This has been given the name of 'Brainerd diarrhoea' after an outbreak in a town in the USA of the same name. It was reported in 1992 when passengers on a cruise ship visiting the Galapagos Islands experienced the syndrome; nearly half who had contracted the disease were still ill a year later.[54]

A severe malabsorption syndrome accompanied by diarrhoea, known as tropical sprue, is sometimes encountered amongst expatriates; the condition fails to improve on returning home. The cause is not fully understood, but is believed to be related to colonisation of the gastro-intestinal tract by aerobic organisms. In the long term, vitamin deficiency and weight loss are observed. The usual antibiotics used in treating TD may temporarily relieve but not resolve the problem. A course of tetracycline 250 mg four times daily, combined with daily folic acid 5 mg for 6 weeks should cure the syndrome.[55]

Another potential scenario is a bout of diarrhoea causing disruption of gut flora which then takes some time to resolve. It is possible that this sort of postdiarrhoeal syndrome is actually made worse by repeated courses of antibiotics. There have also been cases where TD has unmasked a latent IBD.

When the patient presents to a general practitioner, a stool sample would usually be taken. The presence of an organism in the stool does not necessarily mean that it is the responsible organism, e.g. *Entamoeba* cysts may be present even in the absence of clinical dysentery. Likewise, despite a negative stool sample, an infective organism may still be responsible. For *Cyclospora* infection cysts can usually by identified.

Empirical treatment may therefore be indicated if negative results are obtained and, in some circumstances, the physician will wish to commence such treatment while awaiting results. Suitable empirical treatment would begin with a full 5-day course of ciprofloxacin. If this fails, then metronidazole or tinidazole could be used to deal with *Giardia*. Further investigations should be carried out for other causes of persistent diarrhoea; in particular, *Entamoeba* infection should be excluded.

Reinthaler *et al.*[8] calculated in their study that the average cost of antimicrobial therapy per patient was less than a tenth of the cost of investigation of stool samples. They concluded that, in the majority of cases, the pathogen would remain unknown, emphasising the need for empirical treatment.

If a positive culture is obtained then the identified organism should guide therapy, as indicated in Table 2.4.

Entamoeba infection can be hard to eradicate, resulting in reccurrence of symptoms, so a course of the amoebicide diloxanide furoate should be given, following treatment with metronidazole.

Taylor *et al.*[55] have suggested a clinical workup for those travellers presenting with chronic diarrhoea. Their main points are:

- Establish the number of episodes during travel and any symptom-free periods to identify the possibility of multiple infections.
- Ask the patient to describe the presentation of the diarrhoea to help identify a causative organism, as summarised in Table 2.4.
- Carry out physical examination and stool culture.
- Initiate empirical treatment, as described above.
- Undertake malabsorption studies.
- Provide reassurance for those who do not respond to empirical treatment and who have no malabsorption problems that the condition will eventually resolve.
- Other measures, such as avoiding milk products, could be tried.

Summary of main points

- TD usually has an infective origin; ETEC is the most common organism but a number of others may be responsible.
- Most cases of TD will not last longer than 3 days and it is therefore generally considered a self-limiting condition.
- Prophylaxis with antimicrobials is not usually recommended.
- Maintaining fluid intake and the use of loperamide are the mainstays of treatment for adults.
- Self-treatment with antimicrobials is not advocated by all practitioners routinely and self-treatment is not a licensed indication for the quinolones.
- A case could be made for some long-term travellers or those on very important trips to carry antimicrobial self-treatment, ideally for use under medical supervision. A single dose of a quinolone is usually all that is required.

Frequently asked questions

Why does the local population not suffer from diarrhoea to the same extent as the traveller?
The incidence of diarrhoea in local children is very similar to that of travellers visiting the developing country, and is a cause of considerable morbidity and mortality in the very young. Eventually those living in the area will develop a degree of resistance to the organisms causing diarrhoea. However, travellers should not rely on developing such resistance as it could take up to a year, even with ETEC.

What is the ideal drink for adults for rehydration if they develop TD (some say that Coca-Cola is good)?
Coca-Cola should not be used due to its relatively high fructose concentration, that would tend to hold fluid in the bowel. The strategies described in the text should be used, although various experts have their own ideas regarding the best means of maintaining hydration. For instance the following is advocated by Dr C Sherer of Jerusalem:
'After years of treating tourists with TD I have found the best replacement is strong tea, with one teaspoon of glucose per cup, and a pinch of salt covered with some lemon juice. The tea should be as strong as possible. Good Aussie char!'

What is the best way of treating babies and young children who develop TD?
If the baby is being breastfed then this should be continued, supplemented if necessary with ORS. If an infant is vomiting the ORS will need to be given slowly every 5 minutes or so on a teaspoon. Formula milk may need to be stopped for 24 hours while giving oral rehydration. Parents should be aware of the signs of dehydration in babies. Ciprofloxacin is not often used in children, but azithromycin in a single dose of 10 mg/kg followed by half this dosage daily for 4 days may be a suitable alternative for the young if this is thought necessary, but there is little evidence to support such regimens.

Warfarin therapy and TD – is it a problem?
Potentially a severe bout of diarrhoea could affect warfarin absorption and antibiotics such as ciprofloxacin may reduce warfarin metabolism. Those travelling on warfarin therapy should seek to have their international normalised ratio (INR) tested in this situation. Portable testing kits are available but are quite expensive.

Can I use homeopathic or probiotics to protect against TD?
There is no strong scientific evidence that these provide protection, particularly in the case of homeopathic remedies. They can be taken by

individuals but they should not be lured into a false sense of security and the precautions regarding food and water hygiene (Chapter 3) should be followed

Should I take antibiotics such as ciprofloxacin?
The arguments against are that TD is usually self-limiting and ciprofloxacin is not without side-effects. In addition, some are concerned over issues of resistance and that ciprofloxacin is not effective against all causes of diarrhoea.
The arguments for are the greatly reduced time course and the low incidence of side-effects from a single dose.

In my opinion patient preference should prevail to some degree. For those on shorter trips to high-risk destinations antibiotics could be considered for self-administration at the first sign of symptoms. For longer trips of more than 3 months there may be an argument for discouraging use initially, but they may still need to be carried to countries where medical supplies are poor (see Chapter 11). It is likely that they are most effective if taken at the first signs of diarrhoea.

References

1. Caeiro J, DuPont H L. Management of travellers' diarrhoea. *Drugs* 1998; 56: 73–81.
2. Peltola H, Gorbac S L. Travellers' diarrhoea: epidemiology and clinical aspects. In: DuPont H L, Steffen R, eds. *Textbook of Travel Medicine and Health*, 2nd edn. Hamilton, Canada: BC Decker, 2001: 151–159.
3. Ericsson C D, Rey M. Prevention of travellers' diarrhoea: risk avoidance and chemoprophylaxis. In: DuPont H L, Steffen R, eds. *Textbook of Travel Medicine and Health,* 2nd edn. Hamilton, Canada: BC Decker, 2001: 159–164.
4. Castelli F, Pezzoli C, Tomasoni L. Epidemiology of traveller's diarrhoea. *J Travel Med* 2001; 8 (suppl. 2): S26–S30.
5. Ericsson C D. Travellers' diarrhoea: epidemiology, prevention and self treatment. *Infect Dis Clin North Am* 1998; 12: 285–303.
6. Ericsson C D, DuPont H L, Mathewson J J. Epidemiologic observations on diarrhoea developing in US and Mexican students living in Guadalajara. *J Travel Med* 1994; 2: 6–10.
7. Shlim D R, Hoge C W, Rajah R *et al*. Persistent high risk of diarrhoea among foreigners in Nepal during the first two years of residence. *Clin Infect Dis* 1999; 29: 613–616.
8. Reinthaler F F, Feierl G, Stunzner D, Marth E. Diarrhea in returning Austrian tourists: epidemiology, etiology and cost-analysis. *J Travel Med* 1998; 5: 65–72.
9. Sonnenburg F, Tomieporth N, Walyaki N *et al*. Risk and aetiology of diarrhoea at various tourist destinations. *Lancet* 2000; 356: 133–134.

10. Merson M H, Morris G K, Sack D A *et al*. Travellers diarrhoea in Mexico. A propective study of physicians and family members attending a Congress. *N Engl Med J* 1976; 294: 1299–1305.

11. Hill D R. Occurrence and self-treatment of diarrhoea in a large cohort of Americans travelling to developing countries. *Am J Trop Med Hyg* 2000; 62: 585–589.

12. Hoge C W, Shlim D R, Echeverria P *et al*. Epidemiology of diarrhoea among expatriate residents living in a highly endemic environment. *JAMA* 1996; 27: 533–538.

13. Cobelens F G, Leentvaar-Kuijpers A, Kleijnen J, Coutinho R A. Incidence and risk factors of diarrhoea in Dutch travellers: consequences for priorities in pre-travel health advice. *Trop Med Int Health* 1998; 3: 896–903.

14. Stop PPI before travel, expert advises. *Pharm J* 1998; 261: 695.

15 Behrens R H, Taylor R B, Low A S *et al*. Travellers' diarrhoea; a controlled study of its effects on chloroquine and proguanil absorption. *Trans R Soc Trop Med Hyg* 1994; 88: 86–88.

16 Levine M M. *Escherichia coli* that cause diarrhoea: enterotoxigenic, enteropathogenic, enteroinvasive, enterohemorrhagic and enteroadherent. *J Infect Dis* 1987; 155: 377–389.

17. Black R E. Epidemiology of travellers' diarrhoea and relative importance of various pathogens. *Rev Infect Dis* 1990; 12 (suppl. 1): S73–S79.

18. Mattila L. Clinical features and duration of travellers' diarrhoea in relation to its aetiology. *Clin Infect Dis* 1994; 19: 728–734.

19. Mattila L, Siitonen A, Kyronseppa H *et al*. Seasonal variation in aetiology of travellers' diarrhoea. *J Infect Dis* 1992; 165: 385–368.

20. Petruccelli B P, Murphy G S, Canchez J L *et al*. Treatment of travellers' diarrhoea with ciprofloxacin and loperamide. *J Infect Dis* 1992; 165: 557–560.

21. Taylor D N, Connor B A, Shlim D R. Chronic diarrhoea in the returned traveller. *Med Clin North Am* 1999; 83: 1033–1052.

22. Kettlewell J S, Bettiol S S, Davies N *et al*. Epidemiology of giardiasis in Tasmania: a potential risk to residents and visitors. *J Travel Med* 1998; 5: 127–131.

23. Jelinek T, Loscher T. Epidemiology of giardiasis in German travellers. *J Travel Med* 2000; 7: 70–73.

24. Jelinek T, Lotze M, Eichenlaub S *et al*. Prevalence of infection with *Cryptosporidium parvum* and *Cyclospora cayetansis* among international travellers. *Gut* 1997; 41: 801–804.

25. Crowley B, Path C, Moloney C, Keane C T. *Cyclospora* species: a cause of diarrhoea among Irish travellers to Asia. *Irish Med J* 1996; 89: 110–112.

26. Behrens R. Cholera. In: Dawood R, ed. *Travellers' Health: How to Stay Healthy Abroad*, 3rd edn. Oxford: Oxford University Press, 2002.

27. Sack S B, Froehlich J L, Orskov F *et al*. Doxycycline is an effective treatment for travellers diarrhoea. *J Diarrh Dis Res* 1986; 3: 144–148.

28. Thompson M A, Booth I W. Treatment of travellers' diarrhoea: economic aspects. *Pharmacoeconomics* 1996; 9: 82–91.

29. Santosham M, Sack R B, Froehlich JL *et al*. Biweekly prophylactic doxycyline for travellers' diarrhoea. *J Infect Dis* 1981; 143: 598–602.

30. Wistrom J, Layne O, Gentry A *et al.* Ecological effects of short-term ciprofloxacin treatment of travellers' diarrhoea. *J Antimicrob Chemother* 1992; 30: 693–706.

31. Katelaris P, Salam I, Farthing M J G. Lactobacilli to prevent travellers' diarrhoea. *N Engl J Med* 1995; 333: 1360–1361.

32. Dupont H L. *Lactobacillus* GG in prevention of travellers' diarrhoea: an encouraging first step. *J Travel Med* 1997; 4: 1–2.

33. Gorbach S L, Edelman R, eds. Travellers' diarrhoea: National Institutes of Health Consensus Development Conference. *Rev Infect Dis* 1986; 8 (suppl. 2): S1285–S1289.

34. Ostrosky-Zeichner L, Ericsson C D. Travelers' diarrhoea. In: Zuckerman J N, ed. *Principles and Practice of Travel Medicine*. Chichester, UK: Wiley, 2001: 153–163.

35. Behrens R, Barer M. Diarrhoea and intestinal infections. In: Dawood R, ed. *Travellers' Health: How to Stay Healthy Abroad*, 3rd edn. Oxford: Oxford University Press, 2002.

36. Guabdalini S, Fasano A, Rao M C *et al.* Effects of loperamide on intestinal ion transport. *J Paediatr Gastroenterol Nutr* 1984; 3: 593–601.

37. Johnson P C, Dupont H L, Morgan B, Wood L V. Comparison of loperamide with bismuth salicylate for the treatment of acute travellers' diarrhoea. *JAMA* 1988; 255: 757–760.

38. DuPont H L, Hornick R B. Adverse effects of Lomotil therapy in shigellosis. *JAMA* 1973; 226: 1525–1528.

39. Review guidelines for diarrhoea treatment, says pharmaceutical company. *Pharm J* 1999; 263: 9.

40. McIntosh I B, Swanson V, Howell K. Health professionals' attitudes toward acute diarrrhoea management. *Int J Travel Med* 2001; 8: 60–65.

41. Caerio J P, DuPont H L, Albrecht H, Ericsson C D. Oral rehydration therapy plus loperamide versus loperamide alone in the treament of traveller's diarrhoea. *Clin Infect Dis* 1999; 28: 1286–1289.

42. Thillainayagam A V, Carnaby S, Dias J A, Farthing M J G. Evidence of a dominant role for low osmolarity in the efficacy of cereal based oral rehydration solutions: studies in a model of secretory diarrhoea. *Gut* 1999; 34: 920–925.

43. Sack D A, Islam S, Brown K H *et al.* Oral therapy in children with cholera; a comparison of sucrose and glucose electrolyte solutions. *J Paediatr* 1980; 96: 20–25.

44. Pizarro D, Posada G, Sandi L, Moran J R. Rice-based oral electrolyte solutions for the management of infantile diarrhoea. *N Engl J Med* 1991; 324: 517–521.

45. Taylor D N, Sanchez J L, Candler W *et al.* Treatment of travellers' diarrhoea: ciprofloxacin plus loperamide compared to ciprofloxacin alone. *Ann Intern Med* 1991; 114: 731–734.

46. Salam I, Kateelaris P, Leigh-Smith S, Farthing M J G. Randomised trial of single-dose ciprofloxacin for travellers' diarrhoea. *Lancet* 1994; 344: 1537–1539.

47. De Bruyn G, Hahn S, Borwick A. Antibiotic treatment for travellers' diarrhoea. Cochrane Database of Systematic Reviews (computer file) (3):CD002242, 2000.

48. Gallardo F, Gascon R J, Corachan M *et al. Campylobacter jejuni* as a cause of travellers' diarrhoea: clinical feature and antimicrobial susceptibility. *J Travel Med* 1998; 5: 23–26.

49. Adachi J A, Ostrosky-Zeichner L, Dupont H L, Ericsson C D. Emperical antimicrobial therpay for travellers' diarrhoea. *Clin Infect Dis* 2000; 31: 1079–1083.

50. Steffen R. Rifaximin: a nonabsorbed antimicrobial as a new tool for treatment of travellers' diarrhoea. *J Travel Med* 2001; 8 (suppl. 2): S34–S39.

51. Ericsson C, DuPont H L, Mathewson J L. Optimal dosing of ofloxacin with loperamide in the treatment of non-dysenteric travellers' diarrhoea. *J Travel Med* 2001; 8: 207–209.

52. Ala'Aldeen-D A. A microbiologist's guide to travellers abroad: do as I say not as I do. *J Hosp Infect* 1997; 5: 255–257.

53. Dupont H L, Capsuto E G. Persistent diarrhoea in travellers. *Clin Infect Dis* 1996; 22: 124–128.

54. Mintz E D, Weber J T, Guris D *et al.* An outbreak of Brainerd diarrhoea amongst travellers in the Galapagos Islands. *J Infect Dis* 1999; 177: 1041.

55. Taylor D N, Connor B A, Shlim D R. Chronic diarrhoea in the returned traveller. *Med Clin North Am* 1999; 83: 1033–1052.

3

Food and water hygiene for the traveller

Travellers' diarrhoea (TD) is contracted by consuming contaminated food or water. The risk depends on a variety of factors, as outlined in Chapter 2. Contrary to popular belief, food poses a much greater hazard to the traveller than water. The reason for this is that contamination of water by an organism is prone to a dilution effect, so that insufficient organisms are swallowed by an individual at any one time to cause an infection. Some organisms, such as *Shigella* or *Cryptosporidium*, need only be present in small numbers to cause problems, but such infections are comparatively rare in travellers. Occasionally, if a sewage system breaks down, there is a risk of cholera epidemics.

In the case of food contamination, there is an opportunity for organisms to multiply quite rapidly, resulting in large enough numbers being present on a single piece of food to cause an infection if ingested.

This chapter will examine the measures that can be taken by travellers to minimise the risk of contracting a diarrhoeal illness as a result of ingesting contaminated food and water. It is also worth remembering that not all problems are caused by infective organisms and toxins produced by fish and plants can cause serious problems.

Food hygiene

While food hygiene practices are heavily promoted to the travelling public, there is no particular need to miss out on experiencing the local cuisine. It is not necessarily the type of food that poses a danger, but how well it has been prepared and stored. This section considers practical aspects of helping the traveller choose the safest types of foods.

It would logically be expected that travellers who follow the standard advice regarding food hygiene would experience fewer incidences of diarrhoea. However, apart from avoiding very-high-risk foods, e.g. steak tartare or raw oysters,[1] following hygiene advice has not been demonstrated to reduce the risk of TD in most formal studies.[2,3] In one study, despite pre-departure advice, 34% still suffered from TD.[4]

One study of expatriates and tourists in Nepal[5] could find no association between eating high-risk foods and diarrhoea. The best way of avoiding problems appeared to be preparing food at home, rather than eating in restaurants. However, the study did identify some association with foods that had been prepared earlier in the day and left to stand at room temperature.

Bhopal[6] gives a graphic description of a couple on a 'round-the-world' trip who went to the most extraordinary lengths to avoid risky food and yet both developed severe dysenteric disease: 'One developed life-threatening giardiasis, two episodes of diarrhoea and loose stools that persisted for 30 months on returning to Britain.'

It may be tempting to conclude that following dietary advice strictly is unnecessary. However, following the recommendations on food hygiene is supported by a number of compelling arguments:

- It is likely that failure to avoid TD is more due to an inability of travellers to follow food hygiene advice, rather than the advice being ineffective. Only a few per cent of travellers in one study were willing to comply with advice given.[7]
- The trials examining this issue to date have been rather small and therefore not of sufficient power to link incidence to a particular dietary habit.
- Those who do not follow any of the advice given may still be at greater risk of contracting parasites or *Shigella* infections, which give a more serious diarrhoea and to which resistance is not developed. This is supported by studies which indicate that such travellers tend to have multiple episodes, and a more severe TD.[8]

General principles of food hygiene

There is a universally accepted saying to help travellers avoid the riskiest situations: 'peel it, boil it or forget it'. This underlies the principle that cooked, piping-hot food is considered to be the safest. A few other general points should be understood:

- When possible, it is better to prepare food personally, rather than eating in restaurants and hotels. The quality of the restaurant seems to make little difference to the chance of contracting TD.[9] Eating products from street vendors is best avoided unless served hot, e.g. straight from a wok. It may even be the case that staying and eating in five-star accommodation poses a greater risk than lower-quality hotels. The reason for this observation is that the better presentation of food in such restaurants involves greater handling in its preparation and therefore a greater chance of contamination.

- Dry foods are safer as organisms require a moist environment in which to grow. The key message is that bacterial contamination of moist foods, left out in a warm climate, will very rapidly produce a large number of organisms, likely to cause a gastrointestinal infection if consumed.
- Infection can potentially be picked up from contaminated plates or cutlery. Some travellers will carry their own knives, forks and drinking mugs. As an extreme measure, some also use alcohol wipes for swabbing down suspect utensils.
- It is also important to maintain good personal hygiene. If backpacking or living in rough conditions, it is easy to let standards drop. Travellers may need reminding of the importance of clean hands and fingernails when eating or preparing food.
- Even if pre-travel advice does not reduce the incidence of TD, it may help individuals in their understanding of the condition. This was illustrated by a recent study, where those offered such advice tended to be less likely to seek medical help regarding TD.[10]
- Local foods are often safer than attempts by restaurants to produce more westernised foods in a style of cooking with which they are unfamiliar.

Particular types of food

Table 3.1 indicates the types of foods and their relative safety for the traveller. These are now discussed individually.

Salads

These come quite high on the list of high-risk foods.[11] The worst is considered to be broad-leafed vegetables such as lettuce. This is because of

Table 3.1   Choice of foods for the traveller

Usually safe	Risky	Best avoided
Freshly prepared and hot food	Food from street vendors unless fresh and hot	Poorly stored food
Peeled fruit	Unpeeled fruit and salad unless well washed in clean water	Broad-leafed salad
Canned food	Icecream	Shellfish
Dried food and freshly baked bread		Rare meat and fish Unpasteurised dairy products

the large surface area where there is a potential to harbour many organisms, so it must be adequately cleaned. Added to this is the practice of using human excrement, known as 'night soil', as a fertiliser in some developing countries. Other salad items such as tomatoes or cucumber may present a lesser risk if well prepared.

If undertaken personally, preparation of salad or raw vegetables should always include scrubbing with clean water until all visible signs of dirt have been removed and then finally rinsing with sterilised or boiled water. Some travellers like to soak vegetables overnight in a chemical disinfectant. There is little evidence that this offers significant advantage over scrupulous cleaning, but it does no harm. Traditionally, solutions of potassium permanganate were used, but this tends to spoil the quality of the food and vegetables would need a fairly long contact time. Iodine or chlorine used for water purification (as discussed later) can also be used for soaking and manufacturers of these products give recommendations for the appropriate concentrations. It is claimed that eating the salad with a heavy vinegar or lemon dressing might lessen the risk as the organisms survive less well at a low pH.[12]

Fruit and vegetables

The golden rule is that, if fruit and vegetables are not cooked, opt for those that must first be peeled. Therefore, in terms of fruit, bananas and oranges would be ideal, but grapes would be far more risky. Also, any cooked vegetables that have been allowed to stand for some hours could represent a hazard.

Buffets and sauces

These are quite common sources of TD and food poisoning. In the case of open buffets, flies settle on food and can deposit organisms, which in a warm environment multiply very rapidly. Cold sauces that have been left to stand are also a potential breeding ground for microorganisms.

Breads, rice and pasta

Bread, being a dry food, is relatively safe. Rice and pasta, once cooked, should be consumed immediately. Rice in particular may harbour a bacterium called *Bacillus cereus* that produces a toxin, causing severe diarrhoea.

Fish and shellfish

On the list of foods best avoided, fish and shellfish come quite high. Shellfish in particular can present hazards due to their feeding method of filtering large quantities of water for plankton. This results in a high chance of contamination if such fish are exposed to sewage outlets in the shallow waters where they grow. Fish generally require careful storage. Poisoning by specific toxins can be a problem, for instance, ciguatera poisoning is caused by ciguatoxin-producing (neuro- and cardiotoxin) dinoflagellate plankton, which enter the fish food chain.

Meat and poultry

These are not intrinsically any more of a hazard than vegetable dishes, provided that they are well prepared and not reheated or incorrectly stored. When eating out, these conditions may not always be known so they may represent a potential source of infection. Where possible, freshly and thoroughly cooked meat products should be chosen. It may also be wise to avoid more elaborate dishes that have required a lot of handling during preparation.

Dairy

The major problem with dairy products is the potential that they have been made from unpasteurised milk, presenting a risk of brucellosis. Provided milk has been boiled, it can be considered safe. Therefore, Indian chai, which is a widely available brew of tea and milk boiled together in a large vat, presents little danger. Goat's cheese is a particularly notorious cause of problems.

Water hygiene

In many respects it is easier to arrange a source of clean drinking water than to follow strictly the recommendations given concerning food hygiene. In addition, many people in westernised countries now regularly use bottled water as a main source of fluid intake, a practice that can usually be followed when travelling.

The use of bottled water does still carry a risk because in some developing countries there is a trade in 'counterfeit' bottled water that has simply been filled from a tap. Even sealed bottles can be no guarantee of safety. Partly for this reason, it is often recommended to choose carbonated water if available, as this is less likely to be counterfeit. Also, it is claimed that the relative acidity of carbonated water makes it a less hospitable environment for bacteria.[12] Some concern has been expressed over the increased use of bottled water by travellers to developing countries, in that it presents an environmental hazard. It has been observed that discarded bottles cannot be either recycled or properly disposed of due to lack of resources for waste disposal in poorer countries. Thus the litter generated by tourists in some popular tourist destinations has become a problem.

It is generally recommended that ice in drinks be avoided. The biggest danger is ice that has been chipped from large blocks; in some parts of the world these are delivered to restaurants, sometimes being left out in a street and stored in unhygienic conditions. A problem has been reported in cruise ships which take on board water in foreign ports, which is then used to produce ice before being properly chlorinated.[13] A myth that should be dispelled is that alcohol will sterilise fruit juice or water to which it has been added – the quantity required would not be achieved in an alcoholic beverage.[14]

There will be circumstances where the traveller needs to sterilise a supply of water and this will be discussed in some detail. Essentially, parasites tend to be harder to kill than bacteria. *Giardia* cysts are often considered to be the hardest of all to remove. *Giardia* is most likely to be encountered by trekkers using surface waters, e.g. streams and lakes, as a source of drinking water.

There are three methods by which the traveller can prepare clean drinking water: boiling, chemical disinfection and filtration.

Boiling

Boiling should always be recommended as the method of choice for sterilising water. At higher altitudes, water must be boiled for longer than at sea level because of the lower boiling point. To allow for this variable, it is a good idea to boil water for a full 5 minutes at any altitude. Boiled and cooled water tends to have a flat taste due to loss of oxygen content. Cooling with the pan covered and drinking the water cold can improve the taste.[15]

Boiling will kill all organisms and is the most reliable method against *Cryptosporidium*. The main drawback for the traveller is arranging the facilities to boil sufficient quantities. Heating elements are available that can be used to boil water in a suitable cup or mug.

Chemicals

Water purification tablets are often supplied through pharmacies and camping shops and it is important that travellers know how to use them properly. The halogens, chlorine and iodine, are the most commonly used; the only other widely available product is katadyn silver. Their effectiveness will depend on four variables:

1.   concentration of chemical used
2.   contact time
3.   water temperature
4.   water quality (e.g. pH, presence of organic matter)

If the water is clear of particulate matter and at an ambient temperature, it can be left for a shorter time before being safe to drink. However, if the water is heavily contaminated then a higher concentration of halogen should be used. Recommendations on manufacturers' labels should be followed carefully. The concentration of halogen is usually calculated to allow sterilisation in less than half an hour.

In the UK, chlorination has long been used for the preparation of clean water by trekkers and travellers, whereas in the USA iodine appears to be more popular. There is a long-running debate concerning the choice between chlorine- and iodine-based products. Some of these issues will now be addressed.

Spectrum of activity

Both chlorine and iodine have a wide spectrum of activity and are effective against bacteria, viruses and parasites. For iodine, a concentration of around 8 mg/L is quoted[15] as desirable for removal of organisms within less than half an hour. This concentration is required for inactivation of *Giardia* cysts, but for bacterial or viral contamination a concentration of 0.5 mg/L would be sufficient. For chlorine, 8 mg/L is also effective,[16] with the most popular branded product (Puritabs) producing 10 mg/L.

The debate over activity concerns the effectiveness of the two halogens against *Giardia* cysts, which are particularly likely to present a problem to trekkers using surface waters in the wild. Chlorine can inactivate *Giardia* cysts,[17] but a study comparing different chlorine- and iodine-based products found that chlorine removed a lower percentage of cysts than the iodine products over any of the chosen contact times.[18] Interestingly, even the iodine-based products were shown not to remove more than 90% of the cysts unless left for 24 hours.

Stability at high pH

In laboratory studies, chlorine, but not iodine, tends to lose activity at high pH due to the formation of less active hypochlorite ions,[19] requiring an increase in concentration or contact time above pH 7. The relative importance of this effect when higher concentrations of chlorine are used in the field has not been well studied.

Water temperature

Both halogens are less active at lower temperatures[15–17] and an increase in contact time and/or concentration is required, particularly to remove *Giardia* cysts.

Presence of organic matter

Activity of both halogens can be reduced by the presence of organic matter. If the water appears cloudy, it should always be pre-filtered. This can be achieved by passing it through a piece of cloth or muslin. Alternatively, a special canvas bag known as a Millbank bag (Fig. 3.1) can be used to produce large quantities of clear water. These bags are particularly popular with trekkers. If pre-filtering is not possible then a greater concentration of halogen could be used.

Chlorine is claimed to be more sensitive than iodine to such inactivation, particular in the presence of ammonia ions and amino acids, where chloramines tend to be formed.[15,19]

Side-effect profile and contraindications

There are few problems associated with chlorination, and an obvious advantage over iodine, for which certain precautions must be observed:

- An excessive iodine intake could lead to effects on the thyroid. Goitre formation has been reported where iodinated water has been used exclusively for some months. The most recent of such reports occurred among peace corps workers whose purifier was yielding water with a concentration of iodine at 10 mg/L.[20] The goitre does resolve quite rapidly once iodine consumption is reduced.[21] Furthermore, there are no reports of a clinical hyperthyroidism through this practice. It is unlikely that most travellers would use iodinated water exclusively for any length of time, but most products do carry a warning stating that they should not be used continuously for more than a few weeks.

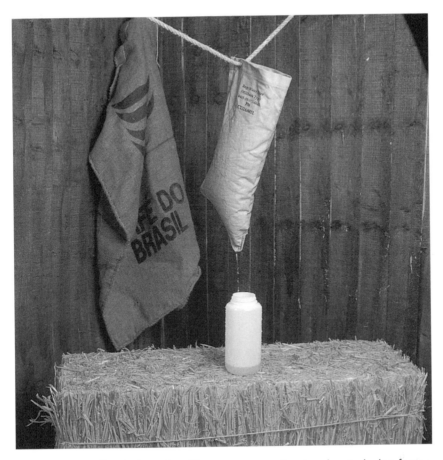

Figure 3.1 Millbank bag for filtering water prior to chemical disinfection. Courtesy of Nomad.

- Because of the theoretical effects on the thyroid, iodination is best avoided in pregnancy and in young children.
- Those people with an allergy to iodine should obviously avoid this method of purification.

Taste

Both halogens impart a taste to the water that some find unacceptable. With the higher concentrations of iodine recommended for *Giardia*, the resultant water is particularly unpalatable. Ascorbic acid is the most convenient neutraliser, removing both the taste and brown coloration of iodinated water. Dispersible ascorbic acid tablets are available for this purpose, but a pinch of ascorbic acid powder would work equally well.

Travellers should be aware that, if a neutraliser is added to the water, then the iodine will be inactivated. Even a small amount of ascorbic acid left in a flask used to sterilise water will reduce the activity of the iodine. Therefore travellers should be advised to add such neutralisers to the final drinking container, e.g. a cup, just before consumption.

The taste of chlorine and iodine can be removed by sodium thiosulphate, although no commercial tablets are available for this purpose. Hydrogen peroxide could be used, but most travellers do not wish to carry bottles of hydrogen peroxide. The taste of chlorine is worse at extremes of pH.

Storage

Once prepared, the presence of chlorine in water may be better at discouraging growth of contaminating organisms than iodine. In either case, it is usually best to consume treated water within 24 hours of preparation.

Conclusion – iodine versus chlorine (Table 3.2)

For most travellers a chlorine-based product would be the most suitable and easily obtainable. Some trekkers and more adventurous travellers

Table 3.2 Comparison of iodine and chlorine as water purification for travellers

	Iodine	Chlorine
Spectrum of activity	Bacteria, viruses and parasites (except *Cryptosporidium*) Possibly more effective than chlorine against *Giardia* cysts	As for iodine
pH	Stable at high pH	Not as active at high pH
Temperature	Less active at low temperature	Less active at low temperature
Presence of organic matter	Less active but more tolerant than chlorine	Less active
Toxicity	Some contraindications; not for continuous use	No special contra-indications; can be used continuously

may wish to use iodine because of the theoretical advantages in certain situations, as outlined. If the water is cold (below about 10°C) it would be wise to let it stand for double the time recommended by manufacturers. Where the treatment time is not made explicit and *Giardia* is suspected, water should ideally be left overnight.

Chlorine-based preparations

Sodium dichloroisocyanurate (Puritabs)   These are one of the UK market leaders and are sold through most pharmacies. They are available in different-strength tablets to treat either 1 or 25 L of water. If used according to the directions on the packaging, they should be effective against *Giardia*, although to date no studies directly investigating their use against this organism have been performed. If the water is heavily contaminated, two tablets should be used. For soaking vegetables, it is recommended to add a total of three tablets to the required quantity of water. A contact time of just 10 minutes is advised. To treat double the quantity of water with the same number of tablets, the time can be increased to 30 minutes.

Household bleach   This can be used provided it is free of additives or disinfectants. Ordinary laundry bleach usually contains 4–6% of available chlorine and one or two drops could be added to a litre of water. This method is probably best reserved for emergency situations where no other products are available. It is also probably not desirable to travel with bottles of bleach as continuous shaking could result in loss of chlorine activity.

Iodine-based preparations

Tincture of Iodine (Alcoholic Iodine Solution BP)   This is the most readily available and cost-effective iodine-based preparation for water purification, containing 2% available iodine. Iodide ions from potassium iodide in the solution are also present; these have no antibacterial activity but double the total iodine concentration.

Directions for using tincture of iodine are somewhat of an anomaly. *Martindale*[22] recommends using five drops per litre, increasing to 12 drops if *Giardia* is suspected. However, the volume per drop would tend to vary to some extent, depending on the type of pipette used. I estimate that one drop of tincture from a standard glass dropper bottle is just 0.02 ml. This would mean that five drops would result in 2 mg/L, more than adequate for removing bacteria and viruses. However, the recommended 12 drops would yield just 5 mg/L, which falls at the lower range of the concentration required for inactivation of *Giardia* cysts. A full 30 minutes or longer (*Martindale* advises 1 hour) at ambient temperatures should be allowed when using tincture of iodine at this dosage if *Giardia* is suspected.

The obvious disadvantage with iodine tincture would be the mess involved with any breakage as it is stored in a glass bottle. The tincture should not be dispensed in plastic bottles because of leaching of iodine. The BP formulation of iodine tincture, which is formulated with ethanol, should always be used. There have been anecdotal reports of other iodine tinctures containing industrial methylated spirits. Povidone-iodine or other forms of aqueous iodine should not be used for water purification. There are a number of commercial pre-packed iodine tinctures in dropper bottles labelled with full instructions and warnings for use.

Tetraglycine hydroperiodide tablet   These are quite widely available in the UK (e.g. Potable Aqua). Each tablet yields 4 mg of available iodine. They are more convenient than the tincture and will give a more reliable dose. However, they do have some disadvantages:

- The tablets can take a long time to dissolve, particularly in cold water.
- They rapidly lose potency once the bottle has been opened.
- They are more expensive than the tincture.

Potable Aqua is also sold in packs containing both tetraglycine hydro-periodide tablets and ascorbic acid tablets for neutralisation of iodine, as mentioned earlier.

Iodine crystals   Most cost-effective of all, and occasionally employed by the more intrepid trekkers, is the system known as the Kahn–Visscher method.[19]

About 5 g of crystals of iodine is stored in a clear glass 30 ml jar with a paper-lined Bakelite cap. This is filled with water to form a saturated solution; the resulting concentration of iodine will vary to some extent with water temperature. The supernatant liquid is then carefully poured off, taking care not to draw off any crystals.

This solution is then used to disinfect water by adding 15 ml to each litre of water. The crystals can therefore generate very large quantities of water, between 250 and 500 L, at little cost.

The procedure is somewhat fiddly, although the system is available in a special cup sold for the purpose (Polar Pur), which gives clear directions on the volume to be added at different temperatures. There is also the risk of inadvertently consuming iodine crystals.

Katadyn silver (Micropure)

The main advantage of katadyn silver tablets (Micropure) is that they impart no taste to water. In addition, water can be stored, once treated, for many months.

There are no particular contraindications to their use. The main drawback is that these tablets are only effective against bacteria and should not be used to treat water where parasites may be a problem. A further disadvantage is that, following addition of the tablets to water, it must be left for 2 hours before drinking. Little published data are available on the effectiveness of katadyn silver.

Pumps and devices

There are a plethora of water purification devices that are marketed as suitable for use by travellers, although there are potential drawbacks with most types. There are two modes by which these devices are able to purify water: by simple filtration or chemically via iodine bound to a resin. Many systems use a combination of both methods.

If a simple filtration method is used, usually with a ceramic filter, the smallest pore size available is around 0.3 μm, which would be too large for removal of viruses (e.g. hepatitis A is 0.03 μm). Therefore, most practical systems that can remove all organisms employ a two-stage device: a filter to remove larger organisms and an iodine-bound resin for viruses. Some also have a third carbon filter to remove chemical contamination and any excess iodine.

The filtering systems that are designed to remove smaller organisms do require a great deal of pumping. Such filters may rapidly become clogged unless water that is free of debris is used. Some devices allow cleaning of the filter system and replacement cartridges to be used. A potential problem is that users may be unaware that the chemical is exhausted, so some purifiers are designed to pass no further water when this stage is reached.

It should be noted that iodine resin could release a high concentration of free iodine, so systems that incorporate a carbon filter are useful.

Those recommending such devices should also note the following points:

- Although it is often stated how many litres a particular system can purify, this may be much reduced if the water is very dirty.
- Be aware of the rate at which water can be produced by the purification system. Some take a great deal of pumping for little reward.
- Although manufacturers may state which organisms are removed, they may not mention the organisms against which the device is not effective.
- For water contaminated by industrial effluent, a device with a carbon filter is required.
- Water produced by purifiers should be used within 24 hours.

Table 3.3 summarises the range of devices currently available in the UK.[23] None is ideal and the price can vary from around £20 for the small-capacity devices up to £250 for the larger katadyn purifiers. The main advantage in their use is that water is available for drinking immediately after it has passed through the system, rather than waiting for a chemical to work or boiled water to cool. They will also impart no taste to the water. Travellers may therefore find them more convenient if the expense and luggage space can be justified. Considering each in Table 3.3:

- The Travelwell is a well-tested range, the PWP version is more compact and robust than the MWP. These work by allowing water to pass by

Table 3.3 Water purification devices

Type of purifer	Maximum amount of water purified (litres)	Type of device
Pocket Travelwell Trekker Travelwell (MWP and PWP)	25 100	Filter and iodine resin
Survival straw	20–40	Filter and iodine resin
Zero B	500	Crystal iodine
First Need Microlite Original	100 400	Filters
Pure cup	500	Filter and iodine resin
Katadyn Mini filter Pocket filter Piston filter pump	7000 10 000+ 10 000+	Ceramic filter and silver

gravity through various filters, thus requiring no pumping to produce drinking water. Two pre-filters remove organic matter, debris and chemical contamination. The water then passes over a resin iodine filter that releases free iodine at 4 ppm. The Travelwell personal purifier has the disadvantage of a somewhat lower yield of water per fill and has a greater tendency to clog up if too much organic matter is allowed to enter the system. On the plus side, it incorporates a final-stage carbon filter that removes any free iodine, improving taste. The MWP model is based on the same principle as the PWP but water must be hand-pumped to pass it through the system so that 200 ml of water can be obtained per minute, unlike the PWP which relies on gravity. Smallest of all is the Pocket Travelwell, which also needs a pump action and is designed for emergency use.

- The travel straw is a small straw containing a pre-filter to remove solid matter, iodine and activated carbon to remove the taste. Water is sucked up directly through the straw and will block off once the iodine is exhausted. It has a very limited capacity and should be seen as a survival aid for trekkers.
- The Zero B is a somewhat fragile gravity filter that uses a crystal iodine filter, but appears not to have an efficient pre-filter for removing debris and other contaminants. It is therefore probably best reserved for treating tap water.
- One of the first purifying devices available to travellers used ceramic filters, which, although very delicate, can be removed and cleaned so that theoretically they will last indefinitely. These ceramic filters are used in the Katadyn range and these are also impregnated with silver to reduce bacterial contamination of the filter. Water must be hand-pumped and a range of sizes are available, from small pocket filters to larger, heavier models suitable for preparing water for small groups of people. A major drawback is that the device cannot be relied upon to remove all viruses.
- The First Need range does not employ any iodine resins, but relies on hand-pumping water through a special purifying cartridge. After being pumped through a 10 μm pre-filter, water then passes through a special matrix that can retain microorganisms, chemical contaminants and any other small particles. Pumping can be quite hard work: the flow rate falls as the filter reaches the end of its life, when it can be replaced. The filter unit is somewhat delicate and easily damaged.

Food and water hygiene in groups and expeditions

There is an even greater imperative for good food and water hygiene amongst those travelling in groups or expeditions as the chance for transmission of diarrhoeal infection can be great. It is common practice amongst such groups for members to design a rota where each will take it in turn to prepare the day's meal. The problem here is that, while individuals may well observe good hygiene in food preparation for small numbers of family or friends, they are not used to preparing food for larger numbers of people, typically in an overland group of 10–20 people. In addition food may be prepared without the availability of running water or adequate sanitation. The following simple rules should be observed.[24]

- Do not let anyone suffering from a diarrhoeal illness be involved in any preparation of food. It is a good idea if just one person is in overall charge of catering to oversee the rota and ensure that good standards of hygiene are maintained.
- Fingernails should be cut and hands scrubbed clean before food preparation. Ideally, separate clean aprons or other outer garments should be available in the food preparation area. Clean, dry utensils should be used and all surfaces should be thoroughly cleaned before food preparation using a suitable chlorine-based disinfectant.
- It may be wise not to include certain foods, such as shellfish, on the menu. Any raw meat should be stored and prepared separately from other types of food.
- Hair should be tied back and any wounds covered with a dressing or plaster.
- Food should be eaten hot and not left out for buffet-style meals (see notes above). If no refrigeration is available then any left-over food most be thoroughly reheated or discarded.

Summary

- Fresh foods: those that are peeled or cooked are the safest.
- Avoid high-risk foods like shellfish.
- Boiling water is the best method of sterilisation.
- Chemicals are useful for preparing safe drinking water but have their limitations.
- Chlorine-based tablets are widely available and will be appropriate for most travellers.
- More intrepid travellers and those planning to use surface waters as a drinking water source should use an iodine-based product.

Frequently asked questions

Is it worth soaking vegetables in solutions of chlorine or potassium permanganate?
Scrubbing the vegetables in soapy water and then rinsing in freshly prepared sterilised water should be the first line of defence. Whether soaking offers any additional protection has not been studied. The contact time for effective treatment may ruin certain vegetables such as lettuce.

Are vegetables safer than meat?
It is true that certain parasitic infections such as tapeworms (Chapter 5) will only be contracted by eating meat. Also food poisoning such as from *Salmonella* may be more likely from undercooked and reheated meat or shellfish. On the other hand, vegetables are a common source of diarrhoea in travellers, particularly in the case of salads. Meat that is freshly and simply prepared, served hot and cooked through can be assumed to be safe.

Is it worth buying a filter device for producing clean water?
On purely economic grounds, for most trips they offer no advantages over chemical methods. In terms of convenience the two big advantages over chemicals are not having to wait while the water boils and leaving no taste in the water. For those using surface waters the devices do not require pre-filtered water. However, the various types on the market all have drawbacks in terms of efficiency, reliability and convenience of use, as discussed in the text.

Is it best to use chlorine- or iodine-based chemicals for water purification?
As discussed in the text, my conclusion is that chlorine is the most convenient method for sterilising tap water, but iodine may have advantages for surface waters. Iodine should not be recommended if this is the sole means of obtaining clean water for a period much greater than a few weeks.

References

1. Mattila L. Clinical features and duration of travellers' diarrhoea in relation to its aetiology. *Clin Infect Dis* 1994; 19: 28–34.
2. Cartwright R Y. Travellers' diarrhoea. *Br Med Bull* 1992; 49: 348–362.
3. Pitzinger B, Steffen R, Tschopp A. Incidence and clinical features of travellers' diarrhoea in infants and children. *Paediatr Infect Dis J* 1991; 10: 719–723.
4. Shlim D R, Hoge C W, Rajah R *et al*. Persistent high risk of diarrhoea among foreigners in Nepal during the first two years of residence. *Clin Infect Dis* 1999; 29: 613–616.

5. Hoge C W, Shlim D R, Echeverria P *et al*. Epidemiology of diarrhoea among expatriate residents living in a highly endemic environment. *JAMA* 1996; 275: 533–538.

6. Bhopal R. Travellers' diarrhoea: difficult to avoid. *BMJ* 1993; 307: 322–323.

7. Steffen R. Epidemiologic studies of travellers' diarrhoea, severe gastrointestinal infections and cholera. *Rev Infect Dis* 1986; 8: S122–S130.

8. Ryder R W, Oquist C A, Greenberg H *et al*. Travellers' diarrhoea in Panamanian tourists in Mexico. *J Infect Dis* 1981; 144: 442–448.

9. Kollaritsch H. Travellers' diarrhoea among Austrian tourists in warm climate countries. *Eur J Epidemiol* 1989; 5: 74–81.

10. McIntosh I B, Reed J M, Power K G. Travellers' diarrhoea and the effect of pre-travel health advice in general practice. *Br J Gen Pract* 1997; 47: 71–75.

11. Merson M H, Morris G K, Sack D A *et al*. Travellers' diarrhoea in Mexico: a prospective study of physicians and family members attending a congress. *N Engl J Med* 1976; 294: 1299–1305.

12. Garelick H. Safe water. In: Dawood R, ed. *Travellers' Health: How to Stay Healthy Abroad*, 3rd edn. Oxford: Oxford University Press, 2002: 71–78.

13. Daniels N A, Neimann J, Karpati A *et al*. Traveler's diahrroea at sea: three outbreaks of waterborne enterotoxigenic *Escherichia coli* on cruise ships. *J Infect Dis* 2000; 181: 1491–1495.

14. Dickens D L, DuPont H L, Johnson P C. Survival of bacterial enteropathogens in the ice of popular drinks. *JAMA* 1985; 10: 953–957.

15. Wilkerson J A, ed. *Medicine for Mountaineers*, 3rd edn. Seattle: The Mountaineers, 1985.

16. Jarroll E L, Bingham A K, Meyer E A. *Giardia* destruction: effectiveness of six small quantity water disinfection methods. *Am J Trop Med Hyg* 1980; 29: 8–11.

17. Jarroll E L, Bingham A K, Meyer E. Effect of chlorine on *Giardia lamblia* cyst viability. *Appl Environ Microbiol* 1981; 41: 483–487.

18. Ongerth J E, Johnson R L, MacDonalds S C *et al*. Backcountry water treatment to prevent giardiasis. *Am J Public Health* 1989; 79: 1633–1637.

19. Kahn F H, Visscher B R. Water disinfection in the wilderness. *West J Med* 1975; 122: 450–453.

20. Kahn L K, Li R, Gootnick D. Peace corps thyroid investigation group. *Lancet* 1998; 352: 1519.

21. Lemar H J, Georitis W J, McDermott M T. Thyroid adaptation to chronic tetraglycine hydroperiodide water purification tablet use. *J Clin Endocrinol Metab* 1995; 80: 220–223.

22. *Martindale: The complete drug reference*, 32nd edn. London: Pharmaceutical Press, 1999: 1494.

23. Goodyer P, Goodyer L. Water purification. In: Warrell D, Anderson S, eds. *Expedition Medicine*. London: Profile Books, 1998: 73–78.

24. Bennet Jones H. Base camp hygiene and health. In: Warrell D, Anderson S, eds. *Expedition Medicine*. London: Profile Books, 1998: 63–72.

4

Malaria

Of the many insect-borne diseases, malaria causes the greatest mortality worldwide. In 2000 there were an estimated 657 million cases of malaria, resulting in 1–2 million deaths,[1] the majority being in young African children. Up to 30 000 travelling from Europe and North America to endemic areas have been estimated to contract malaria every year.[2]

Malaria has long been eradicated from most of Europe and North America, although the mosquitoes capable of transmitting malaria are native to these continents. There have been occasional reports of local outbreaks of malaria as the result of a person, infected with malaria in another country, being bitten by local mosquitoes. If these mosquitoes are allowed to breed, the disease may be transmitted to other people. However, in order to develop a situation where malaria becomes endemic, a critical number of individuals must be carrying the parasites to create a large enough pool to maintain the disease. The other circumstance in which malaria is occasionally observed outside endemic regions is so-called 'airport malaria'. This occurs when infected mosquitoes enter a country via an aircraft, despite the use of knockdown sprays in the cabins. There are reports from time to time of individuals contracting malaria in and around airports.

There are fears that, with global warming, malaria may emerge in more temperate climates. Malaria is at its most active in the broad band between the tropics (Fig. 4.1). For the traveller from the UK, increasing tourism to such areas has resulted in malaria presenting a significant risk. Every year approximately 2000 travellers from the UK contract malaria and up to a dozen deaths occur as a result. This figure has changed little over the past 10 years and, as will be discussed later, over a third of such cases[3,4] occur in people from ethnic groups resident in the UK who have returned to their country of origin for a brief visit. Undoubtedly sub-Saharan Africa poses the greatest risk to the UK travelling public, as of the 100 deaths amongst UK travellers recorded over the last 10 years, 94 were contracted in that part of the world. This is reflected by the numbers of recorded cases of malaria in 2001 as, out of the 2050 cases, 1483 were contracted in sub-Saharan Africa, 1017 from areas of West Africa alone. Furthermore, most of these cases occurred in people who were African or of African descent, identifying travellers visiting family as a particular risk group.

Prevention of malaria in travellers has two major aspects: the use of chemoprophylaxis and the avoidance of mosquito bites, as considered in Chapter 6. Recommendations regarding use of prophylactic agents do vary from country to country and, although the World Health Organization (WHO) issues guidelines regarding the choice of agents to particular areas visited,[5] these are not universally accepted. This situation does tend to cause confusion in travellers when they reach a particular endemic area, to find that others from different countries have not been prescribed the same, or sometimes any, prophylaxis. For the most part this chapter will focus on the current UK guidelines as issued by the UK Advisory Committee on Malaria Prevention.[6] This particular edition of the guidelines offers a useful mnemonic to help health professionals in preventing and treating traveller's malaria:

Awareness: to raise public awareness of the risks of malaria
Bites by mosquitoes: to ensure optimal precautions are taken to avoid bites
Compliance with appropriate chemoprophylaxis
Diagnose and obtain appropriate treatment promptly

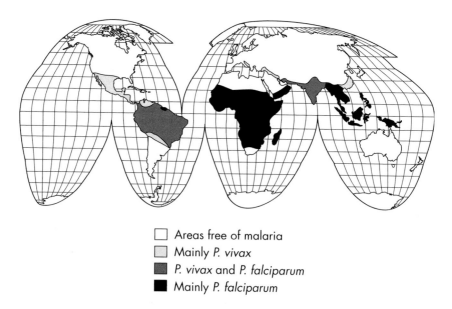

☐ Areas free of malaria
▨ Mainly *P. vivax*
▧ *P. vivax* and *P. falciparum*
■ Mainly *P. falciparum*

Figure 4.1 World distribution of risk of infection from *Plasmodium vivax* and *P. falciparum*.

This chapter will examine various aspects of malaria that are relevant to travellers from non-endemic countries. The treatment of malaria, other than emergency self-medication, will only be briefly described.

Forms of malaria and risk to the traveller

Traditionally, malaria has been defined in two classes: the potentially fatal malignant malaria (caused by *Plasmodium falciparum*) and a less dangerous benign malaria (caused by *P. vivax*, *P. malariae* and *P. ovale*). Figure 4.1 shows the relative distribution of the two most common forms of malaria – *P. vivax* and *P. falciparum*. As can be seen, *P. falciparum* is predominant in sub-Saharan Africa and *P. vivax* causes only 10% of infections. In other areas, such as Haiti, only *P. falciparum* is present. *P. vivax* can be found in more temperate climates and is absent in West Africa. This is because the possession of the Duffy blood group is necessary for *P. vivax* infections and is not present in West Africans. Similarly, possession of sickle-cell trait results in a less severe malaria and glucose-6-phosphate dehydrogenase (G6PD) deficiency offers partial protection. It must be emphasised that there are local variations within the areas shown in Figure 4.1.

P. ovale is mainly found in sub-Saharan Africa, with a further focus in South-East Asia, and *P. malariae* has a patchy distribution in all endemic areas.[7] As will be discussed later, *P. vivax* remains mostly sensitive to chloroquine alone but there is widespread resistance of *P. falciparum*. It is feared that global warming may see a spread of malaria into more temperate climates. Although this has not yet occurred to any significant extent, there is an increased incidence in some parts of the world where endemicity was formerly quite low, as in some central Asian countries experiencing a resurgence of *P. vivax* malaria.

An important aspect of falciparum malaria, in particular, is that those living in highly endemic areas will acquire semi-immunity to it. Therefore, in healthy adults living in endemic countries, life-threatening falciparum malaria might not be seen as often. Young children under 5 years of age have not developed such immunity and mortality in this age group is high. Immunity wanes over a few years once the individual has left the endemic area and is no longer exposed to *P. falciparum*. In a situation where immunity is reduced, for instance during severe illness, resistance may also be lost.[8] Even interruption to exposure to malaria whilst still resident in an endemic areas, for instance due to seasonal variations or local control measures, could result in a loss of semi-immunity.

Malaria is very dangerous in pregnancy and is an important cause of spontaneous abortion and stillbirth in some endemic areas. It is also a particular risk for children. Amongst children under the age of 15 in the UK there were 278 recorded cases of malaria in 2001; again the majority (182) amongst these were African or of African descent. A retrospective study of the period 1975–1999 of childhood malaria treated in St George's Hospital in south-west London[9] found that the incidence had increased over this period, with only 22% accounted for by immigrants arriving in the UK. In only 41% of the cases were children taking malaria prophylaxis and the numbers not taking such prophylaxis seemed to be increasing. So far there have been 10 deaths amongst those under 15 contracting malaria whilst overseas.

Travellers who have no immunity from the disease may receive inadequate treatment from local clinics that are unused to treating non-immune subjects. For instance, it has been common practice for the local population in some countries to receive chloroquine tablets, partly for economic reasons, rather than parenteral quinine, which was generally given to treat falciparum malaria. In recent years the use of chloroquine to treat malaria in many endemic countries has been reduced due to the very high incidence of chloroquine resistance.

As mentioned, a particular at-risk group are immigrants residing in non-endemic areas who return to their country of origin to visit relatives and friends. These individuals will not always take adequate prophylactic measures in the mistaken belief that they still possess a degree of immunity. In one area of London it has been estimated that nearly 90% of travellers having contracted malaria fall into this category. The actual level of risk to an individual will depend upon the proportion of mosquitoes that carry the disease, the number of infected bites received and the time spent in the area. The numbers of mosquitoes carrying malaria will vary between regions and often between times of year relative to the wet or monsoon season.

The risk is often lower in more urban and coastal areas, and is absent above 2000 metres, where mosquitoes cannot survive. A high-risk area is the rainforests of West Africa, where an unprotected individual staying for 1 week has a 2–3% chance per month of contracting malaria. One of the highest-risk areas currently exists in the Solomon Islands, at 8% per month. Incidence can be as low as 0.01% per month in Central America.

Table 4.1 At-risk types of travel for contracting malaria

Contributing to a lower risk	Contributing to a moderate risk	Contributing to a higher risk
Cities or major tourist areas in Latin America or Asia	Business travellers	Most travelling to sub-Saharan Africa, Haiti, Vanuatu, Papua New Guinea and Solomon Islands
Upmarket hotels	Travelling outside the known malaria season in higher endemic areas	Working in rural tropical areas
Less than 2 weeks on organised tour	On organised tours involving rural areas	Backpackers
Not visiting rural areas		Aid workers Immigrants living in non-endemic areas returning for a visit

The type of accommodation, e.g. the presence or absence of air conditioning, will also be an important determinant of exposure to mosquitoes. The most important determinant that can be controlled by the traveller is the preventive measures taken in terms of personal protection against mosquitoes and malarial chemoprophylaxis.

There are therefore quite a large number of interrelated aspects to determining the relative risk of malaria to a particular travel. For instance, although the risk of malaria is general high in sub-Saharan African, this would be considerably less for a business executive visiting a capital city for just a few days compared to a tourist planning a longer safari in rural areas. The particular high- and low-risk groups are summarised in Table 4.1 as an approximate indication of the relative importance of these factors.[10]

Pathophysiology and life cycle

Life cycle

The life cycle of the malaria parasite is described in many medical textbooks, so only a brief summary is given here (Fig. 4.2).

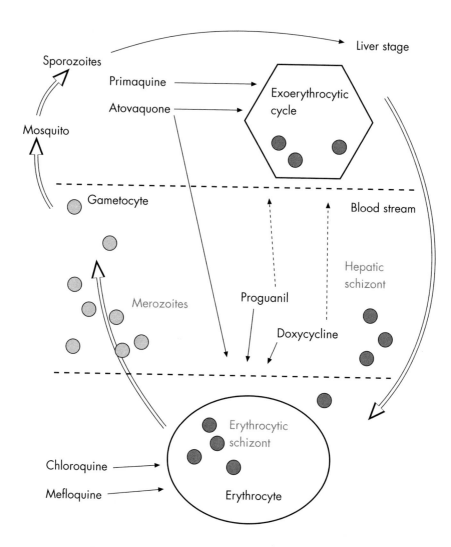

Figure 4.2 Life cycle of malaria parasite and action of chemotherapy.

The insect vectors of malaria are the anophelian family of mosquitoes, of which there are a great many species. For the development of eggs in the female mosquito, a blood meal is necessary. The mosquito lays eggs in still water (anything from a pond to stagnant water in an old tyre) where the free-swimming larvae will eventually pupate. In order to transmit malaria, a mosquito must pick up the sexual state of the malaria parasite, called gametocytes, while biting a human. These mature within the mosquito to asexual sporozoites which can then be transmitted to a human through a bite. These sporozoites will then infect the hepatocytes of the human liver, where further development and multiplication, called extraerythrocytic schizogony, takes place. From the hepatocytes, many thousands of merozoites are released, which then invade red blood cells (RBCs). Once inside an RBC, the merozoite develops into a trophozoite and, following further cell division and multiplication, is termed a schizont (erythrocytic schizogony). The schizonts will form 8–24 mature merozoites which are released into the blood stream to invade further RBCs.

Some of the merozoites will form sexual gametocytes and, if a mosquito takes these up in a bite, the cycle is completed. This, the sexual life cycle, is clinically irrelevant. Symptoms of malaria result from the invasion and rupture of RBCs in asexual reproduction.

P. vivax and *P. ovale* can remain dormant in liver hepatocytes, persisting as hepatozoites.

Pathophysiology

Apart from the fever and malaise associated with release of merozoites into the blood stream, there are few serious complications resulting from the benign malarias, although anaemia will develop over time if the disease is not treated. However, in the case of falciparum malaria in non-immune travellers, there is a high risk of complications resulting from blood vessel damage. In this form of malaria, the surface of the RBCs becomes altered so that they adhere to blood vessel walls. This leads to sequestration of infected RBCs in deep tissues of various organs.[11] Sequestration in the brain can lead to the complication known as cerebral malaria. The tendency to cause vascular damage is further enhanced by the immune response to this form of malaria. It is believed that certain cytokines released by white blood cells, such as tumour necrosis factor and the interleukins, are important in this process and also responsible for the epsiodes of pyrexia associated with the release of merozoites. As it is the immune response to infection that is responsible, more than any direct damage to tissues or red blood cells by the parasite, there is not a very good correlation between the degree of parasitaemia observed and the severity of the disease. Indeed, complications can be experienced despite almost undetectable levels of parasites in the blood.

Although falciparum malaria does not form hepatozoites, the parasites may still be present in the blood at extremely low levels once symptoms have resolved. This can lead to a relapse of the disease, known as a recrudescence, occurring at a later date up to several months after the initial episode. *P. malariae* can display recrudescence 40 years or more after infection. The severity of falciparum malaria is also probably related to the larger numbers of merozoites released on rupture of the schizonts, compared to the other more benign forms. The persistent hepatocyte stages can lead to a recurrence of symptoms for many years.

Clinical presentation

The greatest danger of malaria is that early symptoms tend to be non-specific. Often described as 'influenza-like' (fever, malaise, headaches and joint pains), there may also be associated gastrointestinal symptoms of diarrhoea and vomiting. Attacks of malaria are classically described in three phases: coldness and rigors; feeling hot and flushed; and then intense sweating as the attack resolves. With the benign forms of malaria a synchronicity of fevers can develop as the schizonts rupture within the same time period, classically every 48 hours for *P. vivax* and every 72 hours for *P. malariae*. As with many of the symptoms and complications related to malaria, the fever is a result of the host immune reaction to the parasite. As the schizonts rupture, so the host immune system is activated, and mononuclear white blood cells (e.g. macrophages) release the cytokine tumour necrosis factor-α believed to be largely responsible for the fever.

In the case of severe falciparum malaria, the fevers are irregular, with coma and death sometimes occurring in as little as 24 hours from initial symptoms. For malaria caused by *P. vivax* and *P. ovale*, cyclical fevers and malaise may afflict the individual for many years if not treated, but in healthy adults such infections would rarely be fatal.

Table 4.2 Symptoms and complications of malaria

Presenting symptoms	Complications
Fever and chills	Anaemia
Myalgia and arthralgia	Thrombocytopenia
Diarrhoea	Central nervous system
Headache	Pulmonary
Nausea and vomiting	Renal insufficiency
Malaise	Hypoglycaemia
	Splenomegaly

After being bitten by an infected mosquito, onset of symptoms of malaria will take a minimum of a week to appear. In the case of falciparum malaria 90% of cases would have manifest themselves by 3 months, but periods of a year or more are possible.[1] The other forms of malaria can take longer, sometimes up to a year, to cause symptoms. Hence it is advisable to inquire about travel in the previous year in those presenting with influenza-like symptoms. The presentation of these symptoms can be highly variable and modified by the use of antimalarial and antipyretic drugs. The presence of any pyrexia should immediately alert one to the possibility of malaria.

Malaria is particularly dangerous in pregnancy, resulting in a high risk of abortion and maternal fatalities. Travel to malaria-endemic areas during pregnancy is therefore usually strongly discouraged unless there are compelling reasons.

The issue for the child contracting malaria is that progress of the disease can be even faster than seen in the adult, with symptoms of a greater severity and increased risk of fatality, sometimes within a few hours of onset.[12] There are two reasons for this difference. Firstly, the small body mass and blood volume mean that parasitaemia will be proportionally higher than in an adult. Secondly, an underdeveloped immune system would result in the child being overwhelmed by such an infection. Fever will be present in the majority of cases and often does not follow the pattern of regular fever seen for *P. vivax* in adults. Diagnosis based on symptoms can be very difficult due to the possibility of the occurrence of other very common childhood infections such as otitis media. A range of symptoms may present which are also attributable to other causes in children, e.g. nausea and vomiting, abdominal pain, coughing and irritability. For these reasons WHO has issued a general recommendation that children do not travel to malaria-endemic areas if this can be avoided.

Diagnosis of malaria is based upon the observation of infected RBCs using microscopy – the so-called thick- and thin-plate methods. Potential drawbacks to this method are that non-immune people may develop clinical symptoms before the parasites can be detected and the technique requires skilled personnel. A variety of immunological approaches are also available to help overcome these problems. A detailed discussion concerning the diagnosis of malaria is outside the scope of this book, other than kits used for self-diagnosis in the field by travellers, covered under Diagnostic kits, below.

Chemoprophylactic agents

As shown in Figure 4.2, most antimalarials have their effect on the blood stages of the parasite life cycle, the two exceptions being primaquine and atovaquone. Primaquine is not much used for chemoprophylaxis and will not be discussed further. Both proguanil and doxycycline do have some activity on the liver stages, but this is not thought to contribute significantly to their activity as prophylactic agents.

One of the most important groups of antimalarials is the quinoline group, e.g. chloroquine, mefloquine and quinine. Other antimalarials in common use are the dihydrofolate inhibitors, e.g. proguanil, pyrimethamine, sulfadoxine and dapsone. Doxycycline is becoming more widely used, and ciprofloxacin and azithromycin are being investigated for antimalarial activity. Atovaquone/proguanil (Malarone) is the most recent addition amongst the prophylactic agents. Chloroquine, proguanil and mefloquine are known to offer protection against susceptible strains of both *P. vivax* and *P. falciparum*. There are insufficient data concerning activity against *P. vivax* by atovaquone, but the proguanil content in the formulation would presumably afford satisfactory protection. It has been claimed that doxycycline is less useful against *P. vivax* malaria, although direct evidence for this is lacking.

The mechanisms for parasite resistance to antimalarials are not completely understood. It has been observed that chloroquine is actively excreted by resistant parasites at 40 times the rate of sensitive ones.[13] More is known about the mechanism of resistance for difolate inhibitors and atovaquone than for quinolines, where the specific gene responsible has been identified.

Adverse reactions are an important aspect of antimalarial prophylaxis in that the risks of serious adverse reactions must be clearly balanced against the chance of contracting malaria. However, due to the low doses employed in chemoprophylaxis, the more serious problems encountered when using the agents to treat malaria would rarely be seen. More minor adverse effects are quite common, with a rate of between 12% and 30% reported, no matter what the particular agent used.[14]

The health professional should be in a position to counsel travellers regarding likely side-effects and to screen for potential interactions and contraindications. These are summarised in Table 4.3 and briefly discussed below.

Table 4. 3 Some important adverse reactions and contraindications to antimalarials

Drug	Adverse reactions	Contraindications
Chloroquine	Nausea Visual disturbances Depression Insomnia Dizziness Pruritus Headache	Epilepsy Psoriasis
Proguanil	Mouth ulcers Gastrointestinal disturbance	Renal impairment
Mefloquine	Nausea Headache Dizziness Neuropsychiatric reactions	Pregnancy Psychiatric illness Epilepsy
Pyrimethamine/ dapsone	Blood dyscrasias Cutaneous reactions	Pregnancy Glucose-6-phosphate dehydrogenase deficiency
Doxycycline	Vaginal thrush Photosensitivity	Pregnancy Children
Atovaquone/proguanil	As for proguanil	As for proguanil

Chloroquine and proguanil

Mode of action

The quinolines have activity only at the erythrocytic stages of parasite development; however, the precise mode of action is somewhat contentious. Until recently, the favoured theory was that chloroquine raised pH within the parasite food vacuole. However, some agents that seem to be very efficient at raising pH in this way do not possess good activity against the parasite.[15] The current explanation is that these drugs can inhibit haem polymerase. Free haem, which is toxic to the malaria parasite, is normally detoxified by the action of this enzyme to form haemozoin.

By contrast, more is known regarding the action of the dihydrofolate inhibitors, which have some additional effects on the liver stages of the parasite. Unlike mammalian cells, the malarial protozoa are unable to obtain folic acid as a nutrient and it must be synthesised intra-cellularly, a process which this group of drugs will inhibit.

Adverse effects, contraindications and interactions

Although a fairly long list of adverse events to chloroquine has been presented, only gastrointestinal upset is relatively common.[16] This problem can be relieved to some extent by taking the drug after food. Neuropsychiatric reactions can also occur and up to 2% may discontinue chloroquine prophylaxis either for this reason or due to gastrointestinal effects.[17] Chloroquine also has the potential to cause retinal damage, but this is only apparent at much higher doses than are used for malarial prophylaxis. Prophylactic chloroquine has been observed to cause clonic-tonic seizures and is therefore usually avoided in patients with epilepsy. Likewise, prophylaxis can also result in a flare-up of psoriasis, so should be avoided in individuals with this condition. Chloroquine may suppress the immune response to rabies vaccine if the vaccine is given by the (unlicensed) intradermal route,[18] so the subcutaneous route should be used in such circumstances. Similarly, an inadequate response may result if these antimalarials are taken with an oral typhoid vaccine. There is some racial variation in adverse effects as people with darker skin are more prone to chloroquine-induced pruritus.

Proguanil may increase the effects of warfarin and the international normalised ratio (INR) should be monitored on initiation of therapy. The most frequently observed adverse effect to proguanil is mouth ulcers. Hair thinning has been reported, probably attributable to proguanil, although chloroquine has also been implicated.

Evidence for efficacy

Many efficacy studies have been conducted on chloroquine and proguanil, if only because for some time they were used as a gold standard against which to compare newer agents. As can be seen from the studies described in this section, when used in sub-Saharan Africa they usually prove inferior to such agents. It would be reasonable to assume that a 60–70% efficacy noted 5–10 years ago[19,20] would most certainly correlate with an even lower rate today. It has been argued that the dose of weekly chloroquine used in the UK may not be sufficient, although there is little other than anecdotal evidence to support this view. It has also been claimed that the complication of having to take chloroquine weekly and proguanil daily may reduce compliance, and may even be potentially dangerous if the high dose of chloroquine is taken every day. For this reason a combined daily tablet containing a lower dose of chloroquine with proguanil has been produced, but not licensed in the UK.

Mefloquine

Mode of action

This is as for the quinolines.

Adverse effects, contraindications and interactions

Whether or not to take mefloquine has become a contentious issue since its safety was questioned in the media following anecdotal reports of adverse effects by tourists. An examination of the incidence of adverse effects in a variety of studies indicates a very wide range of between 12 and 90% of participants experiencing adverse events attributable to mefloquine.[19] This variation is probably related very much to the way in which such events are reported and classified as well as the setting in which the study was conducted. For instance, if recording fatigue and sleep disturbance as a potential adverse event, this may well be very high in those studies that involved soldiers undergoing hard physical training in the field. A fairly consistent picture has emerged that in trials where mefloquine is compared directly to another agent, the overall incidence of reported adverse events is similar.[19,20] Even discontinuation of therapy due to adverse effects does not provide a consistent picture of a worse outcome for mefloquine. A recent meta-analysis concluded that the overall incidence of adverse events to mefloquine was indeed no greater than for other agents.[21] There may however be some differences in the type of adverse effects experienced. Some studies indicate a higher incidence of neuropsychiatric effects compared to chloroquine,[22,23] whereas others found no difference in incidence.[19] Compared to atovaquone/proguanil, though, the incidence of such effects and discontinuation of therapy may be higher in those taking mefloquine.[24]

Dizziness is one of the more common reported reactions, which tends to be self-limiting on continuation of treatment. The most contentious issue concerns the neuropsychiatric reaction which includes anxiety, nightmares, abnormal behaviour and psychosis. In a few cases, such symptoms have been claimed to persist long after discontinuation of therapy and appear to be more common in those taking mefloquine than in those taking proguanil and chloroquine.[23]

Of potential concern is that the central nervous system adverse effects of mefloquine may impair performance in certain critical situations, e.g. piloting an airplane or deep-sea diving. There is little in the way of evidence to substantiate such worries and providing the individual appears to tolerate medication it has been suggested that no impairment in ability should be apparent.[25]

Travellers may therefore need careful explanations of the risks/benefits of taking mefloquine. An example of such an assessment is illustrated in Table 4.4. It describes the risk of contracting malaria in the forests of West Africa, which is an area of very high transmission, together with the risk of an adverse event occurring which is serious enough to warrant discontinuation of therapy. The argument is that, for trips of 2 or more weeks, the danger of contracting malaria can outweigh the risk of side-effects of mefloquine, and that the level of protection from chloroquine/proguanil is very much lower. Until recently, for shorter trips the balance was thought to turn in the other direction, making chloroquine/proguanil an acceptable alternative. This was the reasoning in the late 1990s behind the recommendation that mefloquine was not always thought appropriate for short trips to coastal resorts in East Africa. However, the most recent guidelines would indicate the use of mefloquine, even on shorter trips. This is due to the realisation that increased drug resistance to chloroquine would probably result in a level of protection even lower than that indicated in Table 4.4.

Table 4.4 Relative risks of contracting malaria in West and coastal East Africa – late 1990s

	Travellers contracting malaria during a 2-week visit (%)	Travellers contracting malaria during a 4-week visit (%)
West African rainforest		
No prophylaxis	4	8
Chloroquine/proguanil	0.06–1.2	1.2–2.4
Mefloquine	0.02–0.4	0.04–0.8
Coastal East Africa		
No prophylaxis	0.6	1.2

(Neuropsychiatric adverse reactions resulting in discontinuation of mefloquine – 0.5)

Travellers should also be advised that if an adverse reaction is going to occur, then in 75% of cases it will have been noticed by the third dose, emphasising the value of advice to take mefloquine in advance of travel (see below). It has also been observed that neuropsychiatric side-effects are more common amongst women than men.[6]

A further testament to the usefulness of mefloquine is that, after recommendations to use the drug in Kenya in 1993, there was a three-fold reduction in the cases of reported malaria.[26] However, after a reduction in the use of mefloquine following safety concerns, there was a marked rise in imported malaria from East Africa, only partly explained by an increase in malaria transmission.[27]

Mefloquine can potentiate the effect of quinine, and convulsions have been observed when intravenous quinine has been administered to those taking mefloquine prophylaxis. Care should also be taken if administering mefloquine to patients with epilepsy or with certain arrhythmias, and it may potentiate digoxin. It has also been described that partial resistance by some strains may result in a very low level of parasitaemia, so that symptoms are not seen until many weeks after travel – a mean of around 6 weeks for mefloquine compared to 2 weeks for chloroquine/proguanil.[28]

Mefloquine is metabolised in the liver and quite large interindividual variations in elimination and other pharmacokinetic parameters have been noted,[25] some based on ethnic differences, perhaps in part explaining why certain individuals appear to tolerate mefloquine less well than others. Food can also greatly increase the absorption of mefloquine, so it is best taken with a meal. Generic tablets are available in some countries, which may have a different and somewhat lower bioavailability to Lariam. One such generic product had a relative bioavailability about one-quarter less than Lariam,[25] although the clinical significance of these differences is not known.

Evidence for efficacy

There is very good evidence supporting the efficacy of mefloquine as a prophylactic, with trials conducted in a variety of situations and countries involving non-immune subjects. Protection levels of 90–95% are observed in most studies. In all trials where it has been compared to choroquine/proguanil, mefloquine has proved to be superior in efficacy.[19,20] In one trial conducted in Cambodia, mefloquine did not provide particularly good protection – around 85% – due to the presence of resistant strains.[29]

Tetracyclines

Mode of action

The mechanism of action of the tetracyclines, such as doxycycline, is through inhibition of cellular protein synthesis by an action on RNA. It does not have an effect on mammalian cells as, unlike single-celled organisms, they lack an active transport mechanism to take up tetracyclines into the cell.

Adverse effects, contraindications and interactions

Doxycycline can cause a photosensitivity reaction in about 3% of individuals, and protection from this effect by sunscreens has not been assessed. An additional problem for women is the occurrence of vaginal thrush. This may be compounded by the increased incidence of fungal infection when travelling to hot and humid areas. Cases of *Clostridium difficile*-associated diarrhoea have also been associated with doxycyline chemoprophylaxis.[30] There is a tendency for oesophageal inflammation and damage if not swallowed properly, so capsules should always be taken sitting upright with plenty of water. Like all tetracyclines, doxycycline is contraindicated in children, pregnancy and breastfeeding due to staining of developing teeth.

Absorption of doxycycline is impaired by antacid and iron preparations and should not be taken within 3–4 hours of these substances. There is a theoretical interaction with some antiepileptics and also with oral contraceptives. In the case of the latter it is common practice to advise taking additional contraceptive measures for about the first 2 weeks of therapy with any broad-spectrum antibiotic. An increased anticoagulant effect of warfarin has also been reported when taken with doxycycline.

Evidence of efficacy

Doxycycline appears to be as effective as mefloquine in trials conducted in South-East Asia,[31] although less work appears to have been done in Africa. There are a number of trials reported in the literature and in the two double-blind, placebo-controlled trials conducted in Indonesia a 92–100% efficacy was demonstrated against *P. falciparum* and *P. vivax*.[32]

Atovaquone/proguanil

Mode of action

Atovaquone appears to act in a different way to other antimalarials in that it acts directly on the parasite's mitochondrial membrane by inhibiting mitochondrial transport mechanism and thus 'collapsing' the membrane potential. It is also believed that proguanil, but not the metabolite cycloguanil, acts on the mitochondrial membrane, thus explaining the synergism with atovaquone. As well as being a blood schizonticide, unlike other agents, atovaquone also has useful activity against hepatic schizonts. This means that emergence of parasites from the liver stage on discontinuing the antimalarial is less of a problem, so atovaquone only needs to be taken for 1 week after leaving an endemic area, as opposed to 4 weeks for other types. If atovaquone is given alone it has been observed that recrudescence is highly probably, so the commercial product contains both atovaquone and proguanil (Malarone).

Adverse effects, contraindications and interactions

Experience with atavoquone/proguanil is more limited than with some other agents, but to date the side-effect profile seems favourable. The most common adverse events reported have been abdominal pains, headaches and gastrointestinal symptoms. One trial[33] in non-immune travellers described a direct comparison of adverse events to mefloquine, finding that 5% receiving mefloquine experienced adverse drug reaction leading to a discontinuation of therapy, compared to 1% for atovaquone/proguanil. Fewer neuropsychiatric effects were reported for atovaquone/proguanil (14% versus 29%). Also, compared to doxycycline, there are fewer incidents of photosensitivity and gastrointestinal disturbances. Fewer gastrointestinal effects were recorded for atovaquone/proguanil compared to chloroquine/proguanil (10% versus 20%).[34]

Atovaquone is largely eliminated unchanged in the faeces and does not appear to be metabolised. In the presence of rifampicin or rifabutin, blood levels may be reduced by 50%.

Evidence of efficacy

Most of the earlier efficacy studies on atovaquone/proguanil have been conducted using semi-immune travellers, i.e. those in long-term residence in the endemic area.[35,36] For this reason the efficacy of atovaquone/proguanil was questioned[37] and it was suggested that it should not be considered as a first-line prophylactic until further evidence was available. To counter this claim, indirect evidence to efficacy can be seen in a trial examining the incidence of adverse events compared to mefloquine. Although not powered to compare efficacy in the two agents the incidence of malaria in the two groups taking the prophylactics was similar. Furthermore, results of more recent and some as yet unpublished trials have demonstrated the good efficacy of atovaquone/proguanil. Overall, the consensus of opinion is that there is sufficient evidence to warrant first-line use.[38]

The other agents

Pyrimethamine/dapsone (Maloprim) and pyrimethamine/sulfadoxine (Fansidar) have both been associated with severe blood dyscrasias and, apart from increased resistance to these agents, this has been the principal reason for their reduction in use as prophylactics. There is also a risk of sensitivity reactions to their various components.

Use in pregnancy, childhood and various clinical conditions

Only chloroquine and proguanil are currently recommended for use in pregnancy, because the risk of malaria far outweighs the risk of adverse events from medication. It is advisable that pregnant women take folic acid supplements if receiving proguanil (because it is a folate antagonist). There is mounting evidence that mefloquine may be taken in pregnancy as recent case studies have revealed no teratogenicity or other problems.[10,39] WHO has approved the use of mefloquine after the first trimester of pregnancy. However, during early studies in animals, malformations were observed when using high doses for prolonged periods and the current data sheet stringently states that mefloquine should not be used during any stage of pregnancy. If pregnancy should occur during treatment with mefloquine this would not be grounds for considering termination. Very little, if any, of the antimalarials is excreted in breast milk, and only doxycycline should be avoided when breastfeeding. There is insufficient information regarding atovaquone/proguanil to recommend its use in pregnancy and lactation.

Chloroquine is available as syrup for children and is administered just once a week, but proguanil can only be given as tablet formulation daily. Dosage must be calculated according to body weight, not as previously by age, resulting in the need to break up proguanil tablets into halves or quarters and to crush or hide them in food that the child will accept, e.g. jam or peanut butter if they cannot be swallowed whole. There are few data on use for children weighing less than 5 kg. Both drugs appear to have a good safety profile in children at the recommended doses, although just 300 mg chloroquine as a single dose may be lethal for a baby. Doxycycline is contraindicated in children under 12 years of age due to the potential to damage developing teeth and bones. Mefloquine has the advantage of only being given once a week and perhaps is less stressful for the child, but like proguanil tablets, may need to be broken to obtain the correct dose. Central nervous system side-effects such as anxiety and nightmares are reported to be less common in children,[40] but mefloquine should not be given for those with psychiatric conditions or epilepsy. A useful advantage of atovaquone/proguanil for children is that paediatric tablets have recently become available. These are smaller in size than the adult formulation, and are taken as whole tablets depending on the body weight of the child. As absorption is improved by taking with a fatty meal, disguising or crushing the tablets in peanut butter or a chocolate spread may be desirable. At present atovaquone/proguanil is only licensed for those over 11 kg due to lack of data to support prophylaxis at lower body weights and for a maximum of 28 days. If a child on prophylaxis vomits within an hour of administration it has been suggested that the dose be readministered and this general advice could be applied to other age groups.

As both mefloquine and chloroquine could potentially induce fitting in patients with epilepsy they are best avoided in patients with this condition. Doxycycline is a good alternative for such patients, although there is a potential interaction with certain antiepileptics, such as phenytoin and carbamazepine. These antiepileptics tend to induce microsomal enzymes so increasing metabolism of doxycycline and reducing the half-life. Despite this theoretical problem there have been no studies to indicate that the dose of doxycycline should be increased. No interactions between antiepileptics and atavoquone/proguanil have been reported. Maloprim is not susceptible to enzyme induction but has a reduced efficacy if not given together with chloroquine.

As with any medication, those with renal failure or hepatic dysfunction may need special considerations. Of the recommended agents, proguanil is largely excreted unchanged in the urine so dose adjustment may be necessary in renal failure. Both mefloquine and doxycycline rely on hepatic metabolism for elimination and should be used with great care in hepatic dysfunction. There appears to be no significant effect on atovaquone pharmacokinetics in mild to moderate hepatic dysfunction.

Compliance with antimalarials

Compliance is a major consideration, particularly in the scenario where medication needs to be taken regularly over long periods of time. In addition, as such medication is being taken for prophylaxis, even minor side-effects are likely to reduce compliance in an individual.[41]

There have been a few studies examining compliance with anti-malarials. One such study[42] identified that 48% of travellers did not comply with their regimen. Another study[43] found that non-compliance was more likely in the under-55s, in trips of longer duration and non-package tours, and in those who received travel heath advice from more than one source. A similar Dutch study[44] found that compliance rates differed between destinations; from 45% in those travelling to South America to 78% in East Africa. Young age and more adventurous travel were also found to increase non-compliance. Fear of adverse events and belief that medication does not work may be particular reasons why some fail to take prophylaxis.[45] In a study of over 3000 French tourists travelling to malaria-endemic areas, 22% had not sought any advice regarding prophylaxis, and it was estimated the 29% were at risk of contracting malaria due to taking no or inadequate prophylaxis. Whether or not they were using appropriate prophylaxis was dependent upon destination, type of travel and where information had been received. Those visiting family and friends were least likely to take adequate prophylaxis, a well-recognised problem in that there is frequently a false belief in resistance amongst such travellers. In terms of advice it appeared that those who had used pharmacists were most likely to take inadequate medication and the poor knowledge of French pharmacists in this area has been noted in another study.[46]

It may be the case that compliance is better with a weekly rather than a daily regimen, as one trial comparing doxycycline to mefloquine found a poorer outcome with doxycycline attributable to a compliance issue.[47] Despite a higher incidence of neuropsychiatric effects to mefloquine, a German study[48] found that compliance was actually higher with mefloquine than chloroquine/proguanil. Generally, higher levels of compliance are measured when subjects are interviewed regarding medication-taking than by other methods such as tablet counts or estimation of plasma levels. Overall, malaria contracted while taking antimalarials is just as likely to be due to poor compliance as drug resistance.[49]

It may well be that adopting the concordance approach will result in a better outcome than insisting on complete compliance with a regimen with which the traveller is unhappy. Therefore if, for instance, an individual is unhappy taking mefloquine even if it gives the best level of protection, an alternative regimen should be negotiated.

Potential new regimens

Primaquine has been available for many years and is unique in that it only acts on the liver stages, being referred to as a causal prophylactic. It is currently only used in the treatment of vivax malaria, but trials have indicated its potential use as a prophylactic. At present it is not licensed for such an indication; there is some concern about inducing resistance against such a useful agent[50] and it causes severe haemolysis in those with G6PD deficiency.

An analogue of primaquine called tafenoquine seems to possess a very interesting property in that a short initial course may offer many weeks of protection, although, unlike primaquine, it also has activity against the blood stages of the parasite life cycle. In one trial 400 mg taken three times a day for 3 days resulted in over 100 days' protection.[10]

Regimens for prophylaxis

Prophylactic medication must always be taken in advance of travel, both to allow identification of potential side-effects and to allow blood levels to rise sufficiently to inhibit the parasite, as shown in Table 4.5. Both chloroquine/proguanil and doxycycline regimens should be started 1 week before travel, although in the case of doxycycline just 2 days before travel would be acceptable if there was insufficient time. The advice for mefloquine is that it should be commenced 2½ weeks before travel in order to allow three full doses to be taken, for the reasons described above. Atovaquone/proguanil only needs to be commenced 1 or 2 days before travel. Antimalarials should then be taken while away and for 4 weeks on return in case any parasites are emerging from the pre-erythrocytic stage. Again, atovaquone/proguanil is the exception to this rule as it is effective against the pre-erythrocytic stage, so continuing for just 1 week after leaving the endemic area is acceptable.

How long prophylaxis can be taken is sometimes an issue for long-term travellers and expatriates. Prophylaxis with chloroquine/proguanil is believed to be reasonable for up to 5 years. At one time doxycycline was usually only prescribed up to 3 months but may be given for up to

Table 4.5 Regimens for prophylactic agents

Agent	Period of time before departure	Period to continue after leaving endemic area
Chloroquine + proguanil	1 week	4 weeks
Mefloquine	2½ weeks	4 weeks
Atovaquone/proguanil	1–2 days	1 week
Doxycycline	1 week (but 2 days before if insufficient time)	4 weeks
Pyrimethamine/dapsone + chloroquine	1 week	4 weeks

6 months. Mefloquine is prescribed for up to a year and sometimes longer by specialists. Atovaquone/proguanil is only licensed in the UK for 28 days' prophylaxis.

It is important that daily doses of antimalarials are taken at the same time each day and weekly doses at the same time each week. Some antimalarials should be taken with or after food (e.g. chloroquine, proguanil, atovaquone/proguanil and mefloquine) so it may be useful to time doses to coincide with the evening meal. Atovaquone/proguanil absorption is particularly enhanced by food and, where possible, should be taken with food or a milky drink. As pointed out in Chapter 2, there is little evidence that diarrhoea affects the bioavailability of antimalarials. Vomiting soon after taking a tablet could present a problem and it is specifically advised that if vomiting occurs within an hour of taking atovaquone/proguanil, a further dose is taken.

Doses in adults and children are clearly stated in texts such as the *British National Formulary* and useful summary tables are provided in the UK Advisory Committee on Malaria Prevention publication.[6] In the case of chloroquine, calculations should be made on the chloroquine base as there are two different salts available (phosphate and sulphate). It has also been claimed that failure of chloroquine prophylaxis may occur in heavier individuals, i.e. over 75 kg, and that such people should be advised to take the medication (300 mg base) every 5 or 6 days rather than weekly.[17]

Travellers must be made aware that no regimen will offer complete protection. However, if malaria is contracted while taking prophylaxis it is less likely to prove fatal. Because no antimalarial can offer complete protection, bite avoidance measures must always be taken.

Choice of regimen

There are currently six potential regimens described in the UK guidelines:[4]

1. chloroquine or proguanil alone
2. chloroquine + proguanil
3. mefloquine
4. doxycycline
5. atovaquone/proguanil
6. Maloprim + chloroquine

The choice of prophylactic will depend upon the country, the duration of the trip, and sometimes the particular area to be visited, with due consideration to the contraindications, as described above. When making recommendations for chemoprophylaxis, the points to be covered with the traveller are described in Box 4.1. The individual should be happy to take the regimen, which may not necessarily be the most efficacious.

Box 4.1 Checklist of points to be considered when recommending malaria prophylaxis

Details of itinerary
- Countries/areas
- Time of year
- Rural/urban
- Accommodation
- Activities, e.g. expedition
- Style of travel, e.g. business

Traveller's details
- Age
- Pregnancy/breastfeeding
- Previous experience/reactions to antimalarials
- Previous medical history (fits, drug reactions, psychiatric illness, psoriasis)
- Family history (epilepsy, psychiatric illness)

It can sometimes be complex choosing a suitable regimen when an individual is passing through areas where different prophylactics are recommended. The general principle is not to swap regimens but to choose a single one suitable for the whole trip. Therefore, if the traveller is visiting an area where mefloquine is recommended and another where chloroquine/proguanil is recommended, then mefloquine should be chosen throughout.

Current recommendations largely depend on the presence of *P. falciparum* resistant to the chloroquine/proguanil combination. Other forms of malaria remain sensitive to chloroquine, although resistance in *P. vivax* has been reported. In some areas, mefloquine resistance is also present and, in some, only doxycycline or atovaquone/proguanil offers some protection. It must be remembered that within an area the presence of resistance is relative, i.e. there will be some strains that will still be sensitive to a particular agent. It is only when the sensitive strains present fall below an acceptable level that recommendations will be changed. Particularly notorious for multidrug resistance are some parts of Thailand bordering on Cambodia and Myanmar. In this region the risk of actually contracting malaria is not that great if only on a short stay and it may be advisable to take no prophylaxis, whilst being vigilant for the signs of malaria.

The area within a particular country may also be important. Urban areas can carry a smaller risk of malaria than more rural ones, but this rule cannot be generalised. Those going on shorter trips to some countries would not necessarily be recommended mefloquine for the reasons outlined in the section on its adverse effects, above. There may also be seasonal variations in transmission of malaria when the risk may rise from very low to extremely high during the monsoon season.

The duration of the trip is also important, particularly in view of the maximum licensed period for certain malaria prophylaxis, as described in the Compliance with antimalarials section, above. For expatriates and aid workers planning to spend many years overseas, it is common practice to give an initial supply of the recommended regimen. This may be changed after arrival depending on local advice, for instance, only taking medication at times of higher transmission or when travelling to other localities.

Although business travellers may be staying in well-screened rooms and air-conditioned hotels in cities, urban areas in many parts of Africa can still present a risk. The main danger to business travellers is that they may be inadequately protected while making short, unexpected trips to rural areas.

A further confusion for travellers is that recommendations for prophylaxis differ between countries.[51] For instance, proguanil is not available in the USA and mefloquine is more widely prescribed. Travellers from different countries may therefore experience uncertainty when comparing regimens.

For detailed guidelines on prophylaxis for individual countries, the health professional should refer at least to the *British National Formulary* or Communicable Diseases Review (CDR) guide, but more recently updated databases would be ideal, as outlined in Chapter 1.

A few points concerning different destinations are worth making:

- North Africa carries quite a low risk. For many destinations, chloroquine or proguanil alone is sufficient, and is often only required in a few areas at certain times of year. Chloroquine-resistant falciparum malaria is present in a few areas of the Middle East, e.g. Yemen and Oman.
- Much of sub-Saharan Africa carries appreciable risk, particularly the forested areas of West Africa. There are three equal first-line choices available: mefloquine, doxycycline or atovaquone/proguanil. The actual choice of regimen will depend upon itinerary, contraindications and user preference. The combination of chloroquine and proguanil is not now believed to be suitable in this part of the world due to widespread resistance, but is currently still an option only if the other three agents are unsuitable, provided travellers are aware of the lower level of protection.
- In South-East Asia, the situation can become confusing and, in some areas, resistance to many prophylactics is reported. For instance, travellers to Thailand may not require any prophylaxis if visiting the usual tourist areas but should still be alerted to the potential for malaria and to seek treatment if a fever should develop. However, in the areas which border Cambodia and Laos, only doxycycline may be effective. The difficulty arises when travellers are uncertain of their itinerary and indeed these border areas tend to be militarised zones to which it can be difficult to gain access. It may often be best to advise no prophylaxis if the visit to such areas is very short, but to counsel on awareness of the signs of malaria and of the need to take stringent bite avoidance measures. Likewise, there are different recommendations for various parts of Malaysia, varying from very low risk in much of the peninsular to high risk of chloroquine-resistant malaria in Sabah. A similar variable pattern is seen for the various islands that make up Indonesia.
- In most areas of south Asia (e.g. India) or South America, chloroquine and proguanil still offer sufficient protection. The Amazon basin is an area of higher chloroquine resistance where mefloquine or atovaquone/proguanil would be recommended. In some areas of the Pacific, including Papua New Guinea below 1800 metres, Vanuatu and the Solomon Islands, there is a high risk of chloroquine-resistant malaria

and atovaquone/proguanil, doxycycline or mefloquine can be used, with pyrimethamine/proguanil + chloroquine as a possible alternative.

Malaria standby treatment (SBT)

The management of severe or complicated malaria is not covered in this book and would involve the administration of intravenous quinine. In the USA this formulation of quinine is not available and the more cardiotoxic quinidine is used. The only alternative to this is the use of parenteral artemether or artesunate. For uncomplicated falciparum malaria there are a range of oral treatments available and in general they are the same as those employed for standby treatment (SBT), as described below.

If away from medical help for more than 24 hours, some travellers may be advised to take SBT if malaria is suspected, while still trying to find medical attention. There are two broad potential scenarios for requiring such treatment:

1. No prophylaxis has been prescribed because the traveller is visiting a low-risk area.
2. Prophylaxis has apparently failed due to resistant organisms or poor compliance.

The first scenario is contentious, as some practitioners believe that if malaria is endemic at the destination being visited, then prophylaxis should always be prescribed. Others are of the opinion that if the risk is so low, then the benefits of taking regular prophylaxis are outweighed by the risks associated with the side-effects of the medication. Also falling into this category are business executives or others who frequently visit malaria-endemic areas for very short periods of time.

Reasons for supplying SBT under the second scenario are that it is recognised that the chosen prophylaxis may be suboptimal, or that it is felt that compliance is quite likely to be a problem. In this case there may be a concern of an interaction between treatment and prophylactic. In addition there is the likelihood that travellers take medication when it is not needed. Only one study has suggested that this does appear to be the case, where those supplied with self-treatment appear to take it at a greater rate than would be expected for the incidence of malaria normally occurring amongst visitors to the region. At least two other trials have demonstrated an appropriate rate of use amongst travellers supplied with SBT.

Whenever supplying SBT it is important to emphasise that, if it is taken, medical opinion should be sought at the earliest opportunity. Full instructions on administration should be supplied, together with information on recognising malaria and managing symptoms using antipyretics, tepid sponging and a high fluid intake.

There are a number of possible self-treatment regimens, including the use of mefloquine, Fansidar, quinine, co-artemether (artemether/ lumefantrine) or atovaquone/ proguanil (Malarone). The regimens are described in standard textbooks as for the treatment of uncomplicated falciparum malaria (e.g. *British National Formulary*) and will not be discussed further, unless specific differences are recommended for SBT. It must be pointed out that in the UK none of these agents has been licensed specifically for SBT, unlike a number of other European countries. Furthermore, there are few studies directly on the efficacy of using this medication for the treatment of malaria in non-immune travellers, most data being obtained from used a semi-immune population.

The use of mefloquine or atovaquone/proguanil would be precluded if that had been used as prophylaxis. There are an increasing number of areas where Fansidar resistance is a problem and this would not now be much used in SBT.

Quinine

The *British National Formulary* describes a 7-day course of oral quinine, but owing to side-effects, many would find this difficult to complete. The most likely problems would be a dose-related 'cinchonism' consisting of tinnitus, deafness and nausea. More serious side-effects including fitting and hypoglycaemia are less likely to be experienced with oral medication. As compliance may be poor for a full course of quinine, a shortened 3-day course has been recommended by the CDR. If quinine is used, this should always be given together with a course of doxycycline for 7 days. Although mefloquine can increase blood levels of quinine, this does not preclude the use of oral quinine in emergency self-treatment.

Mefloquine

Response to treatment with mefloquine is usually very good, except in the multidrug-resistant areas on the Thai borders. It is widely held that some of the neuropsychiatric side-effects associated with mefloquine use are dose-related, so it would be expected that the higher doses used in treatment could cause problems. The *British National Formulary* recommends a regimen of 20–25 mg/kg (maximum 1.5 g), which can be given as 2–3 divided doses at 6–8-hour intervals to reduce adverse effects. Semi-immune people need a lower dose of 15 mg/kg.

Halofantrine

Halofantrine was at one time used for SBT until it was recognised that it can cause a dangerous prolongation of the QT interval and ventricular arrhythmias. Some fatalities were reported when it was taken with mefloquine. Due to these problems, and the observation that even a prior normal electrocardiogram is not predictive of cardiovascular complications, WHO no longer recommends halofantrine for self-treatment of malaria.

Atovaquone/proguanil

Atovaquone/proguanil is a very useful treatment in SBT and seems to be well tolerated in treatment regimens, with headaches the most commonly reported adverse effect. The self-treatment regimen is relatively simple: four tablets of Malarone daily for 3 consecutive days. Headache, nausea and vomiting and diarrhoea are the most commonly reported problems with this regimen.

Co-artemether

Co-artemether (Riamet) may be another useful drug combination for self-treatment and the clinical data available seem to suggest that it is suitable for this purpose. It is a combination of artemether and lumefantrine. The artemisinin group of antimalarials (including artemether and artesunate) are derived from the herb wormwood that has long been used in Chinese traditional medicine. If used on its own, recrudescence is common, but when combined with lumefantrine this does not seem to be a problem. The recommended treatment regimen is somewhat complex, consisting of a total of 24 tablets to be taken over 60 hours, i.e initially 4 tablets followed by five further doses of 4 tablets taken 8, 24, 36, 48 and 60 hours later.

A potential problem might be anticipated in the similarity of chemical structure of lumefantrine to halofantrine, in that lumefantrine may also have undesirable cardiovascular effects. Two small studies have indicated that lumefantrine does not lengthen the QTc interval when given alone. There also appear to be no problems when lumefantrine is used to treat malaria in those previously taking mefloquine, although again this is based on observations of small numbers of subjects. However, the manufacturers of Riamet do offer a number of warnings in the product data sheet due to a lack of clinical data, that an asymptomatic increase in QTc interval in 5% of patients has been observed, although this has not been observed in other studies. As certain antimalarials, such as quinine, are known to prolong the QTc interval, then caution is advised. This might have implications for those who are treated with co-artemether and subsequently found to require intravenous quinine. Other drugs which lengthen the QT interval such as the quinolone antibiotics and some antihistamines are also advised to be given in combination with caution. The other potential area of concern is that co-artemether has been observed to affect certain microsomal enzymes, inducing CYP3A4 and CYP2C19 whilst inhibiting CYP2D6. Co-artemether itself is metabolised by CYP3A4. Thus there are a number of potential interactions with other drugs which either inhibit CYP3A4 (e.g erythromycin, imidazole antifungals) or are metabolised by CYP2D6 (e.g. tricyclic antidepressants). Atovaquone/proguanil also affects some microsomal enzyme systems but any potential for interaction with co-artemether has not been investigated. Furthermore, grapefruit juice is known to inhibit CYP3A4 and is therefore best avoided. The most common adverse effects of artemether/lumefantrine are headache, dizziness and abdominal pain. It is very poorly absorbed in the absence of food.

SBT for children

For children, side-effects from oral quinine may be unacceptable for self-treatment. Likewise, adverse effects from higher doses of mefloquine make it less desirable as SBT. Atovaquone/proguanil (250 mg/ 100 mg) would be a useful agent in this respect in children over 11 kg as it is generally well tolerated and only needs to be administered once a day for 3 days. Artemether/lumefantrine can be given as whole tablets to children over 12 years of age weighing more than 35 kg, but the regimen is more complicated than for atovaquone/proguanil.

In summary, there does not seem to be any single ideal regimen for SBT. Those involving quinine are somewhat complex and side-effects may well influence compliance. Atovaquone/proguanil has a simple regimen with few reported adverse effects, but could not be used for those already taking this for prophylaxis and treatment failure due to resistance is a concern. Mefloquine would also not be used in those already receiving this for prophylaxis and adverse effects may deter many. Co-artemether has a complex regimen and lack of clinical experience raises some concerns regarding cardiovascular adverse effects and drug inter-actions.

Diagnostic kits

Also available for travellers are blood-testing reagent strips that can be used to detect *P. falciparum* infection from a fingerprick blood sample. These work on an immunological basis by the presence of antibodies in the blood, which can be detected even at very low levels of parasitaemia. This is very attractive for diagnosing non-immune sufferers of malaria who may be experiencing symptoms despite an apparently negative blood film. Studies to date on the use of these kits by tourists have not been encouraging, with reports of false negative readings.[52] In a review of two such kits (Parasight and ICT. Pf) it was concluded that they should not be recommended for travellers routinely, but reserved for special cases when adequate training had been given.[53] An additional problem is that of stability at higher temperatures, making some unsuit-able for long-term travel without refrigeration facilities. New diagnostic kits are being produced to help overcome such problems and may gain more widespread use in the future.

Management of the returned traveller

Recognition of malaria in the returned traveller is a key activity in which all health professionals should be involved, be they doctor, nurse or community pharmacist. This is because a patient is most likely to pre-sent to such workers with non-specific flu-like symptoms which, as dis-cussed, can develop very rapidly to fatal complications. It is sometimes worth reminding both health workers and the travelling public that from initial development of symptoms to death can be as little as 24 hours. When a potential patient presents with malaria the first impor-tant point to establish is when and for how long they last visited a malaria-endemic area. If they were only on a short trip and less than a week has passed since they arrived in the area, malaria could probably be ruled out. If the time has been much greater than 3 months then falciparum malaria is unlikely. All potential cases must be screened for malaria. Reluctance by doctors to screen for malaria in the mistaken belief that the condition is simply flu has in the past led to fatalities. Some patients may have to consider self-referral to a hospital of tropical diseases in such circumstances. It must be emphasised that diagnosis on symptoms alone will be very difficult and many cases of 'mysterious' tropical diseases eventually turn out to be due to malaria.

Once a diagnosis has been made, the next management decision is whether or not complications are present. The most important complications associated with falciparum malaria are neurological, as related to the cerebral malaria previously described. Hypoglycaemia should be screened for, as quinine therapy may lower the blood glucose still further. Pregnancy is a further obvious complication and anyone with extreme pyrexia may need more intensive therapy.

If it is decided that the case is complicated malaria then intravenous quinine remains the gold-standard treatment. A loading dose may be given of 20 mg/kg quinine dihydrochloride infusion over 4 hours, followed by a maintenance infusion of 10 mg/kg 8- or 12-hourly. A plasma level of 8–15 mg/L is felt to be effective and associated with the fewest side-effects.[54] The electrocardiogram should be monitored throughout and therapy discontinued if the QT interval is lengthened by more than 25%, and blood glucose should also be monitored regularly. Once the patient has responded, residual parasites should be eliminated by a 7-day course of doxycycline. Intravenous artemether has been used in the treatment of complicated falciparum malaria but is not licensed for such an indication in the UK and should mainly be reserved for suspected cases of multidrug-resistant falciparum malaria, as might be the case if contracted on the Thai border areas where quinine resistance has been reported.

Management of the complications of falciparum malaria entails many modalities other than antimalarial medication. For instance, fluid and electrolyte balance is critical and phenobarbital may be beneficial in cases of cerebral malaria. This specialised topic will not be discussed further here.

As has been mentioned, the treatment of uncomplicated falciparum malaria employs the same antimalarial regimens as described for SBT. Atovaquone/proguanil has been one of the most popular treatments for returned travellers to the UK. Treatment failures, potentially due to resistant malaria, may lead to other agents being more widely used.

Frequently asked questions

Is mefloquine safe?
As discussed in the text, there are three points to be made:

1. UK experts have identified that 1 in 200 taking mefloquine will experience side-effects that are serious enough to make them discontinue prophylaxis.
2. If the course is started 2½ weeks before travel then in 75% of cases any potential adverse drug reactions will have been identified.
3. There are equally effective alternatives.

Can human immunodeficiency virus (HIV) or hepatitis B be transmitted by mosquito bites?
There are no well-documented cases. Presumably the viruses do not survive well in the insect.

I am going to one area that recommends doxycycline/mefloquine/ atovaquone and another that recommends chloroquine and proguanil, as P. vivax predominates. What should I take?
It is usually best to take doxycycline/mefloquine/atovaquone throughout. Although doxycycline and atovaquone/proguanil are not licensed for prophylaxis against vivax malaria, they will probably still afford protection.

What should I do if I vomit soon after taking my malaria prophylaxis?
If within 1 hour of taking, repeat the dose. Some recommend taking the full dose if within 30 minutes and half the dose if within 30–60 minutes.

Under what circumstances might I need to consider carrying self-treatment for malaria?
If you are away from medical facilities for more than 24 hours in a malaria-endemic area. Even if initiated, still seek medical attention as soon as possible.

It takes 3–4 weeks to reach steady-state levels of mefloquine. Is it necessary to give a loading dose?
If starting 2½ weeks before leaving then there should be no problem. If you are leaving at short notice, or have previously taken mefloquine without any complications and are starting just a week before departure, opinion is divided. Most practitioners do not give a loading dose as mefloquine efficacy may only be reduced by about 10% if half the desirable blood level is attained.[55] Others would recommend a loading dose such as 250 mg of mefloquine for 3 successive days.

I have heard that the area I am travelling to is experiencing a very serious outbreak of malaria – should I consider cancelling my trip?
There is always an increased risk of contracting malaria to higher endemic areas as no measures of prevention are 100% effective. The longer you are away, the greater the chance of eventually contracting the disease. However, increased risk for the endemic population does not necessarily amount to a change in risk for traveller. When malaria incidence rises in an area, for instance due to unusual environmental changes, non-immune populations that do not have the benefit of good prophylactic agents will be harder hit than the traveller taking such medication. A further example is when such climatic changes affect the population living at higher altitudes who are not normally affected by malaria.

Is it safe to take children to a malaria-endemic area?
This is a personal decision, although WHO has recommended such travel should be avoided if possible. For those travelling to highly endemic areas for longer periods, counselling against such travel may be advisable.

If someone is taking minocycline for acne, will that serve as malaria prophylaxis?
In theory a 100 mg dose of minocycline could protect against malaria, but this has never been tested and would be an unlicensed indication. It is better to switch to doxycycline which would also be effective for the acne.

Should mefloquine be given to divers or those ascending to high altitude? What about driving and other skilled tasks?
There have been no well-documented cases of mefloquine central nervous system effects causing problems in divers or others working on skilled tasks. Some may prefer to give an antimalarial that does not result in central nervous system side-effects that could be confused with decompression sickness. Similarly, it may be reasonable to use alternatives in mountaineers in case they confuse a diagnosis of mountain sickness. A 2½ week trial should identify those most likely to experience such problems. Likewise, for driving, there is no evidence of impairment of reaction times.

Malaria prophylaxis can be expensive. Can the medication be bought more cheaply overseas?
This is discussed in Chapter 11. There are a few reasons for discouraging such practice:

- If nothing is taken before departure, then there is a risk whilst supplies are located.
- The antimalarial may not be available at the destination, or hard to find.
- In some parts of the world there is a well-established problem in quality and bioequivalence of antimalarials.

Main points of malaria chemoprophylaxis

- No antimalarial can offer complete protection and bite avoidance measures must always be taken.
- Choice of regimen is largely dependent on the presence or absence of resistance to chloroquine or the chloroquine/proguanil combination. In most destinations where such resistance is a problem, mefloquine, doxycycline or atovaquone/proguanil is recommended.
- Serious adverse reactions to malarial chemoprophylactics are rare, but due care should be taken regarding potential contraindications and interactions. Individuals should be fully informed of potential adverse effects to antimalarials and a 'concordance' approach adopted when identifying suitable therapy in order to maximise compliance.
- All prophylactic regimens are taken before departure, while away and on return. The precise regimen depends on the agent being used.
- Standby antimalarial treatment can be considered for particular groups, but in general should not be a substitute for chemoprophylaxis.

References

1. Sturchler D. Global epidemiology of malaria. In: Schagenhauf P, ed. *Travellers' Malaria.* Hamilton, Canada: BC Decker, 2000: 14–56.
2. Lobel H O, Kozarsky P E. Update on prevention of malaria in travelers. *JAMA* 1997; 278: 167–177.
3. Molyneux M, Fox R. Diagnosis and treatment of malaria in Britain. *BMJ* 1993; 306: 1175–1180.
4. Bradley D J, Warhurst D C. Guidelines for the prevention of malaria in travellers from the United Kingdom. *Commun Dis Rev* 1997; 7: 138–151.
5. *International Travel Guide.* Geneva: World Health Organization, 2003. Available online at: www.who.int/ith/index.html.
6. Bradley D J, Bannister B. Guidelines for malaria prevention in travellers from the United Kingdom for 2001. *Commun Dis Public Health* 2003; 6: 180–189.
7. Lobel H O, Kachur S P. Malaria epidemiology. In: DuPont H L, Steffen R, eds. *Textbook of Travel Medicine and Health*, 2nd edn. Hamilton, Canada: BC Decker, 2000: 184–189.
8. Bell D R. *Lecture Notes on Tropical Medicine*, 3rd edn. Oxford: Blackwell, 1989.
9. Williams J P, Chitre M, Sharland M. Increasing *Plasmodium falciparum* malaria in southwest London: a 25 year observational study. *Arch Dis Child* 2002; 86: 428–430.
10. Shanks G D. Malaria prevention. In: DuPont H L, Steffen R, eds. *Textbook of Travel Medicine and Health*, 2nd edn. Hamilton, Canada: BC Decker, 2000: 192–198.
11. Molyneux M. Malaria in non-endemic areas. *Medicine* 1997; 25: 28–31.
12. Rietveld A E C. Special groups: pregnant women, infants and young children. In: Schagenhauf P, ed. *Travellers' Malaria.* Hamilton, Canada: BC Decker, 2000: 303–324.

13. White N J, Nosten N F. Advances in chemotherapy and prophylaxis of malaria. *Curr Opin Infect Dis* 1993; 6: 323–330.
14. Schlagenhauf P, Phillips-Howard P A. Malaria: emergency self treatment by travellers. In: DuPont H L, Steffen R, eds. *Textbook of Travel Medicine and Health*, 2nd edn. Hamilton, Canada: BC Decker, 2000: 205–213.
15. Schlesinger P H, Krogstad D J, Herwaldt B L. Antimalarial agents: mechanisms of action. *Antimicrob Agents Chemother* 1988; 32: 793–798.
16. Dukes M N G, ed. *Meyler's Side Effects of Drugs: An Encylopaedia of Adverse Reactions*, 13th edn. Amsterdam: Elsevier, 1996.
17. Croft A M, Geary K G. Drugs used in malaria chemoprophylaxis: chloroquine and combinations. In: Schlagenhauf P, ed. *Travellers' Malaria*. Hamilton, Canada: BC Decker, 2000: 163–183.
18. Pappainou M, Fishbein D B, Dreesen D W *et al*. Antibody response to pre-exposure human diploid cell rabies vaccine given concurrently with chloroquine. *N Engl J Med* 1986; 314: 280–284.
19. Lobel H O, Miania M, Eng T *et al*. Long term malaria prophylaxis with weekly mefloquine. *Lancet* 1993; 341: 848–851.
20. Steffen R, Fuchs E, Schildknecht J *et al*. Mefloquine compared with other malaria chemoprophylactic regimens in tourists visiting east Africa. *Lancet* 1993; 341: 1299–1303.
21. Croft A, Garner P. Mefloquine for preventing malaria in non-immune adult travelers.In: Cochrane Collaboration. Cochrane database of systematic reviews. Issue 1. 2001.
22. Schlagenhauf P, Steffen R. Neuropsychiatric events and travel: do antimalarials play a role? *J Travel Med* 2000; 7: 225–226.
23. Barret J, Emmins P D, Clarke P D, Bradley D J. Comparison of adverse events associated with the use of mefloquine and combination chloroquine and proguanil as antimalarial prophylaxis; postal and telephone survey of travellers. *BMJ* 1996; 313: 525–528.
24. Potasman I, Beny A, Seligmann H. Neuropsychiatric problems in 2500 long-term travelers to the tropics. *J Travel Med* 1999; 6: 122–133.
25. Schlagenhauf P. Drugs used in malaria chemoprophylaxis: mefloquine. In: Schlagenhauf P, ed. *Travellers' Malaria*. Hamilton, Canada: BC Decker, 2000: 189–209.
26. Behrens R H, Bradley D J, Snow R N, Marsh K. Impact of UK prophylaxis policy on imported malaria. *Lancet* 1996; 348: 344–345.
27. Marked rise in malaria cases for travellers to East Africa. *Pharm J* 1998; 260: 272.
28. Day J H, Behrens R H. Delay in onset of malaria with mefloquine prophylaxis. *Lancet* 1995; 345: 398.
29. Hopperus Buma A P, van Thiel P P, Lobel H O *et al*. Long term malaria chemoprophylaxis with mefloquine in Dutch marines in Cambodia. *J Infect Dis* 1996; 173: 1506–1509.
30. Colledge C L, Riley T V. *Clostridium difficile* associated diarrhoea after doxycycline malaria prophylaxis. *Lancet* 1995; 345: 1377–1378.
31. Ohrt C, Richie T L, Widjaja H *et al*. Mefloquine compared with doxycycline for the prophylaxis of malaria in Indonesian soldiers. A randomised double-blind, placebo controlled trial. *Ann Intern Med* 1997; 126: 963–972.

32. Beallor C, Kain K C. Drugs used in malaria chemoprophylaxis: doxycycline. In: Schlagenhauf P, ed. *Travellers' Malaria*. Hamilton, Canada: BC Decker, 2000: 210–219.

33. Overbosch D, Schilthuis H, Bienze U *et al*. Atovaquone–proguanil in non-immune travellers: results from a randomised, double-blind study. *Clin Infect Dis* 2001; 33: 1015–1021.

34. Høgh B, Clarke P D, Camus D *et al*. Atovaquone/proguanil versus chloro-quine/proguanil for malaria prophylaxis in non-immune travellers: results from a randomised, double-blind study. *Lancet* 2000; 356: 1888–1894.

35. Shanks G D, Gordon D M, Klotz F W *et al*. Efficacy and safety of atovaquone/proguanil as suppressive prophylaxis for *Plasmodium falciparum* malaria. *Clin Infect Dis* 1998; 27: 494–499.

36. Sukwa T Y, Mulenga M, Chisdaka N *et al*. A randomised double-blind, placebo controlled field trial to determine the safety and efficacy of Malarone for the prophylaxis of malaria in Zambia. *Am J Trop Med Hyg* 1999; 60: 521–525.

37. Atovaquone + proguanil for malaria prophylaxis. *Drug Ther Bull* 2001; 39: 73–74.

38. Shanks G D. Drugs used in malaria chemoprophylaxis: atovaquone/proguanil. In: Schlagenhauf P, ed. *Travellers' Malaria*. Hamilton, Canada: BC Decker, 2000: 227–247.

39. Phillip-Howard P A, Wood D. The safety of antimalarial drugs in pregnancy. *Drug Safety* 1996; 14: 131–145.

40. Mitelhozler M L, Wall M, Steffen R, Sturchler D. Malaria prophylaxis in different age groups. *J Travel Med* 1996; 4: 219–223.

41. Hoebe C, Demunter J, Thijs C. Adverse effects and compliance with mefloquine or proguanil antimalarial prophylaxis. *Eur J Clin Pharmacol* 1997; 52: 269–275.

42. Lobel H O, Phillip-Howard P A, Branding-Bennett A D *et al*. Malaria incidence and prevention among European and North American travellers to Kenya. *Bull World Health Org* 1990; 68: 209–215.

43. Held T K, Weinke T, Mansmaa V *et al*. Malaria prophylaxis: identifying risk groups for non compliance. *Queensland J Med* 1994; 84: 17–22.

44. Coblens F G, Leentvoor-Kuijpens A. Compliance with malaria chemoprophylaxis and preventative measures against mosquito bites among Dutch travellers. *Trop Med Int Health* 1997; 2: 705–713.

45. Chaterjee S. Compliance of malaria chemoprophylaxis among travellers to India. *J Travel Med* 1999; 6: 7–11.

46. Sorge F, Legros F, Goujon C. Pharmacists and travel medicine: needs for training? *Third European Conference on Travel Medicine*. Florence, 2002.

47. Sanchez J L, DeFraites R F, Sharp T W, Hanson R K. Mefloquine or doxy-cycline prophylaxis in US troops in Somalia. *Lancet* 1993; 341: 1021–1022.

48. Huzly D, Sconfeld C, Beurle W, Bienzle U. Malaria chemoprophylaxis in German tourists: a prospective study to compliance and adverse reaction. *J Travel Med* 1996; 3: 148–155.

49. Behrens R H, Taylor R B, Pryce D I, Low A S. Chemoprophylaxis compliance in travellers with malaria. *J Travel Med* 1998; 5: 92–94.

50. Fryauff D J, Baird J K, Basri H *et al.* Randomised placebo controlled trial of primaquine for prophlaxis of falciparum and vivax malaria. *Lancet* 1995; 346: 1191–1193.

51. Waner S, Burrhiem D, Braack L, Gammon S. Malaria protection measures used by in-flight travellers to South Africa game parks. *J Travel Med* 1999; 6: 254–257.

52. Jelinek T, Amsler L, Grobusch M. Self-use of rapid tests for malaria diagnosis by tourists. *Lancet* 1999; 354: 1609.

53. Grobusch M P, Burchard G. Diagnosis of malaria in the returned traveller. In: Schlagenhauf P, ed. *Travellers' Malaria*. Hamilton, Canada: BC Decker, 2000: 393–423.

54. Whitty C, Mweneuanya J. Malaria treatment. In: DuPont H L, Steffen R, eds. *Textbook of Travel Medicine and Health*, 2nd edn. Hamilton, Canada: BC Decker, 2000: 199–204.

55. Lobel H O, Miani M, Eng T *et al.* Long-term malaria prophylaxis with weekly mefloquine. *Lancet* 1993; 341: 848–851.

5

Tropical and other diseases related to travel

With increased travel to the tropics, the subject of tropical medicine has become an important area of travel health. These diseases may be transmitted in one of three ways: via insect, ingestion or by contact with the environment or another individual who carries the disease. The tropical disease spread by insects of most concern to the traveller is malaria, which was discussed in the previous chapter. The subject of travellers' diarrhoea was discussed in Chapter 2 and some further mention will be made of other infections that can be contracted from food and water in this chapter. It also has to be said that some of the diseases discussed here are not limited to tropical areas. With such a wide range of infections that may present a risk to the traveller, it is important that the relative risks of these diseases, and ways in which they can be avoided, are appreciated.

Health professionals should have some understanding of these conditions in order to offer general health advice to travellers and to emphasise bite avoidance measures. A further useful activity is to help put into perspective for travellers the various scare stories concerning such diseases that emerge from time to time. In terms of response to symptoms, it is important to recognise that non-specific symptoms after travel to the tropics can be caused by a number of tropical diseases and referral to a specialist centre may be necessary.

As it is virtually impossible to diagnose many of these tropical diseases in their early stages, malaria should be presumed in the first instance, particularly if there is fever. This point should be emphasised to travellers for consideration both while away and on returning home.

Many of the diseases described in this chapter are more relevant to the local population and to expatriate or other workers living in the area than to tourists on short holidays, as prolonged exposure is necessary. However, travellers on more extended trips may be at increased risk. There are vaccines available to some of the infections described in this chapter and these will be described in further detail in Chapter 7.

The solution to avoiding insect-borne diseases is bite avoidance measures, as will be described in Chapter 6. Some travellers may wish to plan their itineraries to times of low insect activity, e.g. in the dry season to avoid mosquitoes. There are also certain risk groups who may be advised not to travel to certain areas when insect-borne diseases are endemic or experiencing a particularly severe outbreak. Pregnancy needs careful consideration when travelling to such destinations; malaria, Japanese encephalitis (JE) and dengue haemorrhagic fever have the potential to harm both mother and fetus. The elderly are also at risk of the complications from JE and other flaviviruses and may wish to be alerted to the presence of these when travelling to various destinations. In other cases where transmission is not through an insect vector, avoiding certain activities or taking simple precautions can lessen the risk.

The account below does not cover every tropical disease or other infection that could potentially be encountered by the traveller. The focus is on those which might present a greater risk or are well known to the public, who may ask for further information if travelling to certain destinations.

Insect-borne diseases

In this section will be discussed the major diseases, other than malaria, that are transmitted by insects and of potential risk to the traveller. There are a wide range of viral (Table 5.1) and other infections (Table 5.2) that can be transmitted to humans by a number of different insect vectors.

The arboviruses

Meaning literally 'insect-borne virus', the arboviruses are a broad group of viruses that cause a variety of diseases. Some of these viruses are described in Table 5.1. The three main groups (families) of arboviral infections are:

- bunyavirus, e.g. Rift Valley fever, Crimea-Congo haemorrhagic fever
- flavivirus, e.g. yellow fever, JE, tick-borne encephalitis, dengue, West Nile fever
- togavirus, e.g. chikungunya, Ross River fever

Not all forms of arbovirus infection are discussed here and many types will result in mild non-specific symptoms of fever and malaise. The most serious complications of the arboviruses are encephalitis and haemor-

Table 5.1 The arboviruses

Virus	Vector	Type of virus (family)	Distribution
Yellow fever	*Aedes* mosquito	Flavivirus	Tropical Africa, South America and the Caribbean
Dengue fever	*Aedes* mosquito	Flavivirus	Widespread in tropics and subtropics
Japanese encephalitis	*Culex* mosquito	Flavivirus	Asia
Tick-borne encephalitis	*Ixodes ricinus*	Flavivirus	Scandinavia, Eastern Europe, Central Europe, Russia
Rift Valley fever	*Aedes* and *Culex* mosquito	Bunyavirus	Africa
West Nile virus	*Culex* mosquito	Flavivirus	Africa (including Egypt), South-East Asia
St Louis encephalitis	*Culex* mosquito	Flavivirus	North and South America
Nipah virus	*Culex* mosquito	Flavivirus	Thailand
Ross Valley virus	*Aedes* and *Culex*	Togavirus	Australia

rhagic disease and there are over 80 such viruses that can affect humans. Occasionally, outbreaks of arbovirus infections make the headlines, e.g. the recently identified Nipah virus and the West Nile virus (WNV). Many arboviral diseases can cause complications in pregnancy and, together with the risk of malaria, need careful consideration for pregnant women planning a trip to the tropics.

Dengue fever

There are four serotypes of the flavivirus responsible for dengue, which is carried by the *Aedes aegypti* mosquito. After infection lifelong immunity develops to that particular serotype but after a few months reinfection with another serotype becomes possible.

Table 5.2 Insect-borne diseases other than arboviruses

Disease	Organism	Vector	Distribution
Elephantiasis	*Wuchereria bancrofti*	Mosquito	Asia Africa South America Oceania
Onchocerciasis (river blindness)	*Onchocerca volvulus*	Blackflies	Africa Central and South America
Loiasis	*Loa loa*	Chrysops fly	West and central Africa
African trypanosomiasis (sleeping sickness)	*Trypanosoma brucei*	Tsetse fly	Africa
American trypanosomiasis (Chagas disease)	*Trypanosoma cruzi*	Cone-nosed bug	Central and South America
Lyme disease	*Borrelia*	Ticks	USA Europe Australia China
Plague	*Yersinia pestis*	Fleas	Africa Asia The Americas
Typhus	Rickettsiae	Ticks/lice	Africa South America Asia Pacific Islands

The incubation period is about 1 week (range 2–14 days) and the first symptom is fever, which may subside after the initial bout, to recur some days later. The other major symptoms are severe frontal headache, malaise, myalgia, back pain and abdominal tenderness. Joint and muscle pain can be quite severe, the illness is sometimes referred to as 'breakbone fever'.

Around the third to fifth day, a maculopapular rash can appear on the trunk, spreading to the limbs and face but sparing the palms and soles of the feet (Plate 2). After the sixth day, the fever subsides, but convalescence can take several weeks. Only partial immunity to dengue is gained and reinfection with other serotypes remains a possibility. In about 80% of cases of infection in children the disease may be asymptomatic, or present as a mild fever which is difficult to distinguish from common childhood infections.[1] Adults may experience minor bleeding from the gums, nose or vagina.

A potentially fatal immunological reaction, dengue haemorrhagic fever (DHF), can occur, usually in children under the age of 15. A severe attack of DHF results in widespread haemorrhage and extravasation of fluid, leading to hypotension and shock – dengue shock syndrome. A quarter of patients with shock syndrome will die if not treated. In DHF, the immune system causes an abnormal haemostasis and plasma leakage which results in dengue shock syndrome. The mechanism by which DHF occurs is not well understood but is probably related to the formation of virus–antibody complexes, which result in complement activation and vascular damage. It has also been observed that DHF is more likely to occur in children who have previously experienced dengue fever. There may also be an increased risk of DHF among those formerly resident in endemic areas who are returning for a visit.[2] DHF is rarely seen in travellers; in one survey of 294 travellers who had contracted dengue, 7 developed DHF.[3] The explanation of this low incidence is related to previous exposure to dengue.

At one time it was believed that DHF was caused by a specific form of dengue to that causing a dengue fever. What actually appears to happen is that, once an individual is exposed to dengue, then immunity is developed to that particular serotype. When encountering another serotype the immunological response mounted is very much greater and the various cytokines produced are responsible for the haemorrhagic symptoms. This explains why children are prone to DHF, even if no previous exposure has been reported, as the first attack may have been asymptomatic. From this it also follows that when more than one serotype is involved in a particular epidemic, the incidence of DHF rises. One curious aspect is that those who have a less active immune system are less prone to DHF and it is therefore rarely seen amongst malnourished children. In theory at least, travellers making frequent trips to dengue areas could be at increased risk of DHF, but few such cases have been well documented.

Dengue fever is widely distributed in tropical and subtropical areas, often coexisting with malaria from which, in the early stages, it is hard to distinguish (Fig. 5.1). There has been a global resurgence of dengue in recent years, and it is a risk to travellers visiting endemic areas.[4] It is a particular problem in Asia and parts of South America. The most recent large scale epidemic was in Brazil in 2002 when nearly

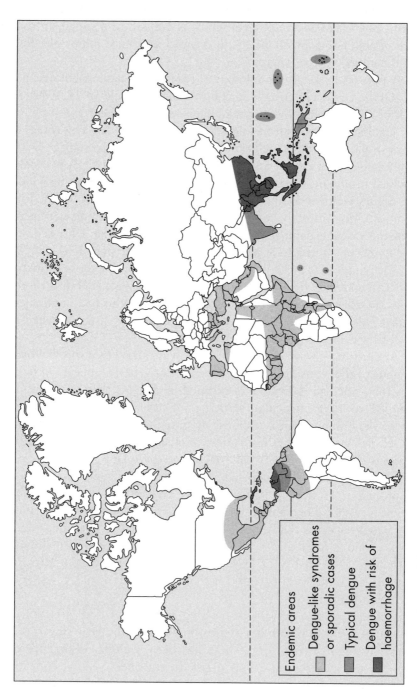

Endemic areas

☐ Dengue-like syndromes
   or sporadic cases

☐ Typical dengue

■ Dengue with risk of
   haemorrhage

Figure 5.1 Distribution of dengue. Courtesy of Eric Caumes.

half a million people were affected and Rio de Janeiro was one of the areas with a high incidence of cases.

Dengue fever is probably greatly underreported because, in many cases, the fever is relatively mild and causes minor symptoms. In addition the virus cannot be identified 5 days after the onset of fever. Thus, in 1998, only 38 cases were listed in the Communicable Diseases Review (CDR) among travellers returning to the UK. However, 465 cases of dengue were diagnosed by the Centre for Applied Microbiology and Research[5] in 1994 and other cohort studies have indicated that 8% of cases of fever amongst travellers to certain endemic areas may be due to dengue. On average the Public Health Laboratory has described reporting of 100–150 probable cases per year.[6] A risk assessment of around one illness per 1000 travellers to some areas has been suggested.[7]

For adult travellers there is little, if any, risk of the more severe DHF. In addition, children travelling to endemic areas would be at little risk if they have not previously been exposed to dengue. For most people, the fever will subside in a week, but a longer convalescence period may well ruin a short holiday.

There is no specific treatment for dengue. In terms of management, travellers should be advised to take paracetamol, rather than aspirin, as an antipyretic because of the risk of haemorrhage. Oral rehydration may also be advisable where there has been excessive sweating and/or diarrhoea. As malaria and dengue often coexist in the same area, it is advisable to assume in the first instance that any fever contracted in such areas is due to malaria.

There is currently no vaccine against dengue and the best protection is bite avoidance, remembering that the *Aedes* mosquito is a daytime-feeding species.

Yellow fever

Like dengue, yellow fever can be transmitted by *A. aegypti*, is caused by the same group of flaviviruses and has seen a resurgence in the last few years. Unlike dengue, yellow fever is a zoonosis, i.e. the disease can be harboured by animal vectors. It is an extremely serious infection and mortality can be between 20 and 50%.

Yellow fever is endemic in many tropical areas of South America and Africa, but is absent in Asia (Fig. 5.2). The majority of cases are reported in Africa and it is estimated that there are as many as 200 000 cases worldwide per year.

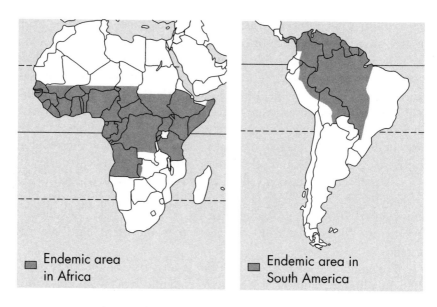

Figure 5.2 Distribution of yellow fever. Courtesy of Eric Caumes.

The mosquitoes capable of transmitting the disease are present in various non-endemic countries. If travelling from an endemic country, a vaccination certificate may be required.

The disease gains its name from the damage caused to the liver, which results in jaundice. Other complications contributing to the high fatality rate are haemorrhage (due to a reduction in clotting factors), renal tubular necrosis, myocardial damage and shock.

Yellow fever is rarely encountered by travellers, not least because visitors to many endemic countries must possess a certificate of vaccination for entry and vaccination is strongly encouraged. There are reports of non-vaccinated tourists contracting yellow fever and, due to haemorrhagic complications, their symptoms have been confused with Ebola. For instance, a sobering story from Germany illustrates the importance of being vaccinated against yellow fever if it is indicated, whether or not a vaccination certificate is required for entry into the country.

A German photographer returned from a trip to the Ivory Coast in 1999, with symptoms of what appeared to be Ebola virus infection. This sparked off a tremendous scare, with fears of an Ebola outbreak in Europe. A perimeter fence was erected around the patient's isolation unit, with security guards patrolling. All his contacts on the airplane were traced and his colleagues and family placed in quarantine. He eventually died and the disease was confirmed as yellow fever and not Ebola, as first thought. Apparently he had never been vaccinated and had somehow managed to gain entry into the country without a certificate.

Japanese encephalitis

JE is also caused by a flavivirus. It is endemic in many parts of Asia and the west Pacific (Fig. 5.3). It is spread by the *Culex* mosquito which tends to breed in rice paddies and, like *Anopheles*, bites from dusk to dawn. It is a zoonosis capable of being carried by birds, although the most important reservoir is domestic pigs. Occasionally, epidemics arise, which result in the culling of the pig population.

There is an incubation period of 4–14 days before clinical signs are apparent. The clinical picture of infection includes a sudden onset of fever, with headaches and vomiting. If encephalitis results, there are neurological disturbances, including convulsions and motor disturbances which may prove fatal or result in permanent disability. However, only around one in 200 people infected by the virus will progress to develop encephalitis, where case fatality is 10–25%. Children and the elderly, in particular[8] are at most risk and form the majority of the fatalities during an epidemic.

The most important consideration for travellers is whether or not it is worth obtaining vaccination when visiting potentially endemic areas. As the outbreaks tend to occur during the monsoon season when mosquitoes are more plentiful, vaccination may be advisable for those travelling on extended visits to rural areas at such times. However, infections of travellers on relatively short excursions into rural areas are not unknown.[9] Reports of JE among travellers are quite rare; in the USA, only 11 cases have been reported since 1981 and an attack rate of one case per 10 000 people per week was estimated for military personnel stationed in Asia.[10] Amongst western travellers only 24 cases were reported between 1978 and 1992[11] and only two cases have ever been documented for UK travellers.[12] For further discussion, see Chapter 7.

Some other arboviruses

Many of the other arboviruses listed in Table 5.1 have reached media attention over the past few years. A common feature of these

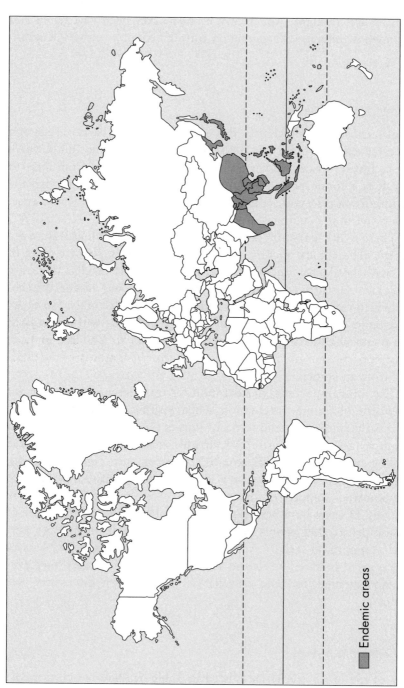

Figure 5.3 Distribution of Japanese encephalitis. Courtesy of Eric Caumes.

Endemic areas

arboviruses is that they are mostly mosquito-borne and have a bird or other animal as a host. Such reports will often unjustifiably deter travel to the affected areas.

Tick-borne encephalitis   Tick-borne encephalitis is found not in the tropics, but in parts of Scandinavia, Eastern Europe and Russia. It is a particular risk to people rambling in the forested parts of these areas and transmission is highest in the months of May, June, September and October. However, only one true travel-related case has been reported and it is considered very rare in this group.[1] Only 1% of cases prove fatal and it seems more of a risk in the elderly.

Nipah virus   Nipah virus caused panic in Malaysia during the spring of 1999, and received media attention around the world. Although it adversely affected the tourist industry, it did not really present a significant risk and no tourists were actually affected.

In the early months of 1999, there were an increasing number of reports of JE emerging from Malaysia. It was noted that this outbreak seemed to be affecting adults, rather than children, which is more usual. Also, some of the affected individuals did not test positive for JE. In fact, in many cases, a completely different virus was involved which gave symptoms very similar to JE. It was described as a 'Hendra-like' virus which was similar to a virus which had originated from fruit bats in Australia. The Australian virus was transmitted to horses and the subsequent infection resulted in the death of two people.

The new virus was called Nipah after the first village it struck near Kuala Lumpur. It is a paramyxovirus transmitted via pigs, and most of the 100 people who died lived on or near pig farms. There was no evidence that it could be passed from human to human, or be caught by eating contaminated pork. Although some horses tested positive to Nipah, they did not appear to be the major source of the disease. The Malaysian government contained the problem with a massive programme of pig culling.

Chikungunya and Ross River fever   Chikungunya is endemic in Africa and Asia whilst Ross River fever is found in Australia, mostly on the eastern seaboard during the rainy season. The main feature is severe polyarthritis, fever and rashes being transmitted by mosquitoes. They are occasionally contracted by travellers; the Australian authorities give frequent alerts as to the localities affected. There are usually no long-term complications, although in some individuals polyarthritis can last for many months.

Crimea-Congo haemorrhagic fever and Rift Valley fever   There are varieties of arbovirus which are harboured by cattle and can be transmitted to humans by an insect vector. Amongst those found in Africa are Crimea-Congo haemorrhagic fever transmitted by ticks and Rift Valley fever, transmitted by mosquitoes. They would not normally be associated with travel-related infections.

West Nile virus   It is worth considering WNV in some detail as it is a good example of an emerging infection that has caused concern amongst the travelling public and has been a subject of intense media interest. It is a flavivirus related to the St Louis encephalitis virus, which actually has a longer history of endemicity in the USA. Also within the same family is JE, found in parts of Asia, and the Murray River encephalitis that is endemic in Australia. Also the Kunjin virus, found in areas of Australasia and South-East Asia, is very closely related. The history of WNV goes back to 1937 when it was identified in the West Nile district of Uganda and has since remained endemic in the eastern hemisphere, causing sporadic, but not particularly widespread or severe, outbreaks in parts of Africa, the Middle East, Asia and Eastern Europe. Elsewhere in Europe an outbreak in southern France in 2000 affected horses but no human cases were reported.[13]

WNV first appeared in the USA in 1999 when 62 documented cases were reported in New York and surrounding areas, resulting in a case fatality of 12% in hospitalised patients. Since that time the virus has returned each year and gradually spread over a wider area; in 2000 there were 21 cases over three states, and in the following year 66 cases over 10 states.[14] Other countries in the eastern hemisphere have also reported outbreaks since 1999, with Israel being one of the worst affected. The emergence of the disease is probably related to changes in climatic conditions resulting in a great increase in the mosquito population. An additional factor in New York was the cessation of a programme to treat potential mosquito-breeding areas with insecticide. The trend seems to have continued in 2002 where most states in the east and mid-west of the USA have reported cases. To the end of September 2002 there were 2206 reported cases and 108 deaths. In 2002 Canada reported 38 cases (10 confirmed) and one death from the virus, but in Israel only eight people were treated and only one death was reported.

The mode of transmission of the virus is through the bite of a mosquito, and the genus *Culex* seems to be the most implicated in its transmission. It is now widely accepted that the virus was carried to the USA by migrating birds. Mosquitoes transmit the virus between these birds and the local bird population, thus amplifying the reservoir of virus. The bird population is itself affected by the virus, with widespread bird die-off, particularly amongst crows and other covids. Eventually mosquitoes will transmit the virus from birds to humans and other mammals, with this tending to occur towards late summer in the USA, with cases falling off over the winter months. Therefore the virus appears well in advance in birds before any human transmission. For this reason special 'sentinel' flocks of chickens over the USA are monitored continuously for the presence of the virus. It is believed that the virus can overwinter in mosquitoes, appearing again the following year. There is some suspicion that it can be transmitted through blood transfusion and organ donation, as a number of cases have been reported of recipients developing infection after receiving blood or organs from donors later being diagnosed as carrying WNV. As all the recipients were living in areas of WNV transmission, this problem has yet to be confirmed and quantified.

Even if the virus is contracted, no symptoms may manifest; only around 20% of people believed to be infected in New York developed a fever.[15] The clinical picture of infection for many is of a fever with a variety of other flu-like symptoms, e.g. gastrointestinal tract symptoms, headache, and these are probably often unreported. A small number of people develop a rash. Based on studies from New York and a Roumanian outbreak, around one in 150 will develop the neurological symptoms that can lead to hospitalisation. The major risk factor for developing neurological complications is advancing age, as those over 50 years of age appear at higher risk than younger adults. Risk of severe neurological symptoms in the New York outbreak was found to be 10 times higher in the 50–59-year-olds and 43 times higher in the over-80s compared to those under 20 years of age.[16] Likewise fatality from infection was nine times more likely in the over-75s. Other risk factors for fatality may be those who are immunocompromised or have diabetes.

The most serious neurological complications are encephalitis or, less frequently, meningitis. Severe muscle weakness has been observed in nearly half of hospitalised patients in the USA, and provides a diagnostic clue to the condition. More rarely, a variety of other neurological signs are observed, including seizures and myelitis. Overall, the case fatality rate in the 1999 New York outbreak was 12% and about half of the hospitalised patients had symptoms such as fatigue, memory loss and muscle weakness 1 year later.[14]

Confirmation of the diagnosis is obtained by immunological tests, through detection of specific immunoglobulin M antibodies to WNV. Treatment is largely supportive; some hospitalised patients require intensive care and mechanical ventilation. Available antiviral agents do not appear to be effective.

Filarial diseases

Filarial worms have a thin hair-like appearance and different species vary greatly in size, causing a variety of diseases.

Elephantiasis (lymphatic filariasis)

Elephantiasis results when a particular filarial worm (*Wuchereria bancrofti*), carried by mosquitoes, invades the lymphatic system, resulting in localised inflammation of the lymph glands. Occasionally, heavy parasitaemia may result, blocking the lymphatic drainage and causing greatly enlarged limbs or scrotum. A low level of parasites rarely does much harm, although some individuals may develop allergic reactions to the worms. It would be unusual for travellers to pick up enough worms to do any harm. Elephantiasis is treated with diethylcarbamazine.

Onchocerciasis

A similar situation to elephantiasis applies to onchocerciasis or river blindness, transmitted by a type of blackfly. While this is an important cause of blindness to the local population in parts of Africa, it rarely causes problems to travellers. There are cases of expatriates or people working on projects in endemic areas needing treatment. It is treated with ivermectin, which stops the reproduction of the worms but must be taken yearly for several years.[17]

Loiasis

One of the most curious filarial diseases is loiasis, also known as African eye worm (Plate 3). The affected individual might notice a slight blurring of the vision in one eye, and on looking in the mirror will be horrified to observe a worm a few centimetres long wriggling just under-neath the conjunctiva. Although it can be removed under a local anaes-thetic, the worm is best left as it will leave the conjunctiva in under an hour, rarely doing any harm. Travellers are rarely affected but loiasis would make an interesting traveller's tale. The only other manifestation of the disease might be transient swellings under the skin called 'Calabar swellings' as the worm migrates through connective tissue.

Protozoal diseases

As with many of the arbovirus infections, protozoal diseases are com-paratively rare in travellers, being of more concern to the local popula-tion.

Leishmaniasis

Leishmaniasis is caused by a small protozoan organism that is trans-mitted by the bite of a sandfly. It is found in areas of Africa, South America and the Mediterranean. Travellers to some tourist areas of the Mediterranean are at potential, if extremely small, risk of the disease. It is often not recognised by physicians unused to seeing the condition. There are rarely more than 20 cases per year reported in travellers from the UK and just 129 cases were reported in travellers from the USA between 1978 and 1990.[18] The risk does vary in different areas, and was estimated as being highest for US travellers to Surinam, at one in 1000 travellers on long-term trips.[19]

The parasite is a zoonosis, being carried by both domestic and wild animals. Bite avoidance is the only method of protection. It was of par-ticular concern among servicemen fighting in the Gulf war, and was the reason why repellents and insecticides of various types were so widely used.

The parasite will invade macrophages and the organism can then potentially be carried around the body. This results in so-called visceral leishmaniasis, or kala-azar, caused by *Leishmania donovani*. The Sudan and India are the most badly affected by this form of leishmaniasis. The symptoms include an enlarged spleen and lymph glands, sometimes appearing months or years after exposure. This form is potentially fatal unless treated with somewhat toxic drugs, such as pentavalent antimony (sodium stibogluconate).

Other species of *Leishmania* will cause a local reaction at the site of a sandfly bite. This is cutaneous leishmaniasis. The lesion will initially appear as a nodule, which eventually develops into a disfiguring but painless chronic ulcer.

Trypanosomiasis

African trypanosomiasis[20] or 'sleeping sickness' is transmitted by bite of the tsetse fly and is due to either *Trypanosoma brucei gambiense* or *T. brucei rhodesiense*. The latter is usually directly transmitted from animals to humans and the former from human to human. After the bite of a tsetse fly, which is notoriously painful, the trypanosomal chancre will appear after about 5 days as a raised inflamed area which can increase in size over a couple of weeks. Travellers should not confuse this with the initial reaction to the bite, which is seen very soon after being bitten. There may be a fever, headaches and enlarged lymph glands. These early signs of the disease can be intermittent, lasting many months, and may be accompanied by anaemia and skin rashes. During early stages of the disease, an acute, rapidly fatal toxaemia can develop. This is more common with *T. rhodesiense*. It can be up to 2 years before central nervous sysytem (CNS) involvement occurs, with psychoactive disturbances and long sleeping periods (from which the disease derives its name).

The disease has a patchy distribution over much of sub-Saharan Africa, with travellers on safari being at greatest risk. The message for the traveller is to watch out for a tryptosomal chancre and any non-specific symptoms because the disease can be treated with suramin in its early stages.

Very few travellers from the UK contract the disease and it would normally be treated before there is any CNS involvement. In Germany, just 11 cases have been reported in travellers since 1970 and, from the USA, only 14 since 1967.[19] In more recent years the incidence of trypanosomiasis in Africa has risen, probably due to poor implementation of control measures due to a failure of the local public health system.

In some parts of South America, another form of trypanosomal infection called Chagas disease[21] (*T. cruzi*) is endemic. This is transmitted by a species of cone-nosed bug, sometimes called the assassin bug, which lives in the walls of dwellings in the more rural areas. Infection can cause chronic renal and gastrointestinal damage. Travellers would be advised not to sleep in the mud (adobe) huts that are common in parts of South and Central America. It is very rare in short-term travellers; just 15 cases have been reported to the US Centers for Disease Control in a 20-year period.[19]

Some other diseases transmitted by insects

Typhus

Typhus is caused by bacteria-like microorganisms called rickettsiae and infection results in skin rashes, fevers and spleen enlargement. It can be transmitted by louse bites from either humans (*Rickettsia prowazekii*) or flea bites from animals (*R. mooseri*) and can present a potential hazard to those working in refugee camps in Africa.

Of a much wider distribution is the form of typhus spread by tick (*R. tsutsugamushi*) or mite bites. Forms of scrub typhus transmitted by ticks are found in parts of the South African veld and in North America, where it is known as Rocky Mountain spotted fever. A scrub typhus transmitted by mites is present in the tropical bush of South-East Asia and the Pacific Islands.

After an incubation period of 3–20 days, local lymphangitis in the area of the bite may be noted, with systemic symptoms such as fever, headache and malaise sometimes accompanied by a rash. If the disease progresses, CNS and vascular complications may result. There are reports of typhus in individual travellers[22] or groups camping out where scrub typhus is present. For instance, a large number of boy scouts in South Africa acquired the infection after just a few nights camping in a rural area. Mild cases may go unrecognised and the condition is treatable by just a single 200 mg dose of doxycycline.[23]

Tick-borne infections

It is not only the tropics that can harbour tick-borne infections. Ticks from deer can transmit Lyme disease, a bacterial infection due to *Borrelia burgdorferi* that can cause chronic joint, cardiovascular and CNS complications. Lyme disease is quite widely distributed round the world, including Europe; at present, it has a low incidence in the UK. In the USA, it is probably the most common vector-borne disease.[24] It is worth removing ticks as quickly as possible, without damaging the tick in the process and causing it to release more bacteria into the wound. This is best achieved by gripping the tick with tweezers, pushing down to disengage the teeth, while gently rocking it from side to side before pulling away.[25]

Plague

Plague transmitted by fleas is endemic in some parts of the world, including areas of North America where it is harboured by some wild animals and is occasionally contracted by humans. Elsewhere, for instance in parts of sub-Saharan Africa, local epidemics of plague occur periodically and this area accounts for the majority of plague cases. A small epidemic of plague hit India in 1994, severely affecting the tourist industry.

The disease is caused by the bacteria *Yersinia pestis*, harboured in rat fleas and passed to humans to cause bubonic plague, where the bacteria is distributed around the body through the lymphatic system, resulting in the typical swelling or 'buboes' of the lymph nodes. This can progress to a fatal septicaemia. It can also be passed between humans by droplet infection, in which case a pneumonic form of the plague, which can be more difficult to manage, can occur.

A vaccine is available, but is rarely used except by those planning to work in areas where plague is endemic. Intramuscular streptomycin is the drug of choice, and oxytetracycline can be effective to treat plague if used in the early stages. Travel need not be deterred, although travellers should be warned that contact with animals, particularly rodents, should certainly be avoided. During the plague scare in India, no travellers contracted the disease.[26]

Skin conditions

The most grotesque of all conditions caused by insects is myiasis, i.e. maggots developing in human skin. The flies responsible are the tambu (tropical Africa) and bot flies (South America) (Plate 4). Tambu flies lay their eggs on clothing hung out to dry and the resulting small larvae are able to penetrate the skin when they hatch. Travellers should be advised to iron clothing left out in this way to destroy any eggs. Placing raw bacon over the maggots' breathing hole is a recognised method of removing them.[27]

Also notorious amongst travellers for causing skin conditions is the burrowing flea *Tunga penetrans*, or chigger, contracted by those who do not wear sufficient foot coverage in jungle areas. The female flea becomes engorged with eggs and forms a small hard nodule in between the toe webs.[28] This can be carefully removed with a needle, taking care not to rupture the flea as this could result in an infection of the skin.

Diseases of contact and environment

This section considers some of the diseases that could be encountered by the traveller, mainly by direct contact either with the environment or with another individual or animal (Table 5.3). A few conditions contracted by drinking contaminated food and water, other than those covered in Chapter 2, will briefly be discussed. The prevention of some of these is discussed under vaccination for travel, in Chapter 7.

Table 5.3   Diseases of environment and person-to-person contact

Condition	Organism	How contracted	Distribution
Schistosomiasis	*Schistosoma haematobium* *S. mansoni* *S. japonicum*	Swimming in fresh water	Africa (mainly) Asia South America
Leptospirosis	*Leptospira interrogans*	Contact with water contaminated by rodent urine	Worldwide
Hepatitis B	DNA hepadnavirus	Sexual	Worldwide
Hepatitis C	RNA flavigroup virus	Contaminated surgical instruments Blood products	
Rabies	Rhabdoviridae	Bite or scratch from infected mammal	Most countries
Anthrax	*Bacillus anthracis*	Infected animals Soil	Many developing countries
Tuberculosis	*Mycobacterium tuberculosis*	Close contact with infected individuals	Many countries
Legionnaires' disease	*Legionella pneumophila*	Droplet infection of contaminated water	Worldwide
Hantavirus	Bunyaviridae	Rodents	The Americas
Worm infestations			
Cutaneous larva migrans	*Ancylostoma braziliense,* *A. caninum*	Through skin	
Hookworm	*Ancylostoma duodenale, Necator americanus*	Through skin	Various
Strongyloidiasis, Larva curens	*Strongyloides stercoralis*	Through skin	
Whipworm	*Trichuris trichiura*	Ingestion	
Round worms	*Ascaris lumbricoides*	Ingestion	

Table 5.3 continued

Condition	Organism	How contracted	Distribution
Tapeworm	*Taenia solium,* *T. saginata*	Ingestion	
Leprosy	*Mycoplasma leprae*	Close prolonged contact	Tropics
Buruli ulcer	*Mycobacterium ulcerans*	Soil	Africa, Australia
Melioidosis	*Burkholderia pseudomallei*	Soil, water	South-East Asia Southern Australia
Ebola	Filovirus	Contact with	Africa
Lassa	Arenaviral	body fluids	

Schistosomiasis

There are some tropical diseases that can be contracted by methods other than insect vectors which may be of concern to travellers. Chief among these is schistosomiasis, also known as bilharzia.

Schistosomiasis is an infection caused by small fluke-like worms that rely upon fresh-water snails as part of their life cycle. Eggs from the worm are passed into fresh water by the urine of infected individuals. In the fresh water, they develop into larvae that enter the snails. These larvae then multiply within the snails and are released as free-swimming circariae, which can penetrate the skin of human bathers. Eventually, the mature worms will find their way to the bladder (*Schistosoma haematobium*) or the intestine (*S. mansoni* and *S. japonicum*). The worms will then lay their eggs in the veins of these organs, causing localised inflammation and tissue damage. This leads to bleeding and, if not treated, a chronic anaemia.

Those who have had previous exposure to *Schistosoma* may experience a rash where the circariae have penetrated the skin. A reaction sometimes seen in travellers is called 'Katayama fever', which represents an acute immunological reaction to the parasite.

Bathers may notice an irritation of the skin after emerging from contaminated water and a few may experience a fever. Otherwise, it can be months or even years before symptoms become apparent. Schistosomiasis is widespread in Africa and is also present in some parts of South America and Asia. A particular problem has been identified in recent years around Lake Malawi (in Africa) and a number of British tourists have been found to be infested after bathing in the lake. There were 133 cases reported to the CDR in 1998; cases were more likely in those individuals on lengthy stays.[29]

Tourists in Africa should be particularly warned against bathing in fresh water. Swimming pools are considered to be safe provided they have been properly chlorinated. If contact with such water occurs, it would be best to rub down with a towel after bathing rather than letting the water dry off in the sun. This manoeuvre cannot give complete protection as penetration of the skin can occur within 10 seconds of contact. Swimming away from the shores of lakes where reeds harbouring the water snails may lessen the risk, but cannot be relied upon. There is some evidence that the use of a long-acting diethyltoluamide (DEET) formulation may prevent the circariae penetrating the skin.[30] Alternatively, another study has demonstrated that applying a DEET-containing product after swimming also provides good protection. It may be worthwhile for some travellers who have had a lot of contact with potentially contaminated water to be tested for the disease. Treatment with praziquantel is very effective.

Leptospirosis

Another disease found in fresh water which is of potential danger to travellers, particularly to those trekking in the wild, is leptospirosis or Weil's disease. The urine of rodents or other animals passes the disease into surface waters. The *Leptospira* enters humans through small breaks in the skin or mucous membranes and causes a severe febrile illness. There may be complications involving liver or renal damage and the disease has a fatality rate as high as 30%. It can be a particular problem in areas of flooding, for instance, following the recent hurricane Mitch. Generally, trekkers should be advised to minimise direct contact with fresh water.

Hepatitis

There are five well-defined forms of viral hepatitis: A, B, C, D and E. Other types do exist, sometimes termed non-A–E virus. Types A and E are transmitted through contaminated food and water, whilst the other three are passed through sexual contact, via blood or contaminated medical equipment. In fact, there have been isolated cases of hepatitis A contracted through the use of contaminated needles. All forms of hepatitis have the following features during the acute phase, but differ in their tendency for chronic sequelae:

- headaches, fever and chills
- malaise
- nausea, vomiting, abdominal pain and anorexia
- jaundice

Hepatitis A and E

Hepatitis A is the form most commonly encountered by travellers, this group being responsible for some 60% of case of hepatitis A seen in the UK. In developing countries, where poor hygiene makes this a common disease, most of the adult population will have developed antibodies whereas in westernised countries the proportion may be as low as 20%,[31] so travellers are at a particular risk. Between 3 and 109/1000 travellers will be at risk of hepatitis A when visiting certain endemic areas.[32] The variation is very much dependent on the area travelled, for instance being relatively lower in Turkey but quite high in India. The incubation period for hepatitis A is 3–5 weeks, and incapacity from the disease ranges from a month in younger adults to many months in older people. Unlike the other forms, it is not associated with chronic liver disease and mortality is low. Young children often have a very mild or asymptomatic infection.

Hepatitis E is very similar to hepatitis A in both aetiology and clinical picture, being endemic in India, Africa and South America and affecting mainly young adults. It does carry a higher risk to pregnancy than hepatitis A. Few figures are available regarding the prevalence in travellers; a rate of 10% of expatriates in endemic areas has been noted.[33] There is currently no vaccine available.

Hepatitis B

This can be contracted in a number of ways and the carrier state is higher in some developing countries. There are a number of quite well-defined activities or situations which could put the traveller at increased risk:

- casual sexual activity
- receiving blood or blood products
- surgical procedures including dental
- other invasive procedures such as tattooing and body piercing

It is also recognised that the longer the residence in countries with high rates of hepatitis B, the more likely infection. One study of expatriates in South-East Asia demonstrated that after 5 years nearly half were seropositive to hepatitis B.[34] The risk to travellers in general has been reported as 20–60 per 100 000 travellers, with those working long-term overseas showing a much higher rate.[32]

The incubation period for hepatitis B is 2–6 months. The consequences of hepatitis B are more chronic than hepatitis A, with an increased risk of liver failure and cancer, although only up to 10% will develop such problems. Both antiviral drugs and α-interferon are used in the management of hepatitis B.

Infection with hepatitis D (or delta hepatitis) seems to be associated with an infection of hepatitis B, either as a superinfection of those with chronic hepatitis B or as a coinfection leading to a more serious outcome.[35]

Hepatitis C

More people appear to suffer some chronic liver damage following hepatitis C than hepatitis B and then progress after many years to cirrhosis. It is contracted in exactly the same way as hepatitis B and is a rising worldwide problem, with no vaccine currently available or even on the horizon.

Typhoid and paratyphoid

There is often confusion in the public mind between *Salmonella typhi* causing typhoid fever and salmonellosis, which is caused by nontyphoid *Salmonella* including *S. enteritidis* and *S. typhimurium* and are quite commonly responsible for food poisoning. The latter is a zoonotic infection, in that the bacterium is present in the living animal and not killed due to poor preparation. Typhoid and paratyphoid are present only in humans passed from person to person by the faecal–oral route, either by those with the active disease or carriers.

S. typhi is an invasive organism, penetrating the gastrointestinal wall and potentially spreading to many parts of the body. Contrary to popular belief, typhoid is just as likely to present with constipation as diarrhoea. In the early stages of the disease, after an incubation period of 1–3 weeks, the patient will be febrile, sometimes with rose-coloured spots appearing on the skin, and provided the condition is identified and treated at this stage no further problems should be seen. If the disease progresses, a life-threatening septicaemia and possible gastrointestinal perforation may result.

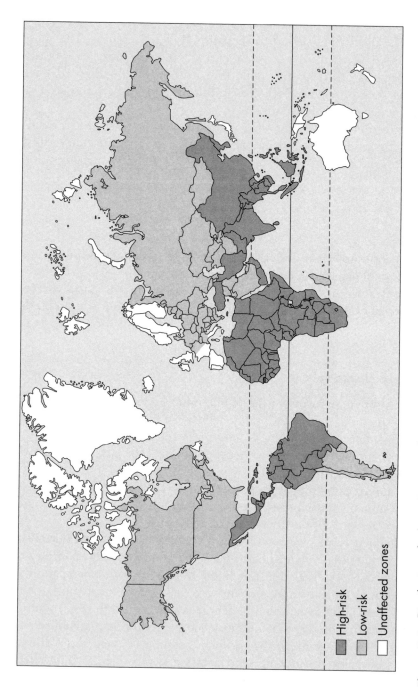

Figure 5.4 Distribution of rabies. Courtesy of Eric Caumes.

High-risk

Low-risk

Unaffected zones

Rabies

This viral infection is one of the most feared and is a major worldwide problem. Only a few countries are completely free of rabies and there are annually 60 000 deaths worldwide,[31] half of them in India (Fig. 5.4). Other areas that have a particularly high incidence include parts of South America, Asia and Africa. There has been some success in eradication in Europe by baiting foxes responsible for harbouring the disease with an oral form of vaccine. Notably France was declared rabies-free in 2001.

The bite from any mammal can transmit rabies and other than dogs the list is quite long, ranging from vampire bats in South America to wolves in arctic areas. It is the presence of stray dogs that probably represents the greatest risk and if these are not controlled outbreaks can reach epidemic proportions. Actual cases of rabies in travellers are rare and tend to make headline news when they occur. None the less, the almost 100% mortality makes pre-exposure vaccination an important consideration (see Chapter 7). Travellers are not always aware of the need to avoid contact with mammals; a study in Thailand demonstrated that 10% of travellers had experienced a dog bite or lick and that nearly 7% of dogs were known to be carrying the virus.[32]

Rabies is a disease of the CNS, where the virus responsible, being passed from the bite of the animal, gains access through the peripheral nerves to the CNS. Once CNS involvement has taken place the well-recognised symptoms of hydrophobia and profound neurological disturbance are seen, resulting almost inevitably in a fatal outcome. How long between being bitten and a point of no return is a question often asked by travellers. The answer is of course simply to find appropriate treatment as soon as possible. It has been suggested that progress is more rapid when the bite is to a highly innervated area, e.g. a bite to the face progresses more rapidly than that to the leg.

After being bitten the first thing that must be done is thoroughly to clean and scrub the wound. Then irrigation with an iodine-based antiseptic is recommended; povidone-iodine solution would be ideal for this situation. If not available, alcohol or even spirit beverages such as vodka or whisky could be used. A major problem for travellers to some parts of the world is the availability of appropriate treatment. For all those who have not received pre-exposure vaccination it is considered essential that passive vaccination with rabies immunoglobulin is given in order to raise antibody titres as the rabies vaccine will take some time to stimulate the body's own immune system. Unfortunately, in poorer countries such immunoglobulin may not be available. Rabies vaccine itself can usually be found but is often of the older cheaper sheep or mouse brain-derived variety, which tends to be less reliable and has a high incidence of adverse reactions. Modern vaccines are much safer and reliable, and there are a number of potential regimens for postexposure treatment given by the intradermal or intramuscular route.

Anthrax

Recent acts of bioterrorism have bought anthrax to the public attention. It is a zoonotic bacterial infection caused by *Bacillus anthracis*. In its most common form, cutaneous anthrax is contracted by contact with contaminated animals or directly with the soil. In the majority of cases this will result in a necrotic ulcer with no further complications; in 20% of cases the bacteria can disseminate, causing a fatal septicaemia and meningitis. Much rarer, and the cause of concern in terms of bioterrorism, is inhalation of anthrax, which carries a high mortality. Rarer still, and also often fatal, is a gastrointestinal infection.

It would only present some risk to travellers if they were handling the hides of animals who were carrying the disease. Anecdotally this has occurred when a tourist purchased an affected hide in Africa and received a small prick from a sharp hair.

Sexually transmitted infections

It is the duty of all health professionals advising travellers to alert them to the possibility of various forms of sexually transmitted disease. This includes not only those planning high-risk sexual activities, but also those who may be involved in any casual sexual relationship. A full discussion of sexually transmitted diseases and the risk to the traveller will not be covered in this book, which does not diminish its importance to the traveller in that it represents a significant risk. This risk is presented by the whole range of such diseases, including human immunodeficiency virus (HIV)/acquired immune deficiency syndrome (AIDS), hepatitis B and C, gonorrhoea, syphilis, herpes simplex and chlamydia. There are two potential situations that may be encountered by the traveller:

1. Sexual encounters concerning prostitution or other high-risk groups in the local population. This is true whether visiting developing or industrialised countries, but high rates of infection, particularly HIV, have

been associated with the former. Such activities may be planned or opportunistic.

2. Sexual relationships with other holiday-makers are probably just as great a risk and more common. Again, these may be planned and the use of recreational drugs or alcohol may contribute to a less than cautious approach.

Counselling before departure may simply be a matter of raising awareness of the dangers. Those who are anticipating casual sexual activities may well respond to such advice and take some measures to plan protection. Condoms, both male and female, are the only effective measure that can be taken during intercourse and the supply of these should be routinely encouraged. It is also worth reminding travellers that condoms may be hard to obtain or of poor quality at certain destinations.

Respiratory tract infections

Travellers would be prone to the same respiratory tract infections encountered in their home countries, i.e. viral or bacterial upper and lower respiratory tract infections. There is a general consensus that upper respiratory tract infections do not require treatment with antibiotics and will be self-limiting without further complications. Travellers should be reassured of this and to be aware of treating symptoms using simple analgesics and maintaining good hydration. Steam inhalations can be useful for cold and chesty coughs. Lower respiratory tract infections can require treatment with antibiotics if presenting as a community-acquired pneumonia. In this case a problem of diagnosis and locating appropriate antibiotics may be encountered by the traveller. For those travelling to destinations with poor medical facilities it may be worthwhile carrying an antibiotic such as amoxicillin.

More exotic respiratory tract infections are rare but need to be considered for certain destinations. For instance, legionnaires' disease has been contracted by travellers, being transmitted through droplets from certain air-conditioning or other cooling systems, though the problem would be difficult to anticipate or avoid.

A good reason for travellers to avoid any contact with environments infested with rodents is the possibility of Hanta virus infection, which can cause haemorrhagic, pulmonary or renal complications. A pulmonary form has been identified in the USA which causes occasional fatalities. It is rarely contracted by travellers.

Tuberculosis is a growing problem and over 10 million people worldwide are infected, but only a few per cent of these are in industrialised countries. The causative organism, *Mycobacterium tuberculosis*, can infect the lung and occasionally other organs such as the gastrointestinal tract. It is transmitted by close and intimate contact and for this reason is not thought be a risk to most travellers, even those travelling to areas of high endemicity. There have been isolated cases of transmission in airlines by close and prolonged contact with a passenger who has tuberculosis, rather than circulation by the air-conditioning systems.[36] Airlines now have guidelines allowing those with tuberculosis to be allowed on board aircraft. Vaccination with Bacillus Calmette-Guérin (BCG) is routinely carried out for children in many countries but is rarely used for travellers, as discussed in Chapter 7. Chemotherapy of those diagnosed with tuberculosis is usually highly effective, despite the rise of multidrug-resistant forms, and those with HIV are a particular group at risk. Details regarding the pathophysiology and management of tuberculosis are outside the scope of this book.

At the time of writing an important new respiratory infection of relevance to travel medicine called severe acute respiratory syndrome (SARS) has emerged. This appears to have originated in the Guangdong province of southern China and spread to other countries in South-East Asia, and then spread to the rest of the world via international travel. The causative agent is undoubtedly a new form of coronavirus, related to that causing the common cold. Those in close contact with infected individuals have a very high chance of contracting the disease, probably through inhalation of aerosol from a cough or sneeze of an infected individual and the virus may well linger for some hours on surfaces. Before the disease was recognised and precautions taken to protect health workers, 56% of health workers caring for SARS patients contracted the disease themselves. Despite this, the chances of contracting SARS during air travel are believed to be low and transmission through air conditioning is not believed to occur. The symptoms are quite typical of pneumonia: fever, shortness of breath, cough. About 10% of those contracting SARS develop a life-threatening disease and the fatality rate is around 15% but higher in older people. By April 2003, 22 671 people had contracted SARS and 103 had died; the disease had spread to 17 countries. There has been some success with treatment regimens employing ribavirin and corticosteroids.

Creeping eruption and other worm infestations

A variety of hookworm, which is usually seen as parasites of dogs, can sometimes cause problems in humans. This arises when larvae are picked up through the skin, usually as a result of walking barefoot, perhaps when walking along a beach. The worms essentially become 'lost' in an unfamiliar host and will move around beneath the surface of the skin, producing an elongated inflamed line on the soles of the feet (Plate 5). This gives the condition the name of creeping eruption or cutaneous larva migrans. It is common on the beaches of the Caribbean, Africa and South-East Asia, but can occur in other parts of the world, including the USA.

Another type of hookworm, *Ancylostoma duodenale*, can penetrate through skin and migrates to the lungs, finally settling in the gut. Light infections will be symptomless, but a heavier parasite load can cause anaemia. More serious is *Strongyloides* infection, referred to as larva currens when seen in the skin. This worm also penetrates skin and can be seen an itchy rash which moves quite rapidly as larvae migrate. The parasite then has the potential to disseminate widely around the body, affecting many organs.

Travellers should therefore be warned against walking barefoot, particularly along beaches above the high-water line. Treatment for cutaneous larva migrans is with thiabendazole, which can be taken orally or formulated as a 1% paste in white soft paraffin for local application.

Other worm infestations of the gut, e.g. ascariasis and tapeworm, can occur as a result of eating poorly prepared food. Amongst the more common worm infestations in travellers are whipworm (*Trichuris trichiura*) and round worm (*Ascaris lumbricoides*). After an initial phase of development in the lungs they will infest the gut. Up to 1% of adults and 2% of children returning from the tropics may carry such worms, although the parasite load is usually not heavy enough to produce overt symptoms.[19] Mebendazole is an effective treatment for these worms.

Tapeworms are contracted through eating contaminated under-cooked meat resulting in either a pork (*Taenia solium*) or beef tapeworm (*T. saginata*) developing in the gut. Beef tapeworms are a potential risk almost anywhere in the world whereas pork tapeworms are more focused in developing countries where hygiene is poor. The most serious complication results from larvae developing in the brain, although this is very rare in travellers. Tapeworms are treated with praziquantel or niclosamide.

Another worm, which is of particular curiosity to the traveller, is the Guinea-worm or *Dracunculus medinensis*. This can be contracted by drinking contaminated water from wells in some parts of the world. The worm will find its way to the skin where it protrudes to release its larvae. Soon after, the worm will die, and it has to be removed by gently wrapping it around a matchstick over a period of some weeks. Dracunculiasis can potentially result in infected ulcers. Worms up to

100 cm in length have been recorded. There has been a fairly successful worldwide campaign of eradication, so it is extremely rare in travellers.

Skin conditions

Chronic skin lesions are a common problem in the tropics and can have a number of causes. It is not uncommon for travellers to return from the tropics with a chronic ulcer which fails to heal, or some other unusual skin lesions which need to be diagnosed and treated by a specialist centre of tropical medicine. One common cause of such problems is a wound which has not been treated effectively using basic wound hygiene measures as described in Chapter 11, allowing pyogenic organisms to penetrate the skin. Such pyogenic infections, caused by streptococcal or staphylococcal organisms, are often initiated by a mosquito bite that is scratched and then becomes colonised by bacteria, but other causes such as blisters or fungal infections may also be responsible.[28] Also as described in the section on Insect-borne diseases, above, a number of tropical diseases transmitted by insects can result in a variety of skin lesions, e.g. leishmaniasis, trypanosomiasis. In addition some parasitic worms, myiasis and skin infestions such as scabies could all present with an unusual lesion or rash.

Leprosy has historically been one of the most feared diseases that can result in horrific disfigurement if not treated. The causative organism is *Mycobacterium leprae*, which, like other mycobacteria, is an intracellular parasite and stimulates cell-mediated immunity in the host. The organism can be present in the body for many years without symptoms. As well as the formation of granulomas that result in the typical skin lesions, the major damage is to peripheral nerves such that paraesthesia and eventually anaesthesia occurs. Any minor wound will tend to go unnoticed and untreated, resulting in the mutilations characteristic of the disease. The disease is transmitted by direct contact but this has to be in the form of quite close contact for a long period of time, so the disease does not really present a risk to travellers. Chemotherapy has resulted in great reductions in the incidence of leprosy and global elimination may be achieved one day.

Buruli ulcer is a growing problem in the tropics[23] and has been described by some as 'the leprosy of the new millennium'. It is found in many tropical areas, including Australia, and is a particular problem in parts of West Africa. Buruli ulcer is caused by *Mycobacterium ulcerans* which is contracted directly though contact with contaminated soil. The result can be a deep and disfiguring ulcer which can grow to involve large areas of tissue, sometimes even penetrating the bone. Antibiotics known to have activity against mycobacteria appear to be ineffective in treating Buruli ulcers. Only surgical excision is effective and this should be done early to minimise the need for subsequent skin grafting.

Sometimes presenting as skin lesions, but also having important systemic effects, is the condition known as melioidosis, caused by the bacteria *Burkholderia pseudomallei,* also called *Pseudomonas pseudomallei.* It is found in the soil and water in parts of South-East Asia, particularly Thailand and also Southern Australia. Incidence tends to rise in the rainy season and it can be contracted through percutaneous absorption through the skin, inhalation and possibly ingestion. It can affect a number of organs, but pneumonia and septicaemia are the most serious outcomes. Many individuals may remain asymptomatic for months or even years, and whilst rare in travellers, it is not unknown. Recognition is important as travellers returning home may not be correctly diagnosed unless it was appreciated that they had travelled to an area where the disease is endemic. The most effective treatment seems to be the third-generation cephalosporin ceftazidime, which can cut fatality by 50%.[37]

Lassa, Marburg and Ebola virus

These viruses are sometimes the source of great panic and give rise to media headlines of 'body-melting diseases'. They are zoonotic viruses that can attack a variety of tissues in the body. Their precise aetiology is not well understood and there is no curative treatment available, so they are considered highly contagious.

Lassa fever is caused by an arenavirus as are the related group of haemorrhagic fevers also found in South America. It is endemic in West Africa and probably harboured by bush rats. It is transmitted by contact with the excretions of such rodents. For instance, it has been claimed that some have caught the disease by sleeping in grass huts where such rats inhabit the rafters; the victim inhales an aerosol of the rat's urine. It can also be transmitted from person to person through contaminated fluids. Death can result from general organ failure. Although the death rate in hospitalised patients in Africa is high, at about 20%, it is believed that there are many cases of mild or subclinical infection. An overall mortality rate of 1–2% has been suggested.[38] The antiviral ribavirin has been used with some success in this condition.

Even less is known in terms of aetiology about the Ebola virus and the related Marburg virus, but they do occasionally cause localised outbreaks in parts of Africa and can carry 50–90% mortality. They are from a group of viruses called filoviruses and the primary reservoir of infection is unclear, being passed from person to person by direct contact of body fluids. The most serious complication is severe bleeding from the gastrointestinal tract, nose and gums. These outbreaks have occurred over the years in various parts of Africa, including Kenya, Zaire and the Sudan. Most recently there have been epidemics in the Congo. The problem is usually identified by the World Health Organization and travel to the affected areas is restricted.

Main points

Insect-borne diseases

- Malaria is the most important for travellers and most others, with the possible exception of dengue, are rarely encountered. In many cases such diseases are of more concern to those living in endemic areas than to the traveller.
- There is a vast range of arboviral infections. Yellow fever is amongst the most serious and vaccination should always be sought if it is known to be endemic. Dengue fever is rarely fatal in travellers, but symptoms are unpleasant and could spoil the itinerary. Vaccination against JE may be warranted in certain situations when travelling to parts of South-East Asia.
- Parasitic diseases other than malaria transmitted by insects include trypanosomiasis, filarial infection and leishmaniasis. Awareness of their presence is particularly important for those staying for longer periods in endemic areas and can be considered for any posttropical screening should this be necessary.
- Bacterial infections can also be transmitted by a variety of insects, including ticks; the best known is typhus.
- Avoiding insect bites is the most practical way of reducing the risk of contracting such diseases.

Diseases from contact with the environment and other individuals

- Avoid swimming in fresh water in Africa due to the risk of schistosomiasis (bilharzia).
- When visiting developing countries consider vaccination against hepatitis A and B. If in close contact with the local population, Mantoux/Heaf test for tuberculosis could be considered pre- and postexposure.
- Observe safe sexual practices.
- Rabies should be considered if bitten by any mammal.

- Avoid blood transfusions or any invasive therapy in developing countries where medical facilities are poor. Consider carrying personal sterile equipment.
- The haemorrhagic diseases such as Ebola carry a very high mortality and are contagious, but extremely rare in travellers.
- Knowledge of these problems and sensible behaviour, with appropriate vaccination in some cases, is the best defence.

Frequently asked questions

A serious outbreak of dengue has been reported at my destination. Should I still travel?
Quite frightening numbers of cases and fatalities can be reported when there is a dengue outbreak. This should not deter travellers as the complications of dengue are extremely rare in this group, as explained in the text. Good counselling on bite avoidance should always be given.

I know about the dangers of schistosomiasis in Africa but I am going on a very long overland Africa trip and am bound to need to swim in fresh water.
If contact with fresh water is inevitable, then the following advice may help to reduce the chances of contracting the condition:

- Try to keep away from the banks of rivers.
- Rub yourself dry with a towel.
- If you can obtain a long-acting cream formulation of DEET, then apply this to exposed skin before bathing. Alternatively rub down with an alcoholic solution of DEET after bathing. This advice is based on some limited experimental data only.

I am going on a safari to a game park where there are tsetse fly carrying sleeping sickness. What should I do?
Sleeping sickness is very rare in travellers. Use bite avoidance measures and if bitten, watch out for the signs described in the text.

I have been in the tropics for 6 months. Should I have a posttropical screen to see if I have picked up anything nasty?
There is no strong evidence that a full posttropical screen is worthwhile, except where a traveller complains of some specific symptoms warranting further investigation.[39,40]

A traveller returning from the tropics is convinced that he has picked up a parasitic worm which he can feel moving inside his stomach and beneath the skin. Hospital tests were negative; and his partner is now complaining of the same problem. What is the probable cause of the problem?

Delusional parasitosis has been reported amongst travellers, and could be viewed as a psychiatric problem. It has also been recognised that the delusion/neurosis can be shared by other household members.

Some months after contracting dengue a traveller still feels tired and depressed. What is the likely diagnosis?
It is unusual for the postinfectious syndrome to carry over longer than a few weeks. In all such cases of recovery from an infectious disease a chronic fatigue syndrome could be considered.

It has been said that living in the rivers of the Amazon is a small fish that can swim up the urethra of men and become lodged in the penis, even swimming up a stream of urine if urinating into water. Is there any truth in this?
The story relates to the infamous candiru fish. Medical opinion is that this is probably a myth as no well-documented and reported cases exist, although there are apparently individuals who attest to its existence.

References

1. Tsia T F, Nimlasson B. Viral and tropical infections: arboviruses and zoonotic viruses. In: DuPont H L, Steffen R, eds. *Textbook of Travel Medicine and Health,* 2nd edn. Hamilton, Canada: BC Decker, 2000: 290–312.
2. Jacobs M G, Brook M G, Weir W R C, Bannister B A. Dengue haemorrhagic fever: a risk of returning home. *BMJ* 1991; 302: 828–829.
3. Jelinek T, Mühlberger N, Harms G *et al.* Epidemiology and clinical features of imported dengue fever in Europe: sentinel surveillance. Data from TropNetEurop. *Clin Infect Dis* 2002; 35: 1047–1052.
4. Rigau-Perez J G, Gubler D J, Vorndam A V, Clark G C. Dengue: a literature review and case study of travellers from the United States 1986–1994. *J Travel Med* 1997; 4: 65–71.
5. Dengue: current epidemics and risks to travellers. *Commun Dis Rev* 1995; 5: 1.
6. Anonymous. *CDR Weekly* 2002; 12: 36.
7. Carroll B, Behrens R. Dengue infection and travel. *Travel Wise (Newslett Br Travel Health Assoc)* 1999; 4: 4–5.
8. Monarth T P. Japanese encephalitis – a plague of the orient. *N Engl J Med* 1988; 319: 641–643.
9. MacDonald W B G, Tink A R, Ouvrier R A *et al.* Japanese encephalitis after a two-week holiday in Bali. *Med J Aust* 1989; 150: 334–336.
10. Tsai T F, Yu. Japanese encephalitis vaccines. In: Putsin S, Mortimer E, eds. *Vaccines,* 2nd edn. Philadelphia: WB Saunders, 1993.
11. Centers for Disease Control and Prevention. Inactivated Japanese encephalitis virus vaccine: recommendations of the advisory committee on immunization practices (ACIP). *MMWR Morb Mortal Wkly Rep* 1993; 42: 6.

12. Viral diseases transmitted by mosquitoes. *CDR Weekly Rev* 2002; 12: 10–13.

13. Shakespeare M. *Zoonoses*. London: Pharmaceutical Press, 2002.

14. Petersen L R, Marfin A A. West Nile virus: a primer for the clinician. *Ann Intern Med* 2002; 137: 173–179.

15. Mostashari F, Bunning M L, Kitsutani P T *et al*. Epidemic West Nile encephalitis, New York, 1999: results of a household-based seroepidemiological survey. *Lancet* 2001; 358: 261–264.

16. Nash D, Mostashari F, Fine A *et al*. The outbreak of West Nile virus infection in the New York City area in 1999. *N Engl J Med* 2001; 344: 1807–1814.

17. Hay J, Burr A. Ivermectin: a novel treatment for onchoceriasis. *Pharm J* 1989; 243: 297.

18. Herwaldt B L, Stokes C L, Juranek D D. American cutaneous leishmaniasis in US travellers. *Ann Intern Med* 1993; 18: 779–784.

19. Wilson M, Loscher T. Parasitic tropical infections. In: DuPont H L, Steffen R, eds. *Textbook of Travel Medicine and Health*, 2nd edn. Hamilton, Canada: BC Decker, 2000: 345–365.

20. Smith D H. African trypanosomiasis. *Medicine* 1997; 25: 42–45.

21. Yasuda M A S. American trypanosomiasis. *Medicine* 1997; 25: 38–41.

22. Thiebaut M M, Bricaire F, Raoult D. Scrub typhus after a trip to Vietnam. *N Engl J Med* 1997; 336: 1613–1614.

23. Carosi G, Matteelli A, Wilde H. Bacterial infections. In: DuPont H L, Steffen R, eds. *Textbook of Travel Medicine and Health*, 2nd edn. Hamilton, Canada: BC Decker, 2000: 325–345.

24. Fry G, Kenny V. Lyme borrellosis imported from Africa. *Lancet* 1993; 342: 689.

25. Robinson R. Fleas, lice, bugs, scabies and other creatures. In: Dawood R, ed. *Traveller's Health*. Oxford: Oxford University Press, 1992.

26. Dennis D T. Plague in India. *BMJ* 1994; 309: 893–894.

27. Bernhard J D. Bringing on the bacon for myiasis. *Lancet* 1993; 342: 1377–1378.

28. Vega-Lopez F, Blackwell V. Tropical skin infections. In: Zukerman A, ed. *Principles and Practice of Travel Medicine*. Chichester, UK: John Wiley, 2001: 128–151.

29. Jelinek T, Northdruft H D, Loscher T. Schistosomiasis in travellers and expatriates. *J Travel Med* 1996; 3: 160–164.

30. Salafsky B, Ramaswamy K, He Y-X *et al*. Development and evaluation of lipodeet, a new long-acting formulation of N, N-diethyl-*m*-toluamide (DEET) for the prevention of schistosomiasis. *Am J Trop Med Hyg* 1999; 61: 743–750.

31. Hatz C F, Thisyakorn U, Thisyakorn C, Wilde H. Viral and tropical infections: other important viral infections. In: DuPont H L, Steffen R, eds. *Textbook of Travel Medicine and Health*, 2nd edn. Hamilton, Canada: BC Decker, 2000: 312–324.

32. Barnett E D, Chen R T, Rey M. Principles and practice of immunoprophylaxis. In: DuPont H L, Steffen R, eds. *Textbook of Travel Medicine and Health*, 2nd edn. Hamilton, Canada: BC Decker; 2000: 232–248.

33. Jaenisch T, Preiser W, Berger A *et al*. Emerging viral pathogens in long-term expatriates (I): hepatitis E virus. *Trop Med Int Health* 1997; 2: 885–891.

34. Dawson D G, Spivey G H, Korelitz J J, Schmidt R T. Hepatitis B: risk to expatriates in South East Asia. *BMJ* 1987; 294: 547.

35. Zukermann A. Virus infections. In: Zukerman A, ed. *Principles and Practice of Travel Medicine*. Chichester, UK: John Wiley, 2001: 39–79.

36. Kenyon T A, Valway S E, Ihle W W *et al*. Transmission of multidrug-resistant *Mycobacterium tuberculosis* during a long airplane flight. *N Engl J Med* 1996; 334: 933–938.

37. Heslop I. Melioidosis – a rare but serious tropical disease that could affect travellers. *Pharm J* 2002; 268: 849–851.

38. De Cook K M. Viral haemorrhagic fevers. *Medicine* 1997; 25: 16–18.

39. Carroll B, Dow C, Snashall D *et al*. Post-tropical screening: how useful is it? *BMJ* 1993; 307: 541.

40. Conlon C, Peto T. Post-tropical screening is of little value. *BMJ* 1993; 307: 1008.

6

Bite avoidance

All travellers to the tropics should be made aware of the importance of bite avoidance in order to reduce the risks of insect-borne diseases, as described in Chapter 5. One large survey of over 100 000 European tourists to East Africa indicated that the risks of malaria are significantly reduced if adequate bite avoidance measures are taken.[1] Biting insects also have a nuisance value and can make life unpleasant for a trekker or walker in many situations. A good example is the infamous Scottish midge that seems to be resistant to most repellents.

Repellents applied to the skin are an important element of any bite avoidance strategy and are widely available through pharmacies, travel stores and a variety of retail outlets. The pharmacist is particularly well placed to offer advice on repellents, as these will be sold on the premises and other bite avoidance measures could also be emphasised. All health professionals with an interest in travel medicine should be in a position to assess and recommend insect repellents and insecticides, as well as offering advice on how they are best used.

This chapter will focus on methods of avoiding mosquito bites, which are responsible for transmitting a variety of tropical diseases, including malaria (Plate 6). There are a number of broad strategies that can be used to reduce insect bites and these will be considered in some detail. They are:

- Reduce general exposure to insects through knowledge of their behaviour and how they are attracted to bite.
- Use repellent applied to the skin.
- Use insecticides which are impregnated into materials such as clothing, mosquito nets or tents.
- Remove insects from the environment using contact insecticides, e.g. knockdown sprays or burners/mats.

A variety of other methods, such as the use of electronic buzzers and vitamin B tablets, will also be discussed.

It is important that travellers are aware that such measures are designed to avoid biting insects rather than stinging insects like wasps and bees.

Reducing exposure to bites from mosquitoes

The key to successful methods of avoiding mosquito bites is to understand the ways in which mosquitoes are attracted to feed from humans.
This is a complex area which is not completely understood.

The bite of the female *Anopheles* mosquito is responsible for transmitting malaria. The male of the species is much more benign, feeding
exclusively on plant nectar. The female's blood meal is important for the
development of mosquito eggs before they are laid. Therefore the tendency to bite is closely related to the reproductive cycle of the mosquito.

Factors that attract mosquitoes

An understanding of some of the factors by which a mosquito is
attracted to feed can help in informing bite avoidance measures.

Attraction to the general vicinity of a blood meal is by products of
metabolism released by a human or other animal. Chemoreceptors on
the insect antennae can detect minute quantities of these substances
released by human skin.[2] The two most important substances are
believed to be lactic acid and carbon dioxide. The quantity produced
may be important, because, as discussed below, larger individuals tend
to be more attractive than smaller people. It has also been reported that
higher concentrations of lactic acid will actually repel mosquitoes.[3]
Mosquitoes can detect carbon dioxide from quite a long range. Some
perfumes or other strong-smelling substances can also act as attractants,
perhaps mimicking chemicals produced by the body.

At a closer range, mosquitoes can find a human by sight or by
detecting movement. They are more attracted by dark clothing, which
validates the wearing of 'tropical whites'. Mosquitoes then rely on body
heat and moisture to determine where to bite once they are within close
range of an individual.

There are some well-defined differences in behaviour of different
species of mosquitoes. *Anopheles* mosquitoes bite at night, with the
most intense outdoor activity being in the early evening. *Aedes*
mosquitoes, which can transmit dengue, are daytime feeders and are
most active in the afternoon. Where the two diseases coexist therefore
longer periods of bite avoidance measures would be required, perhaps
reducing overall compliance, but greater vigilance would be recommended in the later part of the day and evening.

Environmental conditions, such as cold temperature, may reduce
the tendency of insects to bite. Also, as described below, insect repellents

tend to be less effective with a rise in temperature, so it would follow that the warmer the climate, the greater the chance of being bitten. Mosquitoes would also tend to be less likely to bite in a cooler room, so a sealed air-conditioned room would be safe to sleep in without a mosquito net, provided no insects had gained entry during the day. Air turbulence from air-conditioning systems or strong fans also reduces the chances of being bitten. Prevailing wind conditions can influence the number of mosquitoes found in a particular locality. Variations in mosquito numbers are therefore difficult to predict, so travellers may be initially lulled into a false sense of security if relatively few insects are encountered, which could change dramatically with wind strength or direction.

Time of year is perhaps the most important determinant of encountering large numbers of mosquitoes and this is usually linked to the monsoon or wet season. Part of the life cycle of the mosquito is spent as free larvae in fresh, still water that would predominate through such periods. In some areas malaria transmission is quite intense during the wet seasons; at other times of year it may be low or even completely absent. It is quite difficult for the traveller to anticipate these seasonal changes in risk, particularly if they vary greatly by region. This can be a cause of concern to travellers who on reaching a destination are told that the risk of malaria is not present, despite having been advised to take prophylaxis. It is still best for travellers to err on the side of caution and continue their recommended prophylaxis. A further confounding factor is that unusual weather conditions extend the wet season considerably. A recent example was hurricane Mitch that caused a massive increase in insect-borne diseases in Asia and the Pacific region due to widespread flooding. As a general rule, if flooding is reported in a tropical area, it can be anticipated that there will be an increase in mosquito-borne diseases. Whenever possible it is advisable to try and sleep away from areas of stagnant water where mosquitoes might be breeding.

There appears to be a gender difference in attracting mosquitoes, with females getting significantly more bites in trials.[4] In addition, children tend to be bitten less than adults and this may simply be a reflection of the lower quantity of attractants produced by metabolism. Conversely, larger people tend to be bitten more than smaller individuals.

Mosquitoes find it more difficult to bite through loose than tight-fitting clothes. It is particularly important to wear long-sleeved clothing and trousers after dusk to avoid *Anopheles* mosquitoes. Such measures may be less practical for avoiding daytime-feeding species.

There are some species of mosquito that appear to be more attracted to certain parts of the body, the arms and ankles in particular. For instance, in a study in the Kruger National Park, South Africa,[5] *A. arabiensis* was found to bite predominantly on the ankles and repellent applied just to that area afforded a good level of protection. However, other species may not show the same pattern of behaviour.

Reducing exposure to other biting insects

The bite of the tsetse fly can be quite painful (Plate 7). Tsetse flies appear to be attracted by the colour blue and moving objects. They have a tendency to enter through the windows of moving vehicles. Therefore, it is best to keep windows closed when tsetse flies are about. Tsetse flies are less susceptible to insect repellents used to repel mosquitoes.

The sandfly is quite difficult to avoid, apart from by using a mosquito net treated with insecticide (Plate 8). The insecticide is essential because sandflies are small enough to pass through holes in the net. They tend to bite at night or in the early hours of the morning. Sandflies are quite poor flyers, so if sleeping in the open, it may be best to sleep higher up, for instance on the roof of a building.

Of the other biting insects, ticks and fleas can be found in undergrowth in both tropical and temperate climates. Therefore, to prevent bites, ramblers and trekkers should keep trousers tucked into socks.

The key features for avoiding bites are summarised in Table 6.1.

Insect repellents

Insect repellents are the mainstay of bite avoidance strategies. It is important for health professionals to understand their mode of action and limitations in order to advise on correct use. There is sometimes a tendency for the public to view insect repellents in the same way as cosmetics, to be used occasionally to avoid the nuisance of biting insects. Where insects can transmit diseases, they are just as important as any other prophylactic measure and their choice and use should be determined by evidence-based principles. The mechanism of action of repellents applied to the skin is not well understood, but undoubtedly they interfere with the chemical stimuli which attract mosquitoes. Repellents can be thought of as having a vaporising effect: molecules of repellent evaporate from the skin and interfere with the 'homing

Table 6.1 Methods of avoiding insect bites

Insect	Methods
Mosquito	Repellents applied to skin Insecticide applied to clothing Use of knockdown spray or insecticide-impregnated mats to clear room of mosquitoes Avoid night time exposure (*Anopheles*) Cover up arms and legs. Wear light colours and thicker materials Sleep under insecticide-impregnated mosquito net Sleep away from stagnant or other water harbouring mosquitoes Be extra vigilant in the wet seasons Do not use perfume
Ticks	Treat socks with DEET or permethrin Tuck trousers into socks
Tsetse fly	Use DEET repellent Avoid the colour blue Close windows of vehicles
Sandfly	Sleep under insecticide-impregnated mosquito net Sleep above ground level and avoid moving around outside in the early hours of the morning

DEET, diethyltoluamide.

mechanisms' described above, that mosquitoes use to detect a potential blood meal from a distance.

Whether or not a person is bitten while wearing a repellent depends on a large number of variables, partly because of the range of stimuli that attract mosquitoes. It is a common observation that one person may claim a particular repellent does not work while it is of great benefit for other individuals. Therefore, it is worth examining the general factors that affect repellent efficacy.

Kinetics and dynamics of insect repellent activity

There are some interesting parallels between drug pharmacodynamics and pharmacokinetics and the activity of insect repellents. Just as with any drug, there are two important parameters that must be defined: how much is needed to achieve maximum effect and how long that effect might continue. Firstly, there is a linear log dose concentration-dependent relationship between the dose of repellent applied and the

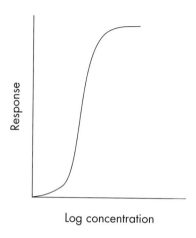

Figure 6.1 A standard log dose–response curve.

percentage protection achieved (Fig. 6.1). This means that it is possible, just as with any drug, to calculate the effective dose to achieve 90% of a maximal effect (ED_{90}). For repellents the ED_{90} could be defined as the amount of repellent that must be applied to the skin to offer 90% protection, or more precisely, to achieve a 90% reduction of the bites that would have taken place if no repellent had been applied. If the ED_{90} cannot be achieved with a reasonable application rate then the repellent would be viewed as having a low potency. The rate of loss of repellent from the surface of the skin, in a constant environment, is believed to follow an exponential decay, as shown in Figure 6.2, which is similar to the rate of fall in blood concentration seen after the administration of many types of drugs, a behaviour known formally as first-order kinetics. The rate of loss of repellent would be determined by the evaporation from the surface of the skin and absorption through the skin. In practice other confounding variables such as wash-off by sweat, abrasion and external temperature would further influence the rate at which the repellent is removed.

A mathematical relationship between percentage protection, amount of repellent applied and length of action was derived by Rutledge et al.[6] for both diethyltoluamide (DEET) and dimethylphthalate, the latter being rarely used now in repellents. Figure 6.3a shows the form of this graph when percentage activity is plotted against time for different concentrations of repellents. There is a plateau, where percentage protection remains at around 100–90% before declining exponentially. The length of this plateau will depend on the initial applied dose,

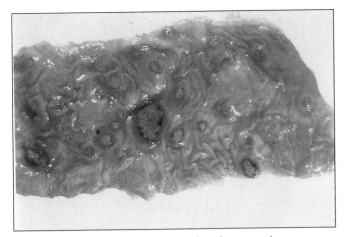

Plate 1 Damaged colon from amoebic dysentry, showing ulceration and haemorrhage. Courtesy of The Medicine Publishing Company.

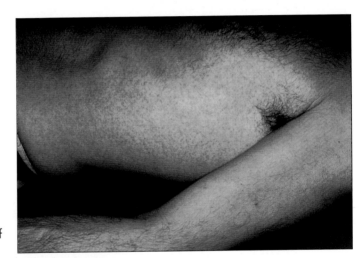

Plate 2 Rash associated with dengue. Courtesy of Eric Caumes.

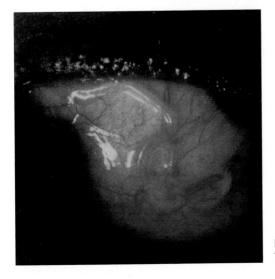

Plate 3 African eye worm. Courtesy of The Medicine Publishing Company.

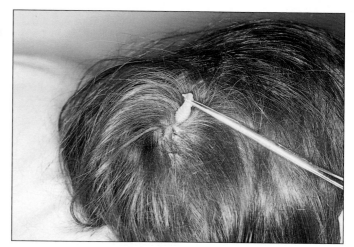

Plate 4 Human bot fly emerging. Courtesy of Eric Caumes.

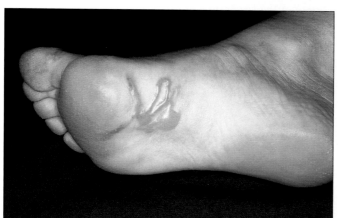

Plate 5 Cutaneous larva migrans on the sole of the foot, showing that the serpiginous lines can be covered by vesiculobullous lesions. Courtesy of Eric Caumes.

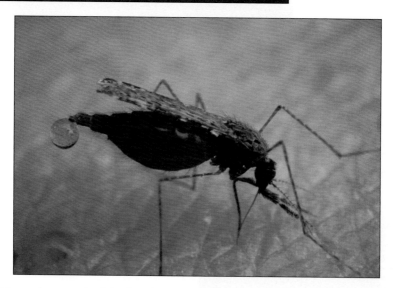

Plate 6 Macrophotograph of the female mosquito *Anopheles balabacensis*, an East Indian malaria-carrying species. The mosquito feeds on human blood while simultaneously depositing the protozoan responsible for malaria, *Plasmodium malariae*. The body is distended with the blood meal and excess fluid is being excreted at the rear. Magnification: ×5 at 35 mm size. Courtesy of Martin Dohrn/Science Photo Library.

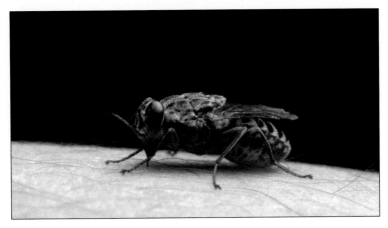

Plate 7 Macrophotograph of a tsetse fly *Glossina morsitans*, a major vector of sleeping sickness, feeding on a human arm. The abdomen of the fly can be seen filling with human blood. Sleeping sickness is mainly a disease of tropical Africa and is caused by the presence in the blood of a parasitic protozoon *Trypanosoma gambiense* or *T. rhodesiense*. These parasites are transmitted to humans through the bite of the tsetse fly. Magnification: ×2 at 35 mm size. Courtesy of Martin Dohrn/Science Photo Library.

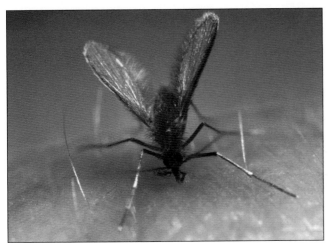

Plate 8 Feeding sandfly. Macrophotograph of a sandfly (*Lutzomyia longipalpis*) feeding on a human. The sandfly feeds on human blood and is a vector for leishmaniasis, a disease which causes breakdown of the tissues in humans. The fly carries the *Leishmania* protozoon in its salivary glands and injects it into the human host as it feeds. Magnification unknown. Courtesy of Sinclair Stammers/Science Photo Library.

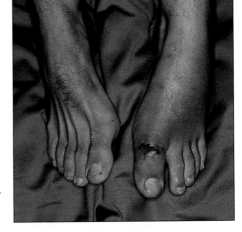

Plate 9 Necrotising cellulitis of the big toe, as a result of poorly fitting walking boots. Courtesy of Eric Caumes.

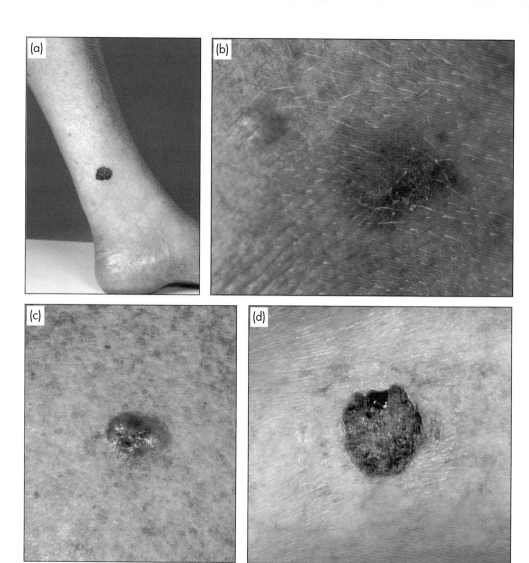

Plate 10 (a) A malignant melanoma affecting the lower part of a leg. Melanomas are highly malignant tumours of the melanocytes, cells which produce a dark-brown to black pigment called melanin. Melanin occurs in the skin, hair, iris and choroid layer of the eyes. In the skin it is contained within special cells called chromatophores, which are found in the dermis. Melanomas usually occur in the skin, but are also found in the eye and mucous membranes. Such tumours may or may not contain the melanin pigment. Spread of this type of cancer to other parts of the body, particularly to the lymph nodes and liver, is common. Courtesy of James Stevenson/Science Photo Library (SPL). **(b)** Ordinary photograph of actinic (solar) keratosis; a well-defined, red, warty growth which occurs in middle or old age and is caused by overexposure to the sun. Courtesy of James Stevenson/SPL. **(c)** Basal cell carcinoma. This is a type of skin cancer also known as a rodent ulcer, which commonly occurs on the face or neck and typically affects fair-skinned people. Direct skin damage from the ultraviolet radiation in sunlight is thought to be the cause in most cases. Basal cell carcinomas usually appear as small, flat nodules and grow slowly, eventually breaking down at the centre to form a shallow ulcer. If untreated they invade deeper tissues but luckily never spread to other parts of the body. They may be removed by cryosurgery or radiotherapy or with a surgical operation. The treatment often results in a complete cure. Courtesy of Dr P Marazzi/SPL. **(d)** Skin cancer: squamous cell carcinoma (cancer), appearing as a red mass on an elderly man's leg. Squamous cell carcinoma is one type of skin cancer. Courtesy of Dr P Marazzi/SPL.

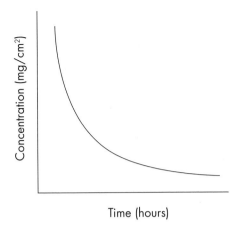

Figure 6.2 Concentration/time plot.

but the rate of decline thereafter is not dose-dependent. The equation can be transformed to give a straight-line plot if probits (the inverse of the normal distribution) are taken and this is useful for making direct comparisons of the rate of decline and calculating the ED_{90} precisely. Although this model was proposed in 1985, there does not seem to have been much work conducted to refine the model further.

The applied doses (mg/cm^2) of repellent shown in Figure 6.3a have been chosen as those most likely to be used by an individual in the field. Very little work has been done to determine how much repellent people actually apply to their skin and, as will be described later, this is very important when comparing different types of repellents.

Duration of action is the single most important factor influencing efficacy, in that repellents may not be applied with sufficient frequency. It must be remembered that, within a short time of applying a repellent, as described above, its efficacy will reduce. When a repellent is advertised as having 'a duration of up to 12 hours' it does not necessarily mean that 100% effectiveness is maintained over the full time period. In fact, there is no accepted standard for expressing length of activity which could be referred to as the time to first being bitten (T_{100}), the time to protection falling by 90% (T_{90}) or by 50% (T_{50}). In situations of high insect density, and where a large number of insects may be carrying malaria, such a fall in efficacy could be unacceptable. For instance, suppose that one is in a situation where, without any repellent applied, 20 bites per hour are experienced. If a repellent is applied when the T_{50} is just 2 hours, then after this time a biting rate of 10 bites per hour will

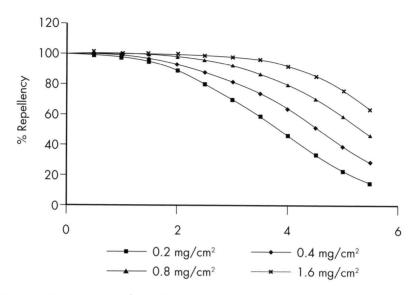

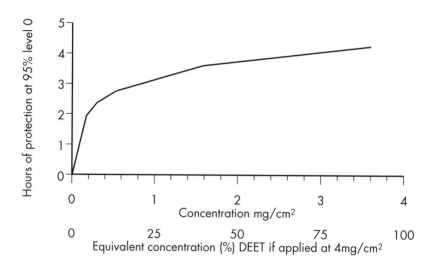

Figure 6.3a   Variation of repellency with time. Derived from Rutledge *et al.*[6]

Figure 6.3b   Hours of protection at 95% level achieved with applied dose of DEET. Adapted from Buescher MD *et al.*[7]

be experienced – unacceptable to users and perhaps putting them at risk of contracting insect-borne diseases. I have talked to many people claiming that a particular repellent is ineffective and on questioning it becomes apparent that they expected no bites to be received over the

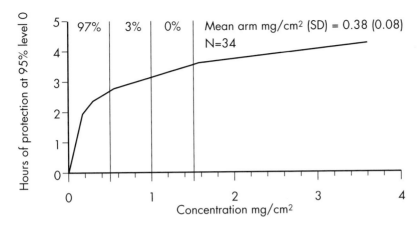

Figure 6.3c Protection time and concentration of diethyltoluamide (DEET), showing % of participants applying at 3 concentration ranges.

entire application period claimed by the manufacturer, despite obviously very high insect density.

The amount of product applied is probably the most critical controllable factor in terms of duration of action. Put simply, up to a certain point the higher the concentration and the greater the amount applied, the longer it will last (with the exception of sustained-release formulations). However, applying twice the amount of repellent does not mean that double the protection time is achieved. In the case of DEET, this has led to a debate concerning the most effective minimum concentration of repellent to be used, and some misunderstandings concerning the mathematical models employed.

It has been suggested that, as the 'protection' given is proportional to the logarithm of the concentration applied, and for DEET a plateau of protection is reached when a concentration of 20% is used, higher concentrations give little added benefit. This may be true in terms of the applied amount needed to achieve protection when a dose of less than 1 mg/cm^2 is sufficient to achieve an ED_{90} for most species but, according to the models described, not really applicable when considering longevity. The important point here is not so much the percentage, but what is actually applied. In the case of alcoholic solutions of DEET, the alcohol evaporates quickly, leaving essentially pure DEET on the skin although the applied total dosage is lower than if a 100% solution had been applied. So a generous application of 20% DEET will achieve the same effect as a sparing 100% DEET and the latter may be more economical. By rearranging the equations proposed by Rutledge for Figure

6.3a, the duration at any protection level against concentration can be plotted as shown in Figure 6.3b. This demonstrates that there is indeed a plateau to the increase in longevity when concentrations around 2–3 mg/cm² have been applied, and this finding was confirmed in an earlier study.[7] The important question is then how much repellent people apply to their skin, an aspect that has not been well investigated. It has been suggested that most people will achieve a maximum of 2 mg/cm² using a 100% solution, and that to apply up to 4 mg/cm² would result in excess liquid simply running off the skin.[8] The quoted figure of a maximum 50% DEET is based on the early study by Rutledge assuming that a full 4 mg/cm² of repellent volume is applied (i.e. 2 mg/cm² of active ingredient) (Figure 6.3b).

The question of how much repellent a traveller would apply to the skin in normal use has been investigated in a small pilot study.[9] In this study 74 volunteers were asked to give a demonstration of how they might apply a repellent if visiting a malaria-endemic area, assuming they were going out at night wearing long trousers and a short-sleeved shirt. They were observed performing this procedure and the repellent container weighed before and after use. The application area was then –measured to calculate the skin surface area. Mean arm application concentration achieved for 50–60% strength products was 0.80 mg/cm² (SD 0.23) and for 20% strength products 0.38 mg/cm² (SD 0.08). The results for the 20% application (Figure 6.3c) indicate the lower protection time achieved. Therefore in normal use it may be that strengths in excess of 50% do indeed offer a significant increase in protection time. The analogy is similar to that described for sunscreens in Chapter 9, where a sun protection factor (SPF) in excess of that theoretically needed may be required to compensate for a low application rate.

Taking all the above arguments into consideration, at the usual application rates discussed there is a general consensus that 30–50% DEET will provide acceptable levels of protection for 3–4 hours in most circumstances, although this is a generalisation. Using higher concentrations of DEET may extend the protection time by another hour or two. Therefore, DEET insect repellents must be reapplied at least every 4 hours. In practical terms, this would mean applying the repellent in the early evening and at least once before retiring, although repellent should not be worn overnight. If there is a high mosquito density and malaria is a risk, it may be prudent to reapply more frequently to achieve better protection. Furthermore, other external factors removing repellent from the skin (e.g. abrasion and water) would be expected to contribute to reducing the amount of the active ingredient. A consideration of duration of activity in a variety of circumstances does not generally seem to be mentioned in manufacturers' instructions.

There are a number of factors that determine duration of activity in terms of the rate at which it is removed from the skin. The analogy to drug kinetics would be those factors which might determine the clearance from the body, e.g. liver or kidney function and rate of absorption from the formulation. These factors are described below, but it would be difficult to quantify the impact on duration from any one if them.

Formulation

Formulation of a product may influence the length of action. Simple liquid or gel formulations evaporate from the skin relatively quickly but there is little evidence that cream formulations last any longer. There are sustained-release formulations which give a longer duration of action, most commonly based on microencapsulated formulations where repellent is gradually released by a rise in temperature from heat supplied by the skin. However, the only sustained-release products that have been developed are based on DEET and none is currently available in the UK, except through specialist stores. For these repellents the important factor is the slow rate of decline in repellency, rather than a maintenance in 100% potency. Furthermore, release of repellent may be retarded, resulting in a somewhat higher ED_{90}. The profile of release of a sustained-release product can be seen from some original data shown in Figure 6.4. This was performed using a standard cage test at the London School of Hygiene and Tropical Medicine on a new 20% microencapsulated formulation, compared to a simple DEET-in-ethanol formulation. Note the similarity in the time to first bite (T_{100}) of the two formulations, but the much slower decline in repellency thereafter. This is further discussed under Insect repellents – what to advise, below.

Sweat

Sweat from the skin which removes the repellent is an important factor, particularly in the humid tropics. Repellents may also be removed through abrasion against clothing or other objects or washing the skin.

Absorption

Absorption through the skin may account for a certain proportion of loss of repellent. This has been reasonably well studied in the case of

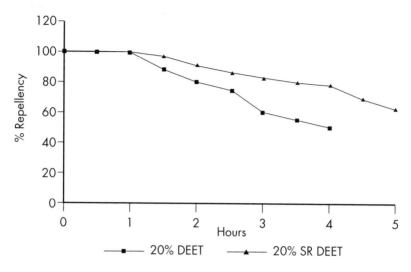

Figure 6.4 A sustained-release (SR) diethyltoluamide (DEET) product compared to standard formulation.

DEET as described under Insect repellents – what to advise, below, but there are few available data for other products.

Ambient temperature

Ambient temperature is known to be quite an important determinant of repellent activity. As temperature increases, protection time is reduced, probably due to increased evaporation of repellent. Protection time may also be reduced in windy conditions.[10]

Other factors affecting insect repellent activity

An important factor explaining the occasional observation by travellers that a repellent works in one locality but not in another is that there is an enormous range of species of mosquito with varying sensitivity to repellents. This variation is even present within species. For instance, DEET is highly effective against *Anopheles stephensi* but much less active against *An. albimanus*.[11] A useful reference species is *An. gambiae*, against which DEET has a reasonable activity. *Aedes* are generally more sensitive than *Anopheles* to repellent.

The individual characteristics of a person may determine the efficacy of a repellent, although this has not been well studied, and probably relates to production of attractants. However, as previously mentioned, female sex and high sweat and lactic acid production reduce repellent efficacy.

Mosquitoes always prefer to bite a person with no repellent on the skin than one wearing a repellent, even if the repellent is not very effective and/or is present in quite low concentrations. Therefore, when travelling in a group, an individual may well be in a better position to avoid bites if others in the group are not using repellents!

Compliance with insect repellents

Compliance is an important factor in determining repellent efficacy. If an insect repellent has to be reapplied every couple of hours throughout the night, just as with any therapeutic regimen, it is highly likely that doses will be missed. In addition, if the repellent is cosmetically unacceptable to individuals, they are unlikely to use it properly. Fears of adverse effects from the repellent may also reduce compliance. Alternatively, poor faith in the efficacy of a repellent may also result in it not being applied. The cost may also influence correct application, with a more expensive formulation being applied too sparingly or infrequently. This area of insect repellent use has not been well studied, but it is known that compliance with bite avoidance measures is in general lower than compliance with malaria chemoprophylaxis.[1] A postal questionnaire to tourists visiting the Kruger National Park in South Africa indicated that, while 80% were using repellents, less than half were following other advice, such as wearing long-sleeved clothing and socks.[12] A survey conducted among servicemen from Singapore found that only half used an army-issued repellent while on exercise.[13]

The most pragmatic answer is a take a concordance approach: any repellent the person is happy to use regularly is better than one they find unacceptable, however efficacious it may be.

Assessment of repellent activity

Before considering the relative merits of the repellents currently available, it is worth examining the way in which they are assessed. This is important from an evidence-based perspective when considering data from manufacturers.

The most convenient methods for assessment in the laboratory are the so-called cage tests. In these, a volunteer is required to place an arm into a cage containing mosquitoes and the number of bites received in a particular time is noted (Fig. 6.5). In a free-flight test, an individual will stand in a large cage containing mosquitoes. Cage test methods are used to calculate the minimum effective dose, i.e. potency of a repellent and also the longevity.

The cage test value which is of greatest use is the longevity of repellent at a particular dose. However, there is little standardisation of the test. One method is to compare two treated arms placed in separate cages. Some tests use the time taken for the first bite (T_{100}), whereas others use the time for repellent activity to fall by 50% (T_{50}) when compared to a control arm with no repellent.

Cage tests do not take into account many of the variables described in the previous section, so the most realistic data might be expected to be obtained from field tests. Again, there are no standardised methods for performing such tests. Field tests are carried out at destinations where mosquitoes are breeding. A count is taken of the number of bites received by volunteers, with and without repellents, in a particular time. In many such field tests the individual remains sitting in a fairly stable environment, without many of the factors present which could reduce efficacy of the repellent, e.g. abrasion, sweat, changes in mosquito density. This could lead to false assumptions regarding actual protection times, but is useful if comparing different products. Larger-scale trials are carried out by the military whilst on

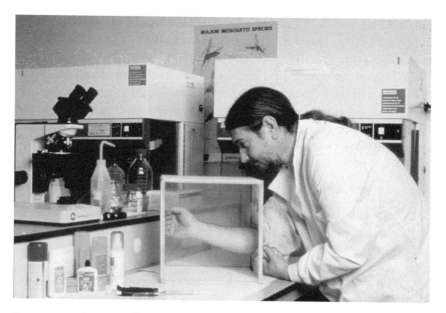

Figure 6.5 Cage test for assessing insect repellents. With permission. Dr Nigel Hill, London School of Hygiene and Tropical Medicine.

manoeuvres in areas where mosquito density is high. Such tests can be difficult to control, but give some indication of actual protection time in certain situations and can usually be viewed as impartial.

There are therefore a number of factors which should be considered by the health professional when presented with data by manufacturers on insect repellent efficacy. In most studies, data are given as a comparison to the 'gold standard' DEET. Indeed, a useful marketing strategy is to present a repellent as 'an alternative to DEET-based products'. Table 6.2 shows a list of the factors to be considered. In practice it can be difficult to ascertain whether, in terms of efficacy, a product is superior, particularly if different dosages are used to those available commercially. Evaluation may not always describe the actual applied dose in terms of mg per body surface area. On the other hand, sometimes an applied dose is quoted which would be difficult to achieve with the commercially available product. As a simple guide, reasonable dose rates and figures to help in their conversion are also shown in Table 6.2. A further area of confusion is that a product may be claimed to be superior in longevity to DEET, when the comparison

Table 6.2 Some factors to consider when assessing efficacy data for insect repellents

Mosquito species	There is great variation in sensitivity to different repellents. As regards DEET, the following is an approximate order of efficacy: *Anopheles albimanus* (least effective) *An. gambiae* *An. stephensi* *Aedes aegyptiae* (but variable)
Location of controls	Control and treated subjects should have adequate distance between them so that controls do not attract insects preferentially. In cage tests, treated and untreated limbs should not be in the same cage
Concentration and application of product	Dose applied should reflect the actual normal application rate of the commercially available product. Approximate reasonable quantities applied of liquid repellent: 1–2 ml leg, 0.5–1 ml arm. Expected dose from a 50% solution: 0.4–0.8 mg/cm^2
Comparison with DEET	Length of action compared with DEET is particularly important. Comparison should be made with both high and low concentrations of DEET

DEET, diethyltoluamide.

has actually been made to a low application rate. Some of the deficiencies in evaluating data will be discussed later when considering individual products.

One helpful study on products available in the UK was a cage test comparison carried out at the London School of Hygiene and Tropical Medicine for *Which?* magazine in which all available repellents were tested and ranked on a star system. Only those products containing concentrations of DEET greater than 30% were recommended as suitable for areas where there was a risk of insect-borne disease (Table 6.3). A similar outcome has been found in studies on US products.[14,15] Most recently, Fradin and Day[16] evaluated repellents available on the US market using a cage test on 15 volunteers; the results are also shown for comparison in Table 6.3. The test used in their study was the time taken before first bite was achieved and involved only 10 mosquitoes per cage, which is somewhat lower than other cage tests. They concluded that a sustained-release product was no better than standard in their test, which is not surprising as the sustained activity might be more accurately measured as a slower decline in percentage protection against time, i.e. a longer time to fall to 50% protection rather than any change in time to first bite. The study tended to use lower-concentration repellents than found on the UK market and the actual dosage applied did not seem to be standardised. Nonetheless, DEET repellents at concentrations greater than 20% did appear to be far superior than others available, particularly compared to some natural products and IR3535. Much publicised in the USA is the moisturiser Skin-so-Soft, which fared particularly poorly.

It is also of interest to note that, unlike in some countries (including the USA), there is currently no requirement in the UK to present efficacy or toxicity data to licensing authorities before marketing a topically applied insect repellent.

Currently available repellents

Below is presented a discussion of some of the more widely available types of repellents on the European and US markets (Fig. 6.6). Not all types can easily be found in different countries.

Diethyltoluamide

Diethyltoluamide (DEET) has been used worldwide as a repellent for over 40 years so it is not surprising that more research has been performed on

Table 6.3 Comparison of repellents available in the UK and the USA[40]

Insect repellent	Effectiveness rating: UK study	Duration (mean) of effect: US study
Synthetic repellents		
Bayrepel 20%	3	
DEET 100%	5	
DEET 27.5–60%	4 (30% stick formulation – 3)	
DEET 20%	3	DEET 20% SR 301 minutes DEET 23% 234 minutes
DEET 10%	3	DEET 7% 112 minutes
Merck IR3535 10–20%	3	IR3535 7.5% 22.9 minutes
DEET/dimethylphthalate	3	
Dimethylphthalate 45%	3	
Plant-derived natural products		
Citronella	2	10–20 minutes
Citradiol 30–50%	3	
Tarconathus camphoratus (extract of wild camphor tree)	2	
Extract of lemon eucalyptus 19%	3	120 minutes
Skin-so-Soft moisturiser		2.8 minutes
Soya bean oil 2%		95 minutes
Bands and patches		
Citronella 90%	2	
DEET 25%	3	
DEET 100%	2	
DEET 9.5%	2	0.3 minutes

DEET, diethyltoluamide; SR, sustained-release.
Adapted, with permission, from *Which?* magazine, June 1999.
UK study: This table was produced in June, 1999. Since then, some formulations may have changed. Jungle Formula aerosol, roll-on and gel appeared in the original table but have not been included here because of a recent formulation change from DEET to Merck 3535.
US study: Based on a mean protection time to first bite of 15 volunteers exposing their arms in a cage containing 10 mosquitoes. Dose application was 'according to manufacturers' instructions'.
Key: effectiveness rating:
5, products containing above 60% DEET. They protect for about 5 hours before needing to be reapplied. Use where there is a risk of malaria or insect-borne disease.
4, products containing 30–60% DEET. They give protection for about 3–5 hours. Also suitable for areas where there is a risk of malaria or insect-borne disease.

continues overleaf

3, products containing 10–30% DEET or other synthetic or natural repellent. Use for European and other malaria-free destinations.

2, suitable for countries where there is absolutely no risk of insect-borne diseases.(The effectiveness of bands and patches was rated according to the level of protection they gave in two test conditions – after 30 minutes and after being worn for 2 hours a day over 5 days. The table was produced from trial results.)

this repellent than any other. There is evidence to suggest that its main mode of action may be through inhibiting lactic acid receptors on mosquito antennae.[17] It has been proposed that lactic acid is an important attractant which orientates mosquitoes to human skin. As it is still regarded as a 'gold standard' repellent, DEET will be discussed in some detail.

Formulation differences

An attractive alternative to reapplying repellents is to use a sustained-release DEET product, based on microencapsulated hydrogel, emulsion or lipospheres.[18] The 3M sustained-release product Ultrathon is no longer widely available, although other sustained-release brands are made in the USA. Ultrathon and some other sustained-release products can be obtained through specialist suppliers in other countries. As less of the DEET is absorbed through the skin from these formulations,

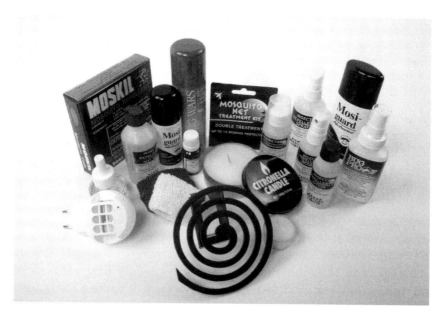

Figure 6.6 Range of insect repellents available in the UK. Courtesy of Nomad.

there are theoretical advantages concerning adverse reactions (see below). They are also formulated with a lower percentage of DEET, at around 20–30%. In cage tests, the length of action has been similar to a high-strength DEET preparation. In the field, some studies have shown better activity than for simple high-concentration DEET, possibly due to resistance to other factors such as wash-off by sweat or water. Nonetheless, claims by manufacturers of lengths of action of 6 hours or more should be taken with caution and more frequent application may be needed in areas of high mosquito activity.

Insect repellents are generally recommended to be applied after sunscreen, as the sunscreen may occlude evaporation of DEET. This was not confirmed in a study comparing the effect of two different sunscreen formulations on the activity of a 33% DEET repellent;[19] no reduction in repellency was observed by the presence of a sunscreen, whether applied before or after the repellent. However, there is evidence of a breakdown in sunscreen efficacy.[20] There are formulations that combine both sunscreen and repellent but these have not been widely tested and should probably not be relied upon in malaria-endemic areas. There may be some rationale for using them when day-biting mosquitoes are a potential problem.

Clothing can be treated with DEET, although this tends to be a somewhat messy procedure. DEET (100%) is diluted one in four with water, with which it is not miscible so the solution must be stirred vigorously to disperse the DEET. Clothing is dipped into the solution. The treated clothing can be expected to retain repellent properties for up to 1 week, providing it is stored in an airtight plastic bag between uses. Clothing treatment with an insecticide such as permethrin is generally preferred.

An alternative way of using DEET is to apply approximately 5 ml of 100% solution to a cotton wrist or leg band. Bands can be worn to give some protection to the areas where mosquitoes might bite. They last some weeks after treatment. Ready-treated bands are commercially available, as are kits to make them. They are not as effective as repellents applied directly to the skin.

In a similar manner, high concentrations of DEET can be applied to the edges of clothes. However, evidence suggests that the repellent action of DEET is observed only 3–4 cm outside the area of application and that different species tend to prefer feeding from various parts of the body. Unfortunately, little work has been performed to define the efficacy of such uses of DEET.

Adverse effects and contraindications

The use of DEET has been the subject of controversy because of perceived disadvantages involving adverse reactions and contraindications in both pregnancy and young children. To a large extent, such fears have been unfounded[21] and the risk of adverse effects in normal use is low.[22] When comparing the benefits of DEET in repellent activity with the risk of adverse events, many experts have concluded that it should still be considered the agent of first choice where there is a risk of malaria. However, the potential adverse events to DEET should be examined.

As for any topically applied agent, allergic skin reactions are occasionally reported. More serious skin reactions have been reported when DEET is left on overnight. It was noticed that soldiers who used high concentrations of DEET on a regular basis just before they went to bed developed a serious skin reaction in the antecubital fossa (the flexure at the elbows),[23] probably related to occlusion of the skin. DEET, or indeed any other insect repellent, should not be applied at bedtime. DEET is irritant to the eyes and mucous membranes and care should be taken when applying it to the face.

A potential drawback in the use of DEET is that it is a plasticising agent, which means that it tends to damage any plastic objects with which it comes into contact. Particular care should be taken regarding plastic glasses and watch faces. In addition, some people find the smell of DEET objectionable but many find it acceptable.[8]

Reported adverse systemic reactions to DEET have resulted in some branded repellents changing formulation to become DEET-free. However, the incidence of systemic reactions must be put into perspective. DEET has been used since the 1950s and it has been estimated that in the USA around 30% of the population use DEET-containing products at least once a year. Until recently, this figure was about 25% for the UK population. With such large numbers of users, the incidence of adverse reactions and toxicity is remarkably low. The low incidence is also attested to by a US survey of reports to poison centres.[24] Unlike in the UK, US reports can be made directly by the public as well as by health workers. The survey found that, of the 3098 adverse reactions to DEET reported between 1985 and 1990, only 44 resulted in a hospital admission and just five were classified as serious adverse reactions. Most of the adverse reactions were due to the inappropriate use of DEET, such as inhalation or ocular contact. The reactions were unrelated to the concentration of DEET in the product. Accidental oral ingestion of large volumes of DEET has led to toxicity of the cardiovascular, respiratory and central nervous systems.[25] Some of the toxicity may be due to the industrial methylated spirits with which DEET is formulated. Quite a large dose (80 mg/kg) accidentally ingested by a child has also been reported to cause neurotoxicity, although in this case the child recovered without further complications.[26] Toxicity from topically applied DEET products in adults, even in high concentrations, is extremely rare.

One of the biggest concerns in recent years has been the safety of DEET in children. This is based on 12 reports of encephalopathy since the introduction of DEET[27] although, in some of these cases, the reaction cannot be positively attributed to the use of DEET. It has been argued that the larger surface area-to-weight ratio in children compared with adults might allow an increased dermal absorption for the same dose if high concentrations are applied. However, studies do not show a high dermal absorption or systemic accumulation of topically applied DEET in humans. One of the studies showed that just 8% of topically applied DEET was absorbed and that it was completely eliminated within 4 hours.[28] Whether or not this kinetic profile would present a risk to children has not been studied. It has been suggested that sustained-release formulations, which have lower dermal absorption, would be a better alternative for children and for pregnant women.[18]

The use of DEET in pregnancy is often discouraged, although there has been only one documented case of harm to a fetus through the use of DEET.[29] A study which examined the use of DEET in 897 women in their second or third trimester of pregnancy[30] could find no associated incidence of harm to the fetus either after birth or at 1-year follow-up, and no adverse effects were reported by any of the women. DEET was detected in only 8% of 50 cord blood samples taken.

There have also been concerns that DEET may have been responsible for Gulf war syndrome (a group of symptoms reported by soldiers who had served in the Gulf war).[31] Again, there is little direct evidence for this hypothesis and no similar symptoms have ever been reported in normal use by travellers.

In summary, DEET is much maligned in terms of toxicity. It would be wise to use it carefully in children and in pregnancy, using a lower-strength sustained-release action formulation if possible.

Bayrepel (Autan)

Autan contained DEET until the late 1990s when it was reformulated to contain Bayrepel, a novel compound. There is only a limited amount of independent published data available on this product. Cage tests have only been reported by the manufacturer for two *Anopheles* species and did not include *An. gambiae*, the most usually studied species. In addition, no studies have been published of laboratory tests comparing the product with concentrations of DEET higher than 20% or with sustained-release formulations.

Data from field tests are also quite limited. One published field test compared Bayrepel to DEET against *Aedes alboticus*,[32] although the design appears flawed in that both treated and untreated limbs were exposed at the same time. The comparison was made to only 10 and 20% DEET, showing equivalence to a similar concentration of Bayrepel. Another field trial using a maximum of 15% DEET and Bayrepel reported an equivalence in activity against a range of mosquito species, including *Anopheles*.[33] Limbs were treated with more than one type of repellent at a time and results are only reported as number of bites, rather than a percentage of protection.

A more recent trial conducted by the World Health Organization,[34] though not published in a peer-reviewed journal, claimed a longer duration of activity for Bayrepel against *An. gambiae* compared to DEET. Various application rates ($0.1–0.8$ mg/cm^2) were examined, and the T_{100} for DEET was reported as 2–4 hours, compared to 3.2–38.7 hours for Bayrepel. The authors admit that, due to the low numbers of subjects bitten at the higher doses, the figures obtained for these higher application rates may be unreliable. They also observed a significantly lower ED_{90} for DEET compared to Bayrepel. It must also be remembered that the commercial products contain a maximum of 20% Bayrepel, so an application rate of 0.8 mg/cm^2 may not be achieved by users.

The product seems acceptable to users and does not possess the plasticising effects of DEET.

Lemon eucalyptus extract (Mosiguard)

An extract of the lemon eucalyptus plant, known as quwenling, has been used for some years in China as an insect repellent. This extract has been marketed as Mosiguard in the UK over the past few years. The main active component of this extract is *p*-methane-3,8-diol, also known as PMD, which is now available as a semisynthetic product and has been incorporated in a number of formulations worldwide. The extract itself contains PMD plus some other less active compounds, ispulegol and citroneliol.

One cage test[35] indicated that a 50% formulation of Mosiguard had a duration of action equivalent to 20% DEET, although the DEET stick used in the assessment was superior to the equivalent Mosiguard formulation (T_{90} = 2.5 hours to T_{90} = 1.8 hours). In practice a higher-concentration formulation of DEET might achieve higher application rates and therefore result in a longer duration of action. The generally higher activity of DEET compared to lemon eucalyptus was demonstrated in an earlier series by Schreck and Leonhardt,[36] who measured time to first bite (T_{100}) against three species of mosquito. A 1 ml application of a 15% solution of DEET had a 4-hour duration against *Aedes aegypti* as against 1.1 hours for 1 ml of 30% lemon eucalyptus. For both products, duration of activity against *Anopheles albimanus* was less than 15 minutes. The findings of a generally lower activity dose-for-dose for lemon eucalyptus when compared to DEET has been observed in other studies[37] One published field test found a similar duration of activity for applied dose of DEET and lemon eucalyptus against *An. gambiae*, although extremely long times to first bite (6–7 hours) were reported, perhaps indicating somewhat low mosquito density.[38]

Generally, though, lemon eucalyptus has been reasonably well studied and, of all the natural-based products, it is probably among the most effective.

Merck IR3535

The manufacturer of Jungle Formula in the UK has recently changed the formulation of its range. All products, except the 50% lotion, have been changed from containing DEET to contain a substance developed by Merck called IR3535 (ethyl butylacetylaminopropionate). Other than the data on file,[39] it is difficult to obtain independent evidence which confirms the efficacy or toxicity profile of IR3535. The UK manufacturer of Jungle Formula suggests that its DEET-based lotion is used when visiting malaria-endemic areas and that the IR3535-based range is reserved for use in areas without insect-borne diseases.

Volatile oils

There are a number of products based on natural products which usually contain a blend of volatile oils as active ingredients. Published literature is only available to any significant extent for citronella which, while effective, has an extremely short length of action, often under 1 hour.[4] There has been interest in the Indian natural product known as neem oil,[40] but there are few trials involving direct comparisons with other repellents. It must also be made clear that just because the product is natural it is not necessarily safe.

Insect repellents – what to advise

It seems a reasonable conclusion that most insect repellents on the market are effective. As regularity of application is one of the most important factors, customer preference is of the highest priority. If users find a product cosmetically acceptable and it has worked for them in the past, then in non-malaria-endemic areas there is little reason to discourage its use. The real debate concerns what to advise as a first-line agent for use in areas where there is a high risk of contracting diseases from biting insects.

Most manufacturers would claim that their product can be used for this purpose but undoubtedly DEET has the backing of the largest body of evidence because of extensive research carried out over the past 30 years. In adults, at least, toxicity of DEET is not an important consideration. Health professionals should encourage correct use of repellents as covered in Box 6.1.

My own feeling is that adults visiting high-risk tropical areas should be offered a high-strength DEET product as a first choice. However, if they are unhappy about the cosmetic properties of DEET or its perceived toxicity, then they should be offered an alternative agent.

Box 6.1   Correct use of insect repellents

- Apply only to exposed skin
- For use on the face, dispense repellent into the palms of the hands, rub together and then carefully apply to the face, avoiding the eyes and mouth
- Do not apply to broken or inflamed skin
- Wash repellent off hands after application to avoid contact with eyes, mouth or genitals. Also, wash off repellent before going to bed
- Apply carefully to children and do not apply to their hands
- If using a repellent for the first time, test the product on a small area of skin in case of allergy
- Follow manufacturers' instructions

Advice points on the correct use of insect repellents are given in Box 6.1. It has been suggested that those who claim to obtain unsatisfactory protection from repellents should be advised to apply them more frequently.[41] Such advice would appear to contradict the usual recommendations of following the manufacturer's instructions, where a specific time interval is often stated as well as directions to apply sparingly to exposed skin. It is quite likely that such a practice could lead to intervals of low protection. It would therefore seem reasonable to recommend a more frequent application should bites be received after an hour or two, particularly in areas of high mosquito density. Also, a more generous than recommended application may be required for some lower-strength products.

It should always be emphasised that repellents cannot be used as a means of protection overnight after retiring, mainly because the length of action gives insufficient protection. Mosquito nets should be used unless sleeping in a sealed air-conditioned room.

Insecticides

Insecticides – products which kill insects – also have an important role in bite avoidance. The organophosphate insecticides are no longer used in products for personal protection and the public should be reassured of this fact. Almost universally, pyrethroids are now used, the most common of which is permethrin. The pyrethroids have a very low mammalian toxicity and permethrin has the additional advantage of a high residue effect on materials, i.e. it has a long persistence on certain fabrics after treatment.

One of the principal uses of permethrin-related compounds is in the treatment of mosquito netting. It is important that netting should be treated for two reasons – to deter insects from biting through the net should a person accidentally touch the side while asleep and to deter insects from entering through a tear in the net. In addition, it helps to prevent the entry of small insects such as sandflies. There are a number of studies that have demonstrated the effectiveness of such nets, and they provide a useful strategy in preventing malaria in the local population.[42] Nets can be purchased ready-treated with insecticides and with treatment kits which can be used to retreat the net every 1–3 months. The principal factors that would reduce the efficacy of permethrin on a treated net are abrasion by constant handling and exposure to sunlight. Legislation regarding application rates to nets does vary from country to country, particularly regarding a maximum applied dose for use in self-treatment kits. It is usually advisable to purchase a ready-treated net, which often contains quite high levels of pyrethroid, and then a retreatment kit if on a trip of more than a few months.

It is claimed that the very highest level of protection can be obtained by using a repellent on the skin and permethrin on clothing, e.g. Bug Proof. Clothing treated with permethrin affords relatively low levels of protection,[10] but when an insect repellent is additionally used on the skin, added protection is obtained.[43,44] The results of one such trial are shown in Figure 6.7. This was carried out in the field by applying 2 g of DEET to the skin of 30 subjects and exposing them to the bites of mosquitoes for a total of 14 hours at various times of the day in humid conditions. Three different species of mosquito were found in the test area. Despite the wide fluctuation in protection over time, probably due to variations in mosquito activity and environment, a consistent picture of additional protection is obtained when permethrin is applied to clothing. Retreatment is only required every couple of weeks even if the clothes are washed. There is evidence that use of an insecticide on clothes will also reduce biting of unprotected individuals when close to the wearer. It is now possible also to purchase clothing that has been treated with pyrethroids and some companies will offer a retreatment service.

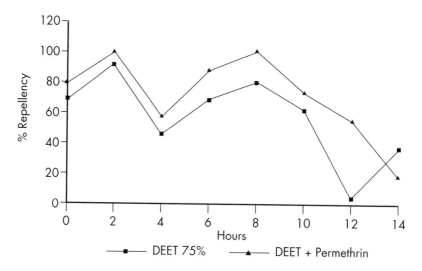

Figure 6.7   Comparison of diethyltoluamide (DEET) and DEET plus permethrin in clothing treatment.[44]

Treating socks and trousers with permethrin is particularly useful for protection against ticks which may be picked up from the undergrowth. This will have the advantage over treating either clothing or exposed skin with DEET, which is also effective against ticks, in that reapplication will not be necessary for some weeks.

Insecticides can be used to clear a room of insects before going to bed. There are three ways that this can be performed:

1. a simple knockdown aerosol spray
2. a small mat inserted into an electronic heating element in the wall socket that will slowly vaporise the insecticide. Alternatively a solution of insecticide in a vial slowly releases the insecticide on to the element
3. coils to burn and release vapour of the insecticide

Coils and mats should be used with care in people with asthma. Manufacturers recommend that coils are only used outdoors.

Some other methods of bite avoidance

There is some anecdotal, but little research-based evidence that thiamine tablets taken at a dose of 50 mg/day can offer protection against mosquito bites. The tablets need to be taken regularly and this method of bite avoidance should not be advised for those visiting malaria endemic areas.

Citronella candles give a pleasant odour and may offer a degree of protection in their immediate vicinity,[45] although burning ordinary candles may also be effective. One of the strangest methods reported for avoiding mosquito bites is using Limburger[46] cheese. When the cheese is placed in a room at night, mosquitoes appear to ignore humans in preference for the cheese. However, this is not really a practicable method of bite avoidance for most travellers. Finally, people should be wary of electronic products claiming to deter mosquitoes by emitting an ultrasonic noise. The evidence supporting these devices is weak or non-existent, and in a controlled trial they were shown to be ineffective.[47]

Main points

There are three major strategies to reducing the risks from biting insects:

1. practical bite avoidance measures, such as covering arms and legs
2. the use of pyrethroid-treated nets and clothing or as knockdown sprays/mats
3. the appropriate skin application of a DEET-based repellent

The conclusion of a review by the British army[48] was that employing all three measures could provide 100% protection against biting arthropods.

The most important points regarding these strategies are as follows.

Repellents applied to skin

- DEET is probably the first choice for malaria-endemic areas, but it is more important that the user finds the repellent acceptable and is willing to use it on a regular basis.
- The toxic effects of DEET have been somewhat overstated and there are rarely any problems if used as indicated in Box 6.1.
- In general, the greater the applied dose of repellent, the longer the action.
- To avoid bites from *Anopheles* mosquitoes potentially carrying malaria, apply repellent to exposed skin between dusk and dawn, but do not apply on retiring. Other species of mosquito, such as *Aedes*, may bite during the day.

Other bite avoidance measures

- Wear long sleeves and trousers of a fairly close-woven material.
- Treating clothing with an insecticide such as permethrin, combined with repellent applied to skin, provides the highest level of protection.
- Sleep under a mosquito net that has been treated with permethrin. Alternatively a well-screened room or one that was sealed and air-conditioned would be safe to sleep in provided any mosquitoes that had entered during the day had been removed. This can be achieved by using a knock-down spray or a plug-in device that releases insecticide.

Frequently asked questions

Is DEET safe?
This question has been raised on numerous occasions in the last decade and is discussed in the text. In summary, the following points could be made:

- It has been the most widely used of all repellents and in that context the number of reports of toxicity are reasonable.
- In normal adult use systemic toxicity is extremely rare, although, as with any topically applied product, allergic reactions do occur.

- Reports of encephalopathy in children would warrant it being used with care on the very young, but again the number of reports of such problems are small compared with the use of DEET.

I have used very-high-strength repellents but still get bitten. Can you advise me what to do?
Travellers should be aware of the factors determining the efficacy of repellents:

- The number of mosquitoes in the vicinity may be large.
- Although the repellent may be reducing the chance of being bitten, 100% efficacy is only maintained for a short period.
- Many factors will reduce the duration of action, as described in the text e.g. sweat, abrasion, temperature
- Individual factors make some people more attractive to insects than others.
- Some species of mosquitoes are less susceptible to repellents than others.

What is the best way to protect babies and children from insect bites?
For very young babies who are not mobile it is best to avoid repellents applied to the skin and to use other methods. This will involve ensuring that at night the cot is protected by an insecticide-treated mosquito net whilst the baby is sleeping. Rooms in the house should be kept free of mosquitoes and the baby clothed as much as is practical when out of doors, minimising outdoor exposure at night.
If the child is mobile then repellents will need to be used. As described in the text, a longer-acting DEET preparation of 20–30% could be used for malaria-endemic areas. It is probably best to avoid application to the hands.

Do I still need a mosquito net if I apply my repellent before going to bed?
Ideally, repellent should be washed off before retiring and should not be used as a means of protection when asleep. Occlusion under bed clothes may lead to a greater chance of skin reactions and the repellent will not last long enough to protect you throughout the night.

What is the best insect repellent on the market?
The best repellent will be the one that the individual is happy to apply on a regular basis. In terms of spectrum of activity and length of action, the evidence base would support DEET as the first-line recommendation for malaria-endemic areas.

What sort of mosquito net should I buy (Fig. 6.8)?
Most travellers will require a net that can be hung relatively quickly in a variety of circumstances. A single-point hanging net that includes a variety

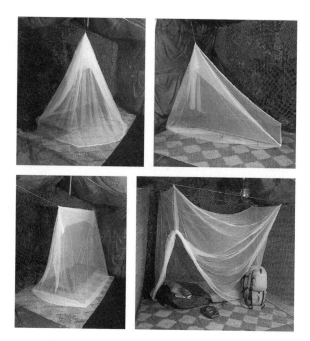

Figure 6.8 A range of mosquito nets suitable for backpackers. Courtesy of Nomad.

of cords and hooks for hanging should be sought. Also for hanging in difficult situations, sticky gaffer tape is useful. The single-point hanging nets are smaller than those requiring a frame system; the latter are also available as double nets and are more suitable when staying in a fixed location.

What formulation of repellent is best?
This has not been well studied, apart from long-acting formulations. It is probable that a roll-on might give the highest and most even level of repellent on the skin. A cream formulation is often the most cosmetically acceptable. Spray and liquid formulations are often the most economical. It is likely that impregnated tissues for single use to rub on the skin may not give very high dose rates.

Can I just apply the repellent to the edges of my clothing?
Again, this has not been well studied. If a large enough dose, say 100% DEET, is applied then this may protect the immediate area around the edges of clothing, but it is possible that mosquitoes are simply driven to unprotected areas.

References

1. Schoepke A, Steffen R, Gratz N. Effectiveness of personal protection measures against mosquito bites for malaria prophylaxis in travellers. *J Travel Med* 1998; 5: 188–192.

2. Fradin M S. Mosquitoes and mosquito repellents: a clinician's guide. *Ann Intern Med* 1998; 128: 931–940.

3. Shirai Y, Kamimura K, Seki T, Morohashi M. L-Lactic acid as a mosquito (Diptera: Culicidae) repellent on human and mouse skin. *J Med Entomol* 2001; 38: 51–54.

4. Golenda C F, Solberg V B, Burge R *et al.* Gender-related efficacy difference to an extended duration formulation of topical N,N-diethyl-*m*-toluamide (DEET). *Am J Trop Med Hyg* 1999; 60: 654–657.

5. Govere J, Braack L E, Durrheim D N *et al.* Repellent effects on *Anopheles arabiensis* biting humans in Kruger Park, South Africa. *Med Vet Entomol* 2001; 15: 287–292.

6. Rutledge L C, Wirtz R A, Buescher M D, Mehr Z A. Mathematical models of the effectiveness and persistence of mosquito repellents. *J Am Mosquito Control Assoc* 1985; 1: 56–61.

7. Buescher M D, Rutledge H C, Wirtz R A, Nelson J H. The dose–persistence of DEET against *Aedes aegypti*. *Mosquito News* 1983; 43: 364–366.

8. Rutledge L C. Some corrections to the record of insect repellents and attractants. *J Am Mosquito Assoc* 1988; 4: 414–423.

9. Thrower Y, Goodyer L I. *Skin Concentration of Insect Repellents Used by Travellers*. New York: International Society of Travel Medicine, 2003.

10. Khan A A, Maibach H I, Skidmore D L. A study of insect repellents II. Effect of temperature on protection time. *J Econ Entomol* 1972; 66: 437–438.

11. Robert L L, Hallam J A, Seeley D C *et al.* Comparative sensitivity of four *Anopheles* (Diptera: Culicidae) to five repellents. *J Med Entomol* 1991; 28: 417–420.

12. Durrheim D N, Leggat P A. Prophylaxis against malaria: preventing mosquito bites is also effective. *BMJ* 1999; 318: 1139.

13. Fai F Y, Lee L. Perceptions and use of insect repellent amongst soldiers in the Singapore armed forces. *Military Med* 1996; 16; 113–116.

14. Chou J T, Rossignol P A, Ayres J W. Evaluation of commercial insect repellents on human skin against *Aedes aegypti*. *J Med Entomol* 1997; 34: 624–630.

15. Anonymous. Buzz off: which repellents work best? *Consumer Rep* 2000; 65: 14–17.

16. Fradin M S, Day J F. Comparative efficacy of repellents against mosquito bites. *N Engl J Med* 2002; 347: 13–18.

17. Dogan E B, Ayres J W, Rossignol P A. Behavioural mode of action of DEET: inhibition of lactic acid attraction. *Med Vet Entomol* 1999; 13: 97–100.

18. Qui H, Jun H W, McCall J W. Pharmacokinetics, formulation and safety of insect repellent N,N-diethyl-3-methylbenzamide (DEET): a review. *J Am Mosquito Control Assoc* 1998; 14: 12–27.

19. Murphy M E, Montemarano A D, Debboun M, Gupta R. The effect of sunscreen on the efficacy of insect repellent: a clinical trial. *J Am Acad Dermatol* 2000; 43: 219–222.

20. Montemarano A, Gupta R K, Burge J R, Klien K. Insect repellents and the efficacy of sunscreens. *Lancet* 1997; 349: 1670–1671.

21. Goodyer L I, Behrens R H. The safety and toxicity of insect repellents [short report]. *Am J Trop Med Hyg* 1998; 59: 323–324.

22. Osimitz T G, Murphy J V. Neurological effects associated with the use of insect repellent N,N-diethyl-*m*-toluamide (DEET). *J Toxicol Clin Toxicol* 1997; 35: 442–445.

23. Reuveni H, Yagupsky P. Diethyltoluamide-containing insect repellents: adverse effects in worldwide use. *Arch Dermatol* 1982; 118: 582–583.

24. Veltri J C, Osimitz T G, Bradford D L, Page P C. Retrospective analysis of calls to poison control centres resulting from exposure to the insect repellent DEET from 1985–1989. *J Toxicol Clin Toxicol* 1994; 32: 1–16.

25. Tenenbien M. Review of toxic reactions and death following the ingestion of DEET containing insect repellents. *JAMA* 1987; 258: 1508–1511.

26. Petrucci N, Sardini S. Severe neurotoxic reaction associated with oral ingestion of low-dose diethyltoluamide-containing insect repellent in a child. *Pediatr Emerg Care* 2000; 16: 341–342.

27. Osimitz T G, Grothaus R H. The present safety assessment of DEET. *J Am Mosquito Control Assoc* 1995; 11: 274–278.

28. Selim S, Ralph E, Hartnagel T G *et al.* Absorption and metabolism of DEET following dermal application to human volunteers. *Fundam Appl Toxicol* 1995; 25 :95–100.

29. Schaefer C, Peters P W. Intrauterine diethyltoluamide exposure and foetal outcome. *Reprod Toxicol* 1992; 6: 175–176.

30. McGready R, Hamilton K A, Simpson J A *et al.* Safety of the insect repellent N,N-diethyl-*m*-toluamide (DEET) in pregnancy. *Am J Trop Med Hyg* 2001; 65: 285–289.

31. Baynes R E, Halling K B, Riviere J E. The influence of diethyl-*m*-toluamide (DEET) on the percutaneous absorption of permethrin and carbaryl. *Toxicol Appl Pharmacol* 1997; 144: 3332–3339.

32. Yap H H, Jahangir K, Chong R *et al.* Field efficacy of a new repellent SBR 3023 against *Aedes albopticus* and *Culex quinquefasciatus* in a tropical environment. *J Vector Ecol* 1998; 23: 62–68.

33. Yap H H, Jahangir K, Zairi J. Field efficacy of four insect repellents against vector mosquitoes in a tropical environment. *J Am Mosquito Assoc* 2000; 16: 241–244.

34. *Review of IR3535 and KBR3023.* Report of the Fourth WHOPES working group meeting. Geneva: WHO, 2003.

35. Trigg J K, Hill N. Laboratory evaluation of a eucalyptus-based repellent against four biting arthropods. *Phytother Res* 1996; 10: 313–316.

36. Schreck C E, Leonhardt B A. Efficacy assessment of Quwenling, a mosquito repellent from China. *J Am Mosquito Control Assoc* 1991; 7: 433–436.

37. Collins D A, Brady J N, Curtis C E. Assessment of the efficacy of Quwenling as a mosquito repellent. *Phytother Res* 1993; 7: 17–20.

38. Trigg J K. Evaluation of a eucalyptus-based repellent against *Anopheles* spp in Tanzania. *J Am Mosquito Control Assoc* 1996; 12: 243–246.

39. Marchia F. Insect repellent 3535. *SOEW J* 1996; 22: 478–485.

40. Prakash A, Bhattacharya D R, Mahapatra P K, Mahnta J. A preliminary field study on the repellency of NEEM oil against anophalose mosquito in Assam. *J Commun Dis* 1999; 32: 145–147.

41. Gossel T. Factors affecting insect repellent activity. *US Pharm* 1984; July: 24.

42. Alonso P L, Lindsay S W, Armstrong J R M *et al.* The effect of insecticide-treated bed nets on the mortality of Gambian children. *Lancet* 1991; 337: 1499–1502.

43. Lillie T H, Schreck C E, Rahe A J. Effectiveness of personal protection against mosquitoes in Alaska. *J Med Entomol* 1998; 25: 475–478.

44. Gupta R K, Sweeney A W, Rutledge L C *et al.* Effectiveness of controlled release personal use arthropod repellents and permethrin impregnated clothing in the field. *J Am Mosquito Control Assoc* 1987; 3: 556–558.

45. Lindsay R L, Surgeoner G A, Heal J D, Gallivan G J. Evaluation of the efficacy of 3 per cent citronella candles and 5 per cent citronella incense for protection against field populations of *Aedes* mosquitoes. *J Am Mosquito Control Assoc* 1996; 12: 293–294.

46. Knols B G. On human odour, malaria mosquitoes and Limburger cheese. *Lancet* 1996; 348: 1322.

47. Kremsner P G. A blinded, controlled trial of an ultrasound device as mosquito repellent. *Wien Klin Wochensch* 2000; 112: 448–450.

48. Croft A M, Baker D, von Bertele M J. An evidence-based vector control strategy for military deployments: the British Army experience. *Med Trop* 2001; 61: 91–98.

7

Travel vaccinations

For the majority of travellers, vaccinations are seen as the most important preparation for a healthy trip abroad. In truth, the risk of contracting many immunisable diseases is quite small. An overemphasis is sometimes placed on vaccinations to the detriment of other diseases which may present a greater risk. Despite this observation, it would not be appropriate to discourage people from obtaining vaccinations, if they are indicated for their destination. Vaccination has another important function – it brings the traveller into contact with the health system, providing an opportunity to educate travellers on wider travel health issues.

This chapter examines the general principles associated with travel vaccinations and gives a more detailed consideration of the vaccines in current clinical use. Childhood vaccinations are not discussed, although it is important to note that, where possible, they should be completed before travel to certain destinations. Those not currently available in the UK, including oral cholera vaccine and a vaccine against Lyme disease, are not discussed.

Role of the health professional and place in the National Health Service

In recent years, UK general practitioners (GPs) have tended to acquire practice stocks of vaccines (rather than obtaining them by prescription) and much of the role of running vaccination clinics has been assigned to a practice nurse. With the advent of patient group directions in the UK,[1] it is now possible for nurses formally to administer travel vaccines without the presence of a doctor. There is a defined format for such proctocols that must be adhered to and they need to be signed off by both a pharmacist and doctor; the main areas that need to be covered are listed in Table 7.1 and these points must be individualised for the specific clinic.

Pharmacists play an important role in giving advice on travel vaccinations. Travellers often make initial enquiries about vaccinations to

Table 7.1 Some points relating to the guidelines concerning UK patient group directions and how they might apply to a nurse-run travel vaccination clinic. This is not an exhaustive guide and serves only as an illustration of principles

Requirements of group direction	Implications for travel vaccination clinic
Name of body, date enforced and expired	Importance of regular review of patient group directions. Attention should be paid to changes in manufacturers of vaccinations and regimen guidelines
Descriptions of medicines and clinical conditions covered	State the vaccine that can be administered under the group direction and its specific indication. The source of information for basing vaccine recommendations to specific areas of travel should be stated, e.g. websites, wall charts and other sources. Make sure that a clear statement is issued regarding risk groups to be administered a particular vaccine, e.g. all those on Haj to be given meningitis ACWY
Arrangements for referral and circumstances for further advice from doctor	Identify all groups that must be seen by doctor, e.g. live vaccines in pregnancy
Dosage, quantity, form, strength, route, period of administration	Write a short monograph covering all these points for every vaccine to be administered. Other important information should also be given regarding use of vaccine, e.g. issue of yellow fever certificates. Pay particular attention to describing regimen.
Relevant warnings/potential adverse drug reactions (ADRs)	All potential ADRs should be listed and any warnings specified. In particular, advise what to tell patient in terms of mild/moderate ADRs that could be anticipated and supply data sheet. Refer to anaphylaxis policy and also syncope (fainting). State time to be spent in clinic after vaccination session, e.g. after Japanese encephalitis vaccine
Details of follow-up	Records of any calls/visits back to clinic by patient after session
Records to be kept for audit purposes	Full records to be kept of vaccination session, including: where travelling, previous vaccination history, details of vaccines administered and any specific questions asked by practitioner. Also keep a record of current medication and medical history

a pharmacist before visiting their GP. Therefore, pharmacists should be in a position to outline travel requirements using the databases described in Chapter 1. An increasingly important role for pharmacists is in practice support, for example, by devising practice protocols or by arranging efficient supply and correct storage of vaccines. Storage procedures apply to all vaccines and the importance of maintaining a cold chain is discussed elsewhere.[2,3]

There is an ongoing debate in the UK about whether it is appropriate for the National Health Service (NHS) to provide travel vaccines. It can be argued that, by supplying such vaccines, the government is, in effect, subsidising an individual's holiday. The only real counterargument to this, in economic terms, is to consider the potential cost of treating disease contracted abroad or spread by travellers on return. If the risks of contracting the disease, and mortality from it, are low then it may be difficult to justify NHS supply. For example, hepatitis A carries a moderate risk in some parts of the world but has a generally low mortality. A pharmacoeconomic analysis of widespread vaccination against hepatitis A has suggested an argument against regular vaccination to some low-risk destinations.[4] The general consensus is that, globally, travel vaccination is not cost-effective but becomes more so when targeted to the highest-risk groups. Economic considerations aside, a possible argument for vaccinating even in a situation of low risk is that vaccinations generally have a good side-effect profile and serious adverse events are very rare, so 'overvaccination' may do no harm. A further consideration is the fear of liability by the health professional if a patient is counselled against vaccination, and subsequently contracts the disease. Finally, there may be ethical issues in charging patients for vaccines that could be perceived as unnecessary.

Vaccinations against diseases which are perceived to be a danger to the UK population are generally provided to travellers on the NHS. However, vaccination for a disease such as yellow fever, which is carried by a species of mosquito not native to the UK, must be obtained privately. In such cases, GPs may charge patients for the cost of the vaccine and enforce an additional administration charge. In some cases, the vaccine can be prescribed on the NHS but an administration charge may be made at the discretion of the practice. This has led to variations in charges between practices, and it may be advisable for travellers to compare charges at different GPs and private vaccination clinics. If travellers receive vaccinations from more than one clinic, it is important that vaccination record books are kept up-to-date.

The characteristics of travel vaccines, including their availability on the NHS, are shown in Table 7.2.

Immunology and types of vaccine used in travel medicine

The principle behind vaccination is that the immune system is stimulated by the introduction of material that it recognises as foreign, i.e. antigenic. If the antigens are the same as, or similar to, those present in the organism responsible for the disease, then cellular (T cell-mediated) and/or antibody (B cell-mediated) immune mechanisms will be directed against the organism. After a primary response to the vaccine, the immune system 'remembers' the antigen and subsequent contact will elicit a more intense immune stimulation. Therefore, the individual will be immune if the pathogenic organism is actually encountered.

Vaccines can be broadly divided into those that contain a live but harmless (attenuated) form of the virus, those which contain a whole killed organism and others comprising a component of the organism that will stimulate the immune system. Live vaccines tend to require only a single dose to elicit the necessary immune response against the disease, although those given orally, such as polio or typhoid, require multiple doses. Other types of vaccine tend to require a primary course of injections, but there are exceptions, such as typhoid and meningitis A and C. After a period of time, immunity declines and a single-dose booster of the vaccine is required. Of particular relevance to travel medicine is that, after the primary vaccination course, the antibody response can take 2–4 weeks to develop, whereas a booster will be effective after just a few days.

The process of immune stimulation is referred to as active immunisation. It is also possible to use passive immunisation, where antibodies (immunoglobulins) are injected to confer immediate protection. Immunoglobulins are usually used for postexposure treatment; the only occasional exception is for the prevention of hepatitis A.

In diseases such as diphtheria and typhoid, the pathological changes are caused by a toxin released by the organisms. Therefore, vaccines against the toxin rather than against the organism are used.

Various methods are employed to produce vaccines. Organisms may be cultured and then inactivated or killed. In other cases, modern techniques using recombinant DNA are used. An antibiotic is sometimes added to vaccines to act as a preservative and potential problems with antibiotic sensitivity should be recognised.

Table 7.2 Characteristics of travel vaccines

Name	Type of vaccine	Available on NHS for travel	Duration until effect
Bacillus Calmette-Guérin (BCG)	Live attenuated strain derived from Mycobacterium bovis	Yes	Full effect after 2 months
Hepatitis A	Formaldehyde-inactivated hepatitis A virus (grown in human diploid cells) adsorbed on to aluminium hydroxide carrier	Yes	Maximum effect 4 weeks after a single dose
Immunoglobulins for passive immunity against hepatitis A	Pooled human immunoglobulins	Yes	Immediate
Hepatitis B	Inactivated hepatitis B virus surface antigen prepared from yeast cells using recombinant DNA technology (also has aluminium carrier)	Yes	Effective after second dose
Japanese encephalitis	Freeze-dried formaldehyde-inactivated virus	No	Full effect after third dose, but should be completed 10 days before travel (see text)
Meningitis A and C Meningitis A, C, W135, Y	Capsular polysaccharide antigens of Neisseria meningitidis	No	10–14 days
Polio (oral)	Live attenuated trivalent	Yes	Effective after third dose (primary course) Immediate after booster

Table 7.2 continued

Name	Type of vaccine	Available on NHS for travel	Duration until effect
Rabies vaccine (Aventis Pasteur)	Freeze-dried inactivated Wistar rabies virus strain cultivated in human diploid cells	For those at occupational risk only	Full effect after third dose
Rabipur	Rabies virus strain cultivated in chick embryo cells		
Tetanus	Toxoid absorbed on to aluminium carrier	Yes	Effective after third dose (primary course)
Typhoid (oral)	Live attenuated *Salmonella typhi*	No	Effective after 7–10 days
Typhoid (parenteral)	Capsular polysaccharide vaccine containing Vi polysaccharide antigens	Yes	Effective after 10 days
Tick-borne encephalitis	Killed virus	No	Effective approximately 1 week after the second dose
Yellow fever	Live attenuated strain grown in developing chick embryos	No	10 days

Note: vaccines for children are only included where they do not form part of the usual childhood vaccination programme or when boosters are needed for travelling.

Regimen planning

It is desirable for travellers to plan vaccinations about 8 weeks before travel but, because this is not always possible, vaccines may need to be given quite close to departure. In such cases, travellers should be made aware that the vaccine has given them reduced immunity, so other measures, e.g. hygiene, should be emphasised. The precise regimens for each vaccine are listed in Table 7.3 and are discussed in some detail below.

In general, inactivated vaccines will not interfere with each other or with live vaccines, so they can be administered at one appointment. Live vaccines can be given together but at different sites, or on separate occasions 3 weeks apart. This is because of the theoretical possibility of

Table 7.3 Dosing schedules of travel vaccines

Name and type/brand	Schedule	Route	Length of protection
Bacillus Calmette-Guérin (BCG)	One dose following Mantoux diagnostic test (using tuberculin purified protein derivative, PPD)	Intradermal	Not known
Diphtheria and tetanus (DT/vac/ads (adult))	Primary – three doses at 1-month intervals	Intramuscular or deep subcutaneous	10 years
Diptheria (Dip/vac/ads (adult))	Booster – one dose		
Tetanus (Tet/vac/ads)			
Hepatitis A Avaxim H.avrix monodose and Havrix Junior for child 1–15 years	Single dose followed by booster after 6–12 months	Intramuscular (deltoid)	6–12 months following first dose, 10 years following booster
Vaqta adult Vaqta paed 2–17 years	Single dose followed by booster 6–18 months (Vaqta paed 6–12 months)	Intramuscular (deltoid)	As above
Normal Immunoglobulins (not recommended in UK)	For normal immunoglobulins, single dose as close as possible to day of departure	Deep intramuscular	Up to 5 months, depending on dose
Hepatitis B Engerix B, Engerix B paediatric HB-Vax II, HB-Vax II paediatric	Three doses at 0, 1 and 6 months Rapid immunisation: four doses at 0, 1, 2 and booster at 12 months Accelerated course – Engerix only (for adults over 18 years only): four doses at 0, 7 and 21 days and at booster 12 months	Intramuscular (deltoid for adults, thigh for children)	Five years. Booster if still at risk of infection

Table 7.3 continued

Name and type/brand	Schedule	Route	Length of protection
Hepatitis A and hepatitis B Twinrix, Twinrix paediatric	Three doses at 0, 1 and 6 months	Intramuscular (deltoid for adults, thigh for children)	Five years for hepatitis B, 10 years for hepatitis A
Hepatitis A and typhoid Hepatyrix VIATEM	Single dose	Intramuscular (deltoid)	Three years for typhoid. 6–12 months for hepatitis A then, following booster, 10 years
Japanese encephalitis	Primary course: doses at 0, 7 and 30 days Quick schedule: doses at 0, 7 and 14 days		Three years
Meningitis Mengivac (A + C) AC Vax ACWY Vax	One dose	Deep subcutaneous or intramuscular	Three years for Mengivac Five years for AC Vax
Polio (oral)	Primary course: doses at 0, 1 and 3 months One-dose booster in immunised adults	Oral	10 years
Rabies Rabies vaccine	Three doses at 0, 7 and 28 days	Deep subcutaneous or intramuscular (deltoid)	Booster at 2–3 years
Rabipur	Three doses at 0, 7 and 21 or 28 days Travellers at low risk: two doses at 0 and 28 days (but need earlier booster at 6–12 months)		Booster at 2–5 years
Typhoid Typherix Typhim Vi Vivotif	One dose. For Vivotif, one capsule on days 1, 3 and 5	Intramuscular Deep subcutaneous or intramuscular Oral (Vivotif)	Three years. For Vitotif, up to 3 years (occasionally, 1 year)

Table 7.3 continued

Name and type/brand	Schedule	Route	Length of protection
Tick-borne encephalitis	Primary course: two doses at 2 weeks to 3 months apart, then booster at 6–12 months	Intramuscular	Three years then single booster
Yellow fever	One dose	Subcutaneous	10 years

Note: vaccines for children only included where they do not form part of the usual childhood vaccination programme or when boosters are needed for travelling.

impaired immune response to both vaccines; however it does not apply to the childhood vaccines measles, mumps and rubella (MMR) and oral polio. There are some theoretical concerns about giving immunoglobulins against hepatitis A with live vaccines, because the immunoglobulins could potentially kill live viruses. However, normal immunoglobulin would not contain antibodies against yellow fever and can also be used at the same time as oral polio vaccine.

A further good reason to plan well in advance of travel is that shortages of vaccines can occur from time to time. Although not used as much in recent times, this was a frequent problem associated with immunoglobulins which must be derived from pooled blood from donors. There have also been supply problems in the UK associated with yellow fever vaccine due to batch failure and transfer of product licences between manufacturers.

The basis for deciding upon a vaccination regimen is the known risk for contracting the disease for travellers. This will be based upon known endemicity, also modified by other factors associated with the itinerary, including:

- length of stay in a particular area increasing possible contact with the infective agent
- contact with the local population when the condition is transmitted person-to-person, e.g. meningitis, tuberculosis and diphtheria
- season and travel to rural areas will influence the risk of contracting some insect-borne diseases, e.g. Japanese encephalitis

Other than yellow fever vaccination, there is no other internationally recognised requirement for a certificate of vaccination. Pilgrims to Saudia Arabia are required to carry evidence of vaccination against

Table 7.4 Local conditions that may necessitate travel vaccination

Condition	Examples of vaccination
Countries where food/water hygiene and sanitation are of a poor standard	Typhoid, hepatitis A
Known presence of insect-borne diseases	Yellow fever, Japanese encephalitis, tick-borne encephalitis
High endemicity/epidemic in local population	Meningitis, tuberculosis
Poor childhood vaccination programme	Polio, diphtheria
Poor medical supplies and facilities	Rabies, hepatitis B

meningitis after outbreaks of the disease during the Haj in recent years. Cholera vaccination certificates have not been required since the late 1980s as the vaccine provided very low levels of protection. However, there are reports of travellers being asked to produce such certificates by customs officials to certain countries, sometimes in lieu of a bribe. The recommendations by country will not be discussed specifically in this book; international guidelines as to the vaccinations which should be considered to certain destinations are described in the World Health Organization (WHO) *International Travel and Health* book.[5] Most developed countries produce own their national guidelines, e.g. the Centers for Disease Control in the USA and the Department of Health in the UK, tailored to local need and vaccine availability. The databases described in Chapter 1 also provide a convenient source of information; the web-based ones are regularly updated. This plethora of sources can lead to some confusion, but advice from official bodies is usually consistent. A few generalisations regarding destination requirements can be made, as summarised in Table 7.4.

Adverse reactions

Reactions are frequently mild, consisting of low-grade fever, muscle pains and fatigue. These symptoms will usually resolve within a day or so and are effectively relieved by paracetamol which could be taken just after receiving vaccinations. Local reactions of pain and swelling around the site of injection are also quite common and can take more than 48 hours to resolve. In most cases, reassurance can be provided to those suffering minor adverse effects of vaccination. A more severe reaction may be observed rarely, and any skin reactions distant from the site of injection should be considered a true allergic-type reaction. More serious systemic allergic responses, e.g. angioedema or anaphylaxis, usually occur very soon after vaccination and need urgent medical attention. Allergy may be anticipated in some cases, for example, yellow fever vaccine is grown in chick embryos and may produce a reaction in people allergic to egg products. Similarly, those who are allergic to antibiotics may be at risk from the traces present in some vaccines. Certain individuals react to thiomersal, which is used as a preservative in a few vaccines.

A problem associated with multiple vaccinations given at the same time is that it may be difficult to identify the cause of an adverse reaction.

There are a few drug interactions or contraindications associated with vaccination. Chloroquine reduces the response to rabies vaccine if this is administered via the intradermal route,[6] probably because of an immune impairment caused by chloroquine. This may also apply to mefloquine, but there is little evidence that such an interaction occurs.[7] Mefloquine and other antibiotics should not be administered at the same time as oral typhoid. Intramuscular injections should be avoided by patients on anticoagulant therapy.

Groups for special consideration

Particular consideration needs to be given to children and this is discussed later in this chapter under each vaccine, although routine childhood vaccinations will not be covered. As a general rule, live vaccines should be avoided in pregnancy and breastfeeding. However, if travel to high-risk areas cannot be avoided, yellow fever and oral polio may be given. Live vaccines should also be avoided in people who are immunosuppressed, for example, people with human immunodeficiency virus (HIV) or leukaemia and people receiving or within 6 months of completing immunosuppressive chemotherapy. They should also be avoided by those on longer term (> 10 days) daily corticosteroids or shorter course at higher doses (> 20 mg/day). The specific guideline in the UK is that live vaccines should not be given to adults who have received the equivalent of 40 mg of prednisolone a day rectally or orally for more than 7 days, and at least 3 months should have elapsed after completing such a course of treatment. People should not be vaccinated while they have moderate or severe fevers because of the possibility of a reduced immune response, and because it may be difficult to distinguish vaccine side-effects from symptoms of fever.

Those who are normally offered vaccination against influenza, e.g. those over 65 years and/or likely to suffer complications from influenza infection, may need to be vaccinated before travel as outbreaks will occur at different times of year than in the western hemisphere, e.g. April–October in the southern hemisphere and throughout the year in some tropical areas.

Individual travel vaccines

Use and administration of vaccines are summarised in Tables 7.2 and 7.3. This section looks at individual vaccines and concentrates on the types of travellers who should be vaccinated, areas of risk for the diseases, effectiveness of the vaccines and special considerations.

Hepatitis A

Among the diseases preventable by vaccination, hepatitis A is one of the most common. For instance, it is 100 times more likely to be contracted by travellers than typhoid. It is possible to test for antibody status in order to avoid vaccination, but this is rarely performed and the vaccine can be given safely to those who have previously contracted the disease.

Until a few years ago, immunoglobulins were widely used for prophylaxis against hepatitis A. Apart from being a blood-derived product which is often in short supply, the resulting passive immunisation affords, at best, 90% protection against hepatitis A.[8] The more immunoglobulin that is administered, the longer the protection but, as only 5 ml can conveniently be given prior to travel, no more than 6 months' protection can be expected. Even for short trips by occasional travellers, hepatitis A vaccine is usually the preferred, but somewhat more expensive, choice. This is an inactivated whole-cell vaccine which may also be given together with hepatitis B, where a synergistic action has been claimed.[9]

A potential drawback of vaccination is that seroconversion may not be reached until 4 weeks after the injection, with around only half of individuals seroconverting at 14 days. The concurrent administration of immunoglobulins in those at high risk and in those vaccinated less than 2 weeks before departure has therefore been advocated. There is evidence that adequate protection is afforded even if given just before departure,[10] as hepatitis A can take a few weeks to develop, by which time the vaccine would have produced adequate levels of antibodies. Normal immunoglobulin is not now recommended for routine prophylaxis in travellers except in those who are immunosuppressed.

It has also been debated whether the vaccine is needed in young children, who are likely to have a subclinical or very mild infection. The counterargument to this is that a few children can suffer a more serious course of infection and that they may transmit the disease to older children and adults.[11] Once contracted, lifelong immunity is developed and immunisation is not necessary. Apart from those known to have contracted hepatitis A, those who have been raised in developing countries or are over 40 years of age may also have immunity. It is possible to measure antibody titres in order to establish such immunity, but this is rarely done as there is no harm in administering the vaccine to those with immunity due to previous exposure. Improved hygiene in developed countries has resulted in a reduced incidence of hepatitis A, hence there is an increased risk to travellers.

Hepatitis A vaccine is indicated for travellers visiting many developing countries including Africa, the Middle East, South America and Asia. After a single injection antibody titres are sufficient to provide protection for up to 1 year. A second booster will provide 10 years' protection and there is some evidence that this may last up to 30 years, but at present further boosters are recommended. At one time it was felt that no more than a few years be allowed to elapse before the second vaccination was given. This has now been revised in the light of further evidence and it would appear that there is no upper time limit to obtain a good response after the primary injection. Hepatitis A vaccine is very well tolerated; any local reaction is more likely to be due to the aluminium included in most formulations.

Hepatitis B

This is now a recombinant yeast-derived vaccine and no longer obtained from human blood products, which in previous years discouraged some people from seeking immunisation. Immunisation is usually mandatory for many health care workers who have contact with patients.

It is not common practice in the UK to vaccinate low-risk travellers against hepatitis B, but in some developed countries it forms part of the routine vaccination programme. Hepatitis B is a disease transmitted through blood products, poorly sterilised surgical equipment and sexual contact. The risk of contracting hepatitis B is at its highest in sub-Saharan Africa and in parts of South-East Asia and South America (Fig. 7.1). In the UK, 12% of all cases of hepatitis B have been attributed to travel.[9] Vaccination should be recommended to long-term travellers, people who routinely visit endemic areas, high-risk groups such as those

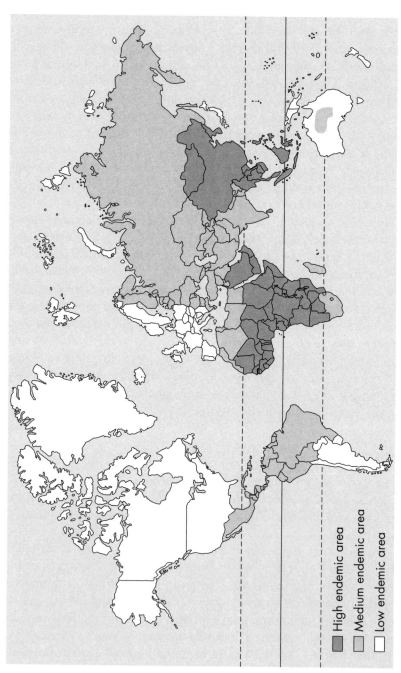

High endemic area

Medium endemic area

Low endemic area

Figure 7.1 Distribution of hepatitis B. Courtesy of Eric Caumes.

likely to engage in unprotected sexual activities, health workers and anyone who might need medical or dental procedures. Worries have been expressed concerning an increased incidence of demyelinating disease associated with hepatitis B vaccine, particularly in France, leading to a suspension of use of the vaccine in their childhood immunisation programme. The WHO and other authorities have found no evidence of such a problem following surveillance of the available data.

Hepatitis C is similar to hepatitis B. It can be caught in the same way and is as big a problem worldwide, but there is no vaccine available. Hepatitis B vaccination will also offer protection against hepatitis D.

From the schedules described in Table 7.3, it can be seen that advance planning of vaccinations 6 months before travel is normally required. This can be reduced to 1 or 2 months for travellers using the rapid schedules and some protection may be afforded after the second injection. It is usual to test for antibodies to hepatitis B in people who work in high-risk occupations because antibody titres can vary and some individuals may require extra or double doses of vaccine. A few individuals fail to respond to even repeated vaccination and the intradermal route (unlicensed) has been claimed to be effective in such circumstances. In general, though, studies have shown lower antibody titres if hepatitis B is administered intradermally compared to intramuscular injection.[12] Apart from those who are immunosuppressed, the elderly, obese, smokers and those receiving renal dialysis may tend to be poor responders.

Revaccination can be performed routinely about every 5 years for those at continued risk. It has been argued that, if antibody titres are low, an infection will effectively act as a booster, giving adequate protection in view of the long incubation period for hepatitis B.[13] The combined hepatitis A + B vaccines may be more convenient for some people and there is good evidence that the accelerated schedule used for hepatitis B vaccine can also be used for the combined vaccine.[12]

Oral polio vaccine (OPV)

In countries with a successful vaccination programme, polio has been virtually eliminated. When health systems break down or when a country is too poor to maintain childhood vaccination programmes, polio becomes a problem. This was witnessed in the early 1980s, when political problems in the old eastern bloc countries resulted in a resurgence of the disease. Primary immunisation will give protection for 10 years and adult travellers to many developing countries would be advised to obtain a booster. OPV consists of live attenuated virus of types I–III, with a high seroconversion rate being achieved for types I–II and 87% for type III. The risk of polio in unimmunised travellers is very low, at 20 per million.[14]

One potential danger associated with OPV is that live vaccine is excreted in the faeces and there have been a few reports of individuals contracting vaccine-associated paralytic poliomyelitis from those who have received OPV. At most risk are the immunosuppressed or elderly and those who have not been previously vaccinated, and these groups should not themselves be vaccinated using OPV: injectable inactivated polio vaccine (IPV) is the method of choice. There are also reports concerning an increased incidence of a wild virus that has been introduced due to widespread use of OPV. This wild virus would not affect immunised individuals, but in developing countries where the immunisation programme is poor this could be a problem. A number of countries, including the USA, now use IPV as the method of choice.

For adults requiring primary immunisation, IPV should always be used because of a risk of vaccine-induced paralysis from OPV. Polio vaccines contain trace amounts of aminoglycoside (e.g. streptomycin) or polypeptide (e.g. polymyxin) antibiotics, and it is prudent to inquire regarding a history of previous sensitivity.

Typhoid

Typhoid fever is caused by *Salmonella typhi* and is contracted from consuming contaminated food or water. The disease causes an initial gastrointestinal upset of diarrhoea or constipation but systemic infection may result, spreading to other organs with serious sequelae. The disease can be treated with antibiotics such as quinolones. Vaccination is recommended for travellers to areas where hygiene may be poor.

Despite being among the most widely administered vaccines, the risk of travellers contracting typhoid is low. In many countries the risk can be as low as one in 30 000, but in India, sub-Saharan Africa and in some parts of South America it can rise to one in 10 000. Despite this level of risk, the majority of cases of typhoid reported in developing countries occur in patients who have contracted the disease overseas; in 1999 150 cases of typhoid were reported in the UK, with nearly 90% being contracted whilst overseas. An additional consideration is that vaccination probably only gives, at best, 70–80% protection against the disease and some studies have indicated that it may be even lower.[15] Furthermore, most trials have been performed on local populations in countries such as Nepal and the benefit for travellers from industrialised countries has not been fully defined. From a study in Nepal[16] it does appear that the risk of contracting typhoid in travellers is reduced by the widespread use of the vaccine, as those groups from countries where immunisation was not normally given appeared to experience a higher rate of infection than those where immunisation was common, such as the USA. It is difficult to quantify the level of protection of the vaccines as attack rates are so low that many individuals are needed for such studies.

The old whole-cell vaccine is no longer used in the UK because the modern polysaccharide vaccine is associated with fewer adverse effects. It is also convenient, requiring just a single dose in advance of travel and is effective after 10 days. However, a meta-analysis indicated that the whole-cell vaccine does offer a superior degree of protection: 73% efficacy for the whole cell, 51% for the polysaccharide and 55% for the oral vaccine.[17]

The oral vaccine contains a short-lived mutant strain of *S. typhi* but is used less because it has a complex dosing schedule, resulting in problems with compliance. It must be taken exactly as described in the schedule outlined in Table 7.3, an hour before a meal, and the efficacy is reduced if taken with antibiotics and some antimalarials. Again, there are limited data concerning the efficacy in travellers.

Due to the somewhat lower level of protection afforded compared to some other vaccines, a large intake of organisms from contaminated foods may well still result in an infection and travellers should be cautioned on the food hygiene measures described in Chapter 3.

Diphtheria and tetanus

In both diseases, a toxin produced by the organisms is responsible for pathological damage. Vaccination is given during childhood using adsorbed toxoid but immunity begins to wane after 10 years. In the UK, it is advisable to have booster injections against tetanus every 10 years until a maximum of five doses in total (i.e. primary plus two boosters) have been given. Extra doses will only be required in the event of an injury where tetanus is a possible danger. An adverse reaction of flu-like symptoms to tetanus is more likely if antibody levels are already high. For travellers to countries where medical facilities are poor it may be worth considering giving booster doses every 10 years, even if more than five total doses have been received.

Diphtheria has been virtually eliminated in many countries because of childhood vaccination schedules, so boosters are not routinely performed. In poorer countries, a similar situation to that described for polio can exist, where the childhood vaccination programme has broken down and diphtheria is a potential danger. For tourists on short stays to such destinations, vaccination against diphtheria is not usually necessary. On longer stays, particularly if there will be contact with the local population, boosters for adults over 20 years of age would be recommended. It is important that adults and children over 6 years of age receive an adult formulation of diphtheria vaccine which contains a lower dose than that used for younger children.

Yellow fever

Yellow fever is a dangerous arboviral disease which is endemic in parts of Africa and South America. Yellow fever remains one of the few diseases for which a vaccination certificate is required for entry into some countries, although certificates may only be needed if entering from a yellow fever-endemic area. The vaccine is live freeze-dried, cultured on chick embryos and can only be supplied by registered yellow fever centres. This is partly historical because the vaccine can be sensitive to poor storage conditions and refrigeration equipment must be of a high standard and stored at 2–8°C. It is relatively easy for GPs to become yellow fever centres and increasing numbers are now registered. Once reconstituted, the vaccine must be used within a few hours.

A yellow fever vaccination certificate is not valid until 10 days after vaccination, so good planning is essential. Even if a certificate is not required for entry, the vaccine should be given if the disease is a risk. A single dose may provide lifelong immunity, although a booster is required every 10 years in order to renew the vaccination certificate.

It should not be given to children under the age of 6 months because of a potential risk of encephalitis. Travel should be delayed, if possible, until infants are over 12 months of age, although most countries will allow exemption of a certificate for children younger than 12 months. Although yellow fever vaccine is theoretically contraindicated in pregnancy, no fetal malformations have been reported and the benefits may outweigh the risks.

Minor adverse reactions are experienced in up to 5% of individuals and serious reactions are rare. Care should particularly be taken that patients do not have a history of sensitivity to eggs in view of the method of culture. In recent years there have been some reported cases of encephalopathy after administration.

Tuberculosis

Tuberculosis is of greatest risk to travellers working or living with local populations in developing countries. Until the 1980s, most children in the UK were vaccinated with Bacillus Calmette-Guérin (BCG) at the age of 12. In more recent years, some health authorities have stopped carrying out this programme so that some younger adults have no immunity.

There are a number of problems associated with the routine use of BCG in travel vaccination. First, it is important that individuals are tested for immunity before the vaccine is given because of a danger of an exaggerated immune response. This is complicated by the fact that reactions to the Mantoux/PPD (tuberculin purified protein derivative) skin test may be lost in later life, despite immunisation. In addition, it takes 2 months following the BCG vaccine for immunity to develop. Another problem is that, while BCG gives an adequate response in young adults and children, whether immunity is conferred to older adults is a matter of debate. It has been claimed that BCG does not actually prevent infection, but helps to prevent complications and disease spread.[14]

It is sometimes useful to test whether a traveller has become infected with tuberculosis using a Tine or Heath test. Such skin tests are positive when the individual has either contracted tuberculosis or has been immunised, so a test would really have to be performed both prior to travel and on return if previously negative. In practice, vaccination clinics would mainly consider testing those at most risk, e.g. people living in high-risk areas, especially where multidrug resistance is common, and those who have not been previously vaccinated.[18] Skin testing should be done either before or 4–6 weeks after giving a live vaccine, as these can interfere with the test. As described in Chapter 6, testing could also be performed on return to identify those who may have contracted tuberculosis and then receive appropriate treatment. Some take the view that it is worth vaccinating adults at higher risk of tuberculosis if the test is negative and they have not previously received a vaccination in childhood.

Meningitis

Meningococcal infection can be contracted in both industrialised and developing countries. In the UK, recent localised outbreaks have been of particular concern among young adults attending colleges. The strains of *Neisseria meningitidis* which have been most frequently responsible for infection in Europe are of the serogroups B and C, whereas in other regions, such as Africa, serogroups A, C, Y and W135 are more common. In Africa, there is a 'meningitis belt' extending from Mauritania to Ethiopia where an increased incidence of meningitis A can be expected during the dry season (December to June). Epidemics can occur almost anywhere in the world, and are often associated with dry seasons. In India outbreaks of meningitis A will sometimes warrant vaccination. There is a greater risk of infection where many people are living in close proximity. For instance, during Haj pilgrimages to Mecca, serious outbreaks of meningitis have been reported in recent years. It is now an entry requirement to Saudi Arabia that those attending the Haj must possess a vaccination certificate against meningitis, issued not less than 10 days before arrival and expiring 3 years after vaccination. Therefore, those travellers most commonly requiring vaccination are visitors to certain parts of Africa, to areas where an epidemic has been reported; in particular, those planning to live in close proximity to local populations. It is also worth considering vaccinations in other parts of the world experiencing local epidemics, an example being Northern India around Delhi where quite serious outbreaks have occasionally been reported.

The only vaccine currently available in the UK until recently was effective against the A and C strains only and gives protection for 3–5 years, probably less than 3 years in younger children, and is effective about 2 weeks after vaccination. The C component is not effective in young children. This vaccine may not be adequate for protection in some situations, e.g. during the Haj in the late 1990s some pilgrims may have developed the W135 strain of meningitis.[19] It is therefore now advised that such pilgrims are given the new meningitis vaccine that provides protection against ACY and W strains. A new conjugate vaccine against the C strain is being employed in a childhood vaccination programme, but it gives no protection against other forms and the polysaccharide vaccine may need to be given in addition. If the conjugate form is given first, an interval of 1 month should be left before giving the polysaccharide form. This is because of a reduced response to the conjugate vaccine and an increased incidence of side-effects. If the polysaccharide form has already been given, then a 6-month interval should be left, although a 2-week gap is adequate for children under 5.

Rabies

Rabies has an almost 100% fatality rate so, despite the fact that only an extremely small number of travellers have ever contracted the disease, pre-exposure vaccination is an important consideration for those at risk. Rabies is transmitted by the bite of any mammal and is only completely absent in a few countries, e.g. the UK and Australia. In most industrialised countries where there is effective control of dogs and other mammals that might carry the disease, the risk of rabies is low and pre-exposure vaccination is unnecessary. In developing nations where control policies cannot be effectively enforced, the risk of being bitten by a mammal carrying rabies might be considerable. For instance, in recent years, there has been a particular problem of poor control of stray dogs in Nepal. Therefore, travellers visiting countries in Africa, Asia and South America for longer than a month may be advised to have pre-exposure vaccination.

Individuals must be aware that, if they are bitten by an animal that may be carrying rabies, medical advice and postexposure treatment must be sought immediately, even if they have had rabies pre-exposure vaccination. People often ask why they should bother with pre-exposure vaccination if such treatment is necessary. The main reason is that, in many parts of the world, postexposure treatment cannot be assured. In addition, pre-exposure vaccination may 'buy time' for those at a distance from medical help, and treatment is simpler in vaccinated individuals.

Treatment for rabies consists of immunoglobulins followed by a course of vaccinations of the same type used for pre-exposure. The immunoglobulins are sometimes unavailable and there have been worldwide supply problems. The human immunoglobulin in particular can be very difficult to locate; horse serum-derived immunoglobulin is more widely available in developing countries but carries a high incidence of adverse effects. The modern human diploid cell (HDCV) or other purified vaccines, such as the chick embryo vaccine, available in developed countries, are very different from the older type that required a series of painful abdominal injections. However, in some countries, only the older brain-derived tissue vaccines are still produced locally and are generally viewed as inferior.

Rabies vaccine is only available on the NHS for people with occupational risks, e.g. veterinary surgeons, and the course of three subcutaneous injections can cost almost £100. Vaccination clinics often offer cheaper vaccines given by the unlicensed intradermal route which requires 0.1 ml instead of the usual 0.5 ml. If given by the intradermal route, the course must be completed at least 1 month prior to travel. Note also the warnings given in Chapter 4 concerning the use of the intradermal route if certain antimalarials are also being taken, and that the concurrent use of even low doses of corticosteroids may result in failure to seroconvert. Although responses to the vaccine administered by this route are good, some have suggested that individuals should be tested for seroconversion prior to travel.[20]

For travellers at lower risk where postexposure treatment can be obtained, a two- (0, 28 days) rather than three-dose intramuscular schedule may be offered; a booster should be administered at 6–12 months. There is a further unlicensed regimen which involves multiple intradermal injections at different sites for when vaccination is required at short notice.

Reactions to rabies vaccine are relatively frequent; around 5% of recipients receiving boosters can develop a delayed type 3 (immune complex) systemic hypersensitivity which consists of an urticarial rash and malaise. Local and other milder systemic reactions such as headache and nausea are reported in 10–40% of individuals.

Japanese encephalitis

Japanese encephalitis is an arboviral infection which is rare in travellers, with an estimated incidence of just one per million;[14] this may rise to one in 500 per month if travelling to rural endemic areas. Travellers at greatest risk are those on trips lasting longer than 2–4 weeks, and those visiting certain rural areas in Asia during the monsoon season, particularly pig-breeding regions because pigs are important intermediary vectors for the disease.

Japanese encephalitis vaccine is currently unlicensed in the UK and a full course is expensive. There are currently two available types; the Biken vaccine from Aventis Pasteur and that imported from Japan through the company Denka Seiken. The main limitation of the vaccine is a high incidence of both local and systemic adverse drug reactions. Local reactions have been reported in as many as 30% of individuals vaccinated. Systemic reactions, including angioedema and urticarial rash, occur in one in 1000 people but may be delayed for up to 2 weeks following injection.[18] Therefore, it is advised that individuals are observed for 30 minutes after injection and that the course is completed 10 days prior to departure in order to identify these problems.

Studies in children in Asia have indicated that a reasonable response is obtained after two injections. However, studies in US travellers demonstrated that only 30% of individuals had adequate levels of antibody after the second dose, so a full three-dose schedule is now recommended. These studies were carried out on the Biken vaccine, but the Denka Seiken vaccine is licensed in Japan as a two-dose schedule. There do not appear to be any published studies supporting this reduced schedule in travellers, but it has been claimed that a two-dose schedule (given at 1–2 weeks apart with the second dose at least 10 days before travel) will give immunity to 80% of individuals, lasting between 3 and 12 months.

Tick-borne encephalitis

Tick-borne encephalitis is present in many parts of Europe, except for Portugal and the Benelux countries, and has the highest incidence in the Baltic regions. It is contracted through bites from ticks that thrive best in clearings in wooded areas. Vaccination is advisable for forestry workers and travellers planning to trek extensively in the countryside.

Frequently asked questions

The chart for yellow fever states that a 'certificate is required if travelling from an endemic area'. Is this needed if I am flying from the UK?
This statement on wall charts and databases does result in some confusion. If flying from the UK straight to the country, then no certificate is required. If visiting another country en route where yellow fever is present, even if that particular country does not require a certificate, then a certificate must be obtained. However it should be noted that if visiting any yellow fever-endemic area vaccination should be given, whether or not an international certificate is mandatory.

As typhoid vaccine is only partially effective, is it worth having it for destinations where this risk is very low, e.g. certain parts of Central America?
Some of the general points regarding necessity of vaccines are discussed in the text. For typhoid the considerations are:

- Mortality is low if appropriately diagnosed.
- The vaccine has a very low incidence of adverse drug reactions and only a single injection is required.

- Cost may be an issue, but it can be given on the NHS.
- The longer the trip, the more likely the chances of contracting the problem.

On balance it would probably be worth recommending to most tourists.

Is meningitis vaccination necessary for India?
Given that the incidence of meningitis is probably in the single figures per 100 000, it would not be an important consideration for shorter trips and where there would be little close contact with the local population. Local outbreaks, such as have occurred in and around Delhi might warrant vaccination.

In view of the very low risk of Japanese encephalitis for travellers, under what circumstances is it worth vaccinating with this unlicensed expensive vaccine, with a relatively higher incidence of adverse drug reactions?
The subject has recently been reviewed by Shlim and Solomon,[21] who were unable to provide a definitive answer to this question.

The overall risk to travellers visiting Asia of contracting Japanese encephalitis has been reported at just 1 000 000 to 1. On the other hand it is a serious disease if contracted and these two facts have to be balanced against the potential side-effects of the vaccine, so opinion amongst practitioners of its necessity is often divided. Even figures concerning incidence in particular parts of the world can provide very little guide. For instance, in Kathmandu a relatively high incidence is observed in the local population, but no cases have been reported in travellers. This compares to Bali, where three cases of Japanese encephalitis infection have been reported amongst tourists in 1989–1995 but none since that date. It is felt that, while certain catagories of travellers with high exposure in rural areas may warrant vaccination, for others bite avoidance measures are probably sufficient. Who is at risk will have to be identified on an individual basis.

A child under 1 year needs to travel as the family are relocating. There are some vaccinations indicated not licensed for children under 1 year: rabies, yellow fever and typhoid. How should the family be advised?
It is advisable to counsel against travel to a yellow fever area under 9 months of age. If travel is unavoidable, then the risk of disease may outweigh the possibility of encephalopathy from the vaccine.

Response to typhoid vaccine is poor under 18 months of age. Oral vaccine should not be used.

Remember to complete as many as possible of the childhood vaccines.

How many vaccines can be administered in any one session?
There is no upper limit and theoretically five or six types could be administered, but this can be reduced by the use of some of the combined vaccines.

Are vaccinations safe if a woman is breastfeeding?
There seem to be no theoretical reasons to contraindicate the travel vaccines or reports of any adverse effects on children being breastfed.

A tourist from overseas has brought in his vaccination booklet, but I do not recognise the names of his vaccines. Where can I find information?
The following websites will be useful for identifying vaccines given in other countries: www.health.state.mn.us/divs/dpc/adps/forgnvac1.pdf and for translations www.health.state.mn.us/divs/dpc/adps/forgnvac2.pdf

A child of 5 months of age is due to travel to a developing country in 8 weeks' time for residence of a year. What vaccination should he receive?
All childhood vaccines administered by accelerated schedule: IPV, diphtheria, pertussis, tetanus (DPT), *Haemophilus influenzae* type B (HIB). Also hepatitis B for the first two doses at least. Give MMR just before departure. Also give rabies just before departure. Pneumococcal vaccine could also be considered.

There are reports that border officials in a particular country are demanding cholera vaccination certificates. You are asked to issue one for a traveller to this area: what should you do?
Neither the vaccine not the certificate is available any longer, for the reasons discussed in the text. Likewise, the country in question cannot officially demand such vaccination. To avoid problems at entry, one approach is to stamp and sign an official-looking vaccination record book or yellow card, stating that either cholera vaccine is unavailable or that it has been 'contraindicated' for the traveller. A letter could also be issued on clinic paper to the same effect. Most practitioners would be wary of issuing documents stating falsely that vaccinations had been given.

A woman who is 3 months' pregnant must travel to a yellow fever-endemic area. How should you advise her?
Waiting until the end of the second trimester may theoretically be advisable. Otherwise the risk/benefit ratio should be considered. Although there are documented cases of possible complications in pregnancy caused by the vaccine, the small-scale studies that have been undertaken are reassuring. However, one study noted low antibody titres in pregnancy. Estimating risk is not easy as official figures from some parts of the world may be liable to underreporting. Due to the dangers of contracting yellow fever, in many situations the danger would outweigh risk. It may also be advisable to ask patients to sign a statement to the effect that the risk of vaccination and the disease has been explained and that the outcome is their own decision. This has been summarised by I Dale Carroll MD, USA (personal communication).[22–25]

How important is rabies vaccination if you are careful about contact with animals? Is the intradermal route effective?

As described in Chapter 5, the risks can be higher in countries with a stray-dog problem; also postexposure treatment can be difficult. The intradermal route is not licensed but provided it is given by those experienced in the technique, it gives a good response.[19] Note that most studies for this route have been performed on the HDCV. A further consideration is that when seeking postexposure treatment, some clinics may not recognise the intradermal route as having given sufficiently reliable protection and still administer the full postexposure protocol, which will include immunoglobulins if available.

A traveller has missed an appointment for a second dose of hepatitis B vaccine. Does the course need to be started again? Would the same rules apply to second doses of rabies vaccine?

There is some evidence that second and third doses of hepatitis B do not need to be given on exactly the dates specified.[26]

However, in the case of rabies it is recommended that interrupted courses follow the schedule below (Aventis Pasteur MSD):

- If interrupted after day 0 by more than 3 months, restart course.
- If interrupted after day 7 by more than 6 months, restart course.
- If interrupted more than 5 years after three-dose primary course, restart course.

For a two-dose course, restart if more than 2 years have elapsed between the primary (0.28) and the 6–12-month booster.

Is a booster of hepatitis B necessary for travellers 5 years after travel?

Current UK guidelines suggest a single booster at 5 years for those who continue to be at risk of infection – which could be taken to apply to certain travellers. In the USA it is felt that routine reimmunisation is not necessary for those who have responded to the primary course in view of the very long immunological memory for the vaccine.

Further reading

1. Department of Health. *Health Information for Overseas Travel 2000*. London: Stationery Office, 2000.
2. Salisbury D, Begg N, eds. *Immunisation Against Infectious Diseases*. London: Stationery Office, 1996.
3. Kassianos G C. *Immunisation: Childhood and Travel Health*. Oxford: Blackwell Science, 1998.

References

1. Raffaitin J. Patient group directions and the law. *Pharm J* 2000; 265: 851.
2. Grassby P F. The safe storage of vaccines: problems and solutions. *Pharm J* 1993; 251: 323–327.
3. Thakke Y, Woods S. Storage of vaccines in the community: weak link in the cold chain. *BMJ* 1992; 304: 756–758.
4. Behrens R H, Collins M, Bott O B, Heponstall J. Risk for British travellers of acquiring hepatitis A. *BMJ* 1995; 311: 193.
5. *International Travel and Health*. Geneva: World Health Organization, 2003. Available online at: www.who.int/ith/index.html.
6. Pappaioanou M, Fisien D B, Dressen D W *et al*. Antibody response to pre-exposure human diploid cell rabies. *N Engl J Med* 1986; 314: 280–284.
7. Lau S C. Intradermal rabies vaccine and the concurrent use of mefloquine. *J Travel Med* 1999; 6: 140–141.
8. Anonymous. Prevention and control of hepatitis A. *Drug Ther Bull* 1994; 32: 9–16.
9. Loscher T, Keystome J S, Steffen R. Vaccination of travellers against hepatitis A and B. *J Travel Med* 1999; 6: 107–114.
10. Sagliocca L, Amoroso P, Stroffolini T *et al*. Efficacy of hepatitis A vaccine in prevention of secondary hepatitis A infection: a randomised trial. *Lancet* 1999; 353: 1136–1139.
11. Warson I. What type of traveller would benefit from combined vaccination against hepatitis A and hepatitis B? *J Travel Med* 1998; 5: 80–83.
12. Zuckerman J. Vaccine-preventable disease. In: Zuckerman J, ed. *Principles and Practice of Travel Medicine*. Chichester, UK: Wiley, 2001: 165–183.
13. Weidermann G, Kollaritsch H. Vaccine preventable diseases: the commercially available vaccines. In: DuPont H L, Steffen R, eds. *Textbook of Travel Medicine and Health*, 2nd edn. Hamilton, Canada: BC Decker, 2000: 219–229.
14. Klugman K P, Gilbertson I T, Koornhoff H J *et al*. Protective activity of Vi capsular polysaccharide vaccine against typhoid fever. *Lancet* 1987; 2: 1165–1169.
15. Schwartz E, Shlim D R, Eaton M *et al*. The effect of oral and parenteral typhoid vaccination on the rate of infection with *Salmonella typhi* and *Salmonella paratyphi* among foreigners in Nepal. *Arch Intern Med* 1990; 150: 349–351.
16. Engels E A, Falagas M E, Lau J, Bennish M L. Typhoid fever vaccines: a meta-analysis of studies on efficacy and toxicity. *BMJ* 1998; 316: 110–116.
17. Barnett E D, Chen R T, Rey M. Principles and practice of immunoprophylaxis. In: DuPont H L, Steffen R, eds. *Textbook of Travel Medicine and Health*, 2nd edn. Hamilton, Canada: BC Decker, 2000: 232–248.
18. Ryan E, Kain K. Primary care: health advice and immunisation for travellers. *N Engl J Med* 2000; 343: 1716–1725.
19. Anonymous. Meningococcal infection in pilgrims returning from the Haj. *Commun Dis Rep Weekly* 2000; 10: 125.
20. Lau C, Sisson J. The effectiveness of intradermal pre-exposure rabies vaccination in an Australian travel medicine clinic. *J Travel Med* 2002; 9: 285–288.
21. Shlim D R, Solomon T. Japanese encephalitis vaccine for travelers: exploring the limits of risk. *Clin Infect Dis* 2002; 35: 183–188.

22. Nasidi A. Yellow fever vaccination and pregnancy: a four-year prospective study. *Trans R Soc Trop Med Hyg* 1993; 87: 337–339.

23. Robert E. Exposure to yellow fever vaccine in early pregnancy. *Vaccine* 1999; 17: 283–285.

24. Nishioka S de A. Yellow fever vaccination during pregnancy and spontaneous abortion: a case-control study [see comments]. *Trop Med Int Health* 1998; 3: 29–33.

25. Tsai T F, Paul R, Lynberg M C *et al.* Congenital yellow fever virus infection after immunization in pregnancy. *J Infect Dis* 1993; 168: 1520–1523.

26. Mangione R, Stroffolini T, Tosti M E *et al.* Delayed third hepatitis B vaccine dose and immune response. *Lancet* 1995; 345: 1111–1112.

8

Environmental hazards

Until recently, the dangers of exposure to extremes in environmental conditions were mainly of concern to people undertaking scientific or military expeditions, those involved in special outdoor pursuits, such as mountaineering, and to expatriate workers. However, the 'adventure holiday' is becoming increasingly popular and a wider range of travellers may be exposed to extremes of temperature and high altitudes.

This chapter outlines the appropriate advice that health professionals can offer to travellers to reduce the physiological risks associated with exposure to such conditions. The drug management of altitude sickness will be examined as an area of particular interest to pharmacists. Travelling to cold environments and diving will also be briefly considered.

There are three broad themes that run through this review:

1. the prevention of potential problems by careful preparation and by observing some simple rules concerning acclimatisation
2. avoiding situations that could overwhelm normal temperature control homeostatic mechanisms (it is particularly important that those who might have impaired homeostatic mechanisms, such as the elderly, are aware of such problems)
3. management of conditions caused by environmental extremes

Acclimatisation to hot climates

Those travelling from temperate to hot climates may be unaware of the dangers associated with exposure before acclimatisation has occurred and of the long-term risks associated with undertaking a great deal of physical activity. It sometimes helps to consider the various types of hot climate to devise strategies to minimise the risk.[1]

In hot, wet climates such as the tropics, particularly rainforests, there is little variation in day- and night-time temperatures, combined with high humidity. In hot, dry climates, such as deserts, the temperature can fall dramatically at night, and humidity is low.

The body possesses the ability to survive in these types of climate; however, the necessary thermoregulatory mechanisms can take some time to develop if travelling from temperate regions. When environmental temperature exceeds body temperature, the most effective means of heat loss is evaporation of sweat from the surface of the skin. It is failure of the sweating mechanism that causes most problems for travellers. After arriving at a destination with a high ambient temperature, the sweat glands adapt and start to increase their output. On continued exposure to high temperatures, the kidney will begin to retain more sodium, and hence more water.

The key point is that time is required for these adaptations to take place. Acclimatisation is crucial in hot, wet climates where evaporation of sweat is more difficult and, unlike desert conditions, there is no period of rest for the sweat mechanism at night. Factors associated with heat-induced illness, which are particularly important in the first week of exposure, are summarised in Table 8.1. It should be noted that full acclimatisation can take up to 3 weeks to occur.

The result of poor acclimatisation may be heat stroke/exhaustion, discussed in the next section. There are other more minor heat-related problems that may be encountered by the traveller. Heat syncope (fainting) is not an uncommon occurrence in those exposed to a hot climate. It is largely a vasomotor response combined with a degree of dehydration, which will usually respond well to reclining and oral fluids. Muscle cramps are also quite common amongst those undertaking heavy physical exertion, and although often attributed to insufficient salt intake, this aetiology has been questioned.[2] A further common problem if not acclimatised is swelling around the feet and ankles (heat oedema), possibly related to vasodilation in the skin. Simple elevation will help relieve the problem.

Heat stroke and heat exhaustion

Heat stroke and heat exhaustion are sometimes confused and actually represent a broad continuum of problems. They describe a breakdown in the body's thermoregulatory mechanisms, either caused by these mechanisms becoming overloaded or by poor acclimatisation.

Heat stroke, which is sometimes incorrectly referred to as sunstroke, is a dangerous condition in which the sweat and other thermoregulatory mechanisms suddenly stop functioning. Body temperature rapidly rises in excess of 40°C and the subject will sweat very little and appear flushed. Sufferers may initially complain of headache and will later become confused. Delirium and convulsions will follow with death occurring in just a few hours if measures are not taken to cool the

Table 8.1   Factors associated with heat-induced illness and preventive measures

Factor	Preventive measure
Recent arrival	Graded physical activity in the first few weeks of arrival. Avoid long periods of continuous exertion
Lack of fitness and obesity	If strenuous activity is to be undertaken, build up fitness before travel
Inappropriate clothing	Advance planning of clothing and equipment
Certain drugs (diuretics, sympathomimetics) and alcohol	Avoid
Salt loss	Replace in food and/or beverages
Any skin condition that reduces sweating	Extra vigilance is recommended
Insufficient fluid intake	Consume a good supply of clean water, even if not thirsty

patient. The condition carries about a 25% mortality.[3] The younger fit person suffering from a more 'exertional' type of heat stroke may exhibit the signs of heat exhaustion (see below) before progressing rapidly to coma, with only half of such people exhibiting a reduction in sweat output.[2] A further danger to be aware of is that some of these symptoms could also represent cerebral malaria. The exact physiological cause of heat stroke has not been well defined, but will almost certainly be triggered by the factors listed in Table 8.1.

Heat exhaustion carries a lower mortality than heat stroke. However, some forms of heat exhaustion are associated with impairment of sweating and can progress to heat stroke if not treated. Heat exhaustion can be difficult to differentiate from heat stroke, but elevation in body temperature and central nervous system (CNS) disturbances tend to be less profound.

Heat exhaustion can simply be caused by water deficiency. Surprisingly large amounts of fluid (in excess of 10 L/day) may need to be consumed in some hot conditions. If fluid intake is restricted in such circumstances, dehydration can result and insufficient sweat will be produced to cool the body. Initially the patient will be thirsty with dry lips and mouth. Urine output is reduced and there will be mild CNS disturbances, such as giddiness and neuropathy. With a slight rise in body temperature (to no greater than 40°C), breathing becomes rapid and the patient appears cyanosed. Coma and death can follow if the patient is not rehydrated.

Salt deficiency is another cause of heat exhaustion, particularly in those undergoing strenuous activity where there is profuse sweating. The subject may have maintained fluid intake but not replaced the salt lost in sweat. Signs of salt deficiency include lethargy and muscle or 'heat' cramps. Another, rarer form of heat exhaustion is called anhidrotic heat exhaustion, which can appear many months after living in a hot climate. In a similar way to heat stroke, the sweat glands appear to malfunction, the problem being mainly in the trunk and upper arms.

Prevention and treatment of heat-induced illness

Prevention of the problems outlined above is summarised in Table 8.1. Acclimatisation is particularly important.[4] Efficient acclimatisation involves not only exposure to the hot environment but also maintaining a level of exercise. Such acclimatisation can take up to 10 days. On the other hand, whilst acclimatising to a warmer climate, the individual should take care not to undertake too high a level of prolonged physical exertion; about an hour a day is ideal. When acclimatised, the individual will respond much more efficiently to heat stress, with both an earlier onset of response and more profuse sweating. One important aspect of acclimatisation is that far less sodium tends to be excreted in the sweat; this retained sodium causes a rise in serum osmolarity. The result of this raised osmolarity is that thirst tends to be more readily stimulated and the individual will tend to drink at the appropriate time to prevent dehydration. Until such time as acclimatisation occurs there is an increased risk that simply drinking when thirsty is insufficient to prevent such dehydration. Acclimatisation could equally well be lost, for instance if returning largely to an air-conditioned environment.

Apart from diuretics, which cause salt and water loss, other medication can affect sweating and heat regulation. For instance, phenothiazines can suppress sweating, and tricyclics can increase heat production.[3] Similarly, medicines with anticholinergic properties, including some antihistamines, can adversely affect sweating mechanisms. Those on β-blockers should also take care when travelling to warmer climates. The reason for this is that peripheral vasodilation and increased heart rate, a process that can be inhibited by β-blockers, are important physiological responses to a hot environment, bringing more blood to the skin surface for cooling. Other stimulants that tend to

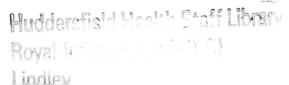

increase activity, e.g. cocaine, amfetamines and PCP, could also present problems related to heat-induced illness in a hot environment.

It is also important to stress that travellers to warmer climates should have an adequate intake of water and realise that simply drinking enough to quench thirst may not be sufficient (as above). Alcoholic beverages, in particular, should not be used as a source of fluid intake and many commercial drinks contain too much sugar, so should be diluted before drinking. An early danger-sign of insufficient fluid intake is reduced urine output that is dark in colour. Therefore, vigilance is required that greater than usual amounts of fluids are consumed: individuals should not just wait until they feel thirsty before drinking.

Other problems experienced when undertaking heavier physical exercise can be avoided by ensuring a sufficiently high salt intake. Pharmacists are sometimes asked to supply salt tablets, but these should generally not be provided for this purpose. Apart from causing gastrointestinal disturbances, the tablets themselves neither provide an adequate daily intake of salt nor often disperse sufficiently in the gastrointestinal tract. Instead, travellers should be advised to use extra salt on food. Alternatively, water can be pre-salted (about half a teaspoonful per litre[1]) and then can be used to make beverages.

Heat exhaustion must be treated with rehydration therapy. If the patient is not comatose, about half a litre of water should be given every 15 minutes until urine output returns to normal. Some authorities advise against using isotonic electrolyte solutions for treating heat exhaustion, because a high water intake is more important than salt intake.[4] In the case of salt-induced deficiency problems, the body's reserves must be made up relatively quickly. If given orally, about two teaspoonfuls of salt are needed per litre of water and about half a litre of this salted water should be given every hour for 6 hours.[1] Following heat exhaustion, it is advisable to keep in the cool for 3 days and only gradually return to strenuous activity. For anhidrotic heat exhaustion, such recuperation can last up to a month. In all cases, admission to hospital is recommended.

Any strategy to cool a patient with heat stroke should be used while urgent transfer to hospital is made. This will involve shelter from the sun, removing all clothing and covering with a wet sheet or similar material. Cold-water immersion is probably the most efficient way to cool the patient down but would be difficult to perform in the field. Easier to organise is cooling by evaporation, i.e. keeping wet material in contact with the skin. If available, ice packs can be placed around the groin and axillae. Fluid replacement is also essential, and will need to be given intravenously if the patient is unconscious.

Cold climates

It is not possible to acclimatise the body to cold environments. Those exposed to very cold climates should ensure that they maintain good general health, e.g. adequate nutrition and physical fitness. It is sometimes not appreciated that dehydration can be a risk even in cold climates. This can arise when an individual is undertaking physical activity over quite a prolonged period of time, e.g. skiing and not taking adequate fluid as the subject may not feel particularly hot and sweaty in cold dry conditions. It is important to recognise the particular risk posed to children who are more prone to hypothermia due to their larger body surface area and may be less aware of exposing skin to freezing conditions. Travellers with babies and toddlers should be encouraged to check them regularly for hypothermia, even if apparently well clothed and insulated.

Appropriate clothing and equipment help to avoid potential problems, such as hypothermia and frostbite. These conditions are more likely to occur on expeditions to cold climates where prolonged exposure to extreme conditions is expected, e.g. polar regions. However, health professionals would rarely be in a position to advise these travellers, who should consult a practitioner experienced in polar medicine. By far the largest group of travellers in this category would be those undertaking skiing holidays, where suitable clothing, equipment and knowledge of the rules concerning safe skiing are of the greatest importance.[5]

Problems associated with the peripheral circulation

During prolonged contact with a cold environment there are a series of potential conditions that reflect the degree of damage/impairment to peripheral circulation: trench foot, chilblains, frostnip and frostbite. The principle here is that, in contact with the cold, circulation to the periphery will be reduced as part of a homeostatic mechanism to preserve core temperature. If this is prolonged or inappropriate then tissue ischaemia and potentially damage by freezing of the tissue will occur.

Trench foot due to microvascular damage may be seen if the feet are in prolonged contact with cold water over many days or weeks. The foot is numb and swollen and can be painful, associated with muscle cramps, but there is less chance of permanent damage than for true frostbite. Chilblains on the toes may also be a result of reduced microvascular circulation from contact with the cold and the small red nodules produced about 12 hours after rewarming can be quite uncomfortable and pruritic. Finally, at the milder end of the spectrum, frostnip, where vasoconstriction results in pale cold skin, could be a warning of impending frostbite.

Frostbite is a potentially serious condition in which, due to cold and vasoconstriction, ischaemia has resulted in tissue destruction. The affected tissue will appear white, frozen and with blue patches, accompanied by a loss of sensation. The strategy here is to warm the affected part and allow blood to circulate. However, great care must be taken not to allow skin affected by frostbite to refreeze as this will greatly worsen the extent of tissue damage. In some situations it may be advisable to delay thawing the affected area until it is certain that the victim will not be exposed to the cold and potential refreezing. The thawing process is best performed by immersion into a bath of water at 40°C, resulting in a great deal of pain that may require narcotic analgesics. The damaged tissue requires specialist wound care and may eventually lead to amputation of an affected limb.

Hypothermia

This potentially life-threatening condition is defined as a core temperature below 35°C. Above 32°C the condition is defined as mild hypothermia, where the homeostatic mechanisms of shivering and peripheral vasoconstriction can still maintain body temperature. Below this temperature severe hypothermia will result in the individual becoming extremely drowsy, with cessation of shivering and eventually coma. Life-threatening cardiac arrhythmia may result if rewarming is not achieved. Hypothermia of sudden onset will develop when falling into freezing water: survival is greatly prolonged if the subject is wearing clothing as insulation and a life jacket to keep the head above water and can remain quite still in the water. The other scenario of a more gradual onset of hypothermia can occur when trekking for prolonged periods in cold and wet climates.

In the case of mild hypothermia, after removing any wet clothing the person should be insulated from the cold using whatever materials are to hand and offered warm sweet uncaffeinated drinks until transported to a warm environment. Survival blankets can be useful and the most convenient source of heat may be that of another person in contact within a sleeping bag. For severe hypothermia minimising heat loss is even more critical, and vital signs of life can be difficult to detect in order to carry out cardiopulmonary resuscitation, should that be required. Emergency transport to an appropriate medical centre is the only option for saving the life of those with severe hypothermia.

For those recovering from any degree of mild hypothermia it is good practice to ensure that the individual does not return to the cold, despite feeling warm, as peripheral warmth may not reflect a true rise in core temperature. This principle is reflected in the advice to avoid alcohol in the common misapprehension that it can help to warm you up, because alcohol is a vasodilator, increasing blood flow to the periphery. The individual may therefore experience warmth from the alcohol, but this is simply at the expense of diverting blood form the core and so causing a fall in body temperature. Tobacco is a vasoconstrictor and can worsen the affects of frostbite. The other important strategy in those who are at risk from hypothermia is to keep them dry and away from water.

High altitudes

There are many popular tourist destinations at higher altitude that could present the traveller with various health issues. A reduced exercise tolerance is expected to be very noticeable before acclimatisation. Other common minor complaints include a troublesome dry cough and disturbed sleeping patterns with frequent waking. Travellers should be assured that such symptoms are not related to acute mountain sickness (AMS), which is associated with travelling to high altitudes, and is a potential problem for travellers to many destinations. A high altitude is considered to be anything over 1500 metres, and a very high altitude over 3500 metres. AMS most commonly occurs at altitudes of greater than about 3000 metres, although cases have been reported at as low as 2000 metres. It has been reported to affect 50% of trekkers at altitudes above 4000 metres.[6] A more recent study[7] estimated a 25% incidence at 2000–3000 metres and identified that people who were younger, less fit and with lung problems were more likely to develop symptoms. However physical fitness is not believed to affect susceptibility and there does seem to be a wide variation in the general population of those who are less and more prone to developing the problem.

A particularly important contributory factor to AMS is the speed of ascent to high altitudes. Thus, people travelling to high altitudes by road or rail, rather than walking and allowing the body to acclimatise, have a greater chance of encountering problems. Similarly, when flying straight to destinations that are over about 3000 metres above sea level, as may be the case when travelling to some destinations in South America and the Himalayas, travellers risk high-altitude problems.[8] For instance, nearly 85% of those flying from Kathmandu to a popular tourist destination near Mount Everest at 3740 metres developed AMS.[9]

There are a few chronic conditions that are contraindicated for travel to high altitude: for patients with sickle-cell disease travel to destinations over 2000 metres is absolutely contraindicated as is acute or decompensated heart failure, unstable angina or a recent myocardial infarction. Mild to moderate stable heart failure (New York Heart Association class I–II) may be fit to travel to altitude, but not those with more severe forms. Those with more severe chronic obstructive pulmonary disease (COPD) may find dyspnoea worsens, but those with mild to moderate COPD or asthma seem to fare quite well providing optimal medication is maintained. Similarly, stable ischaemic heart disease does not seem to present any particular problems with travel to higher altitudes, though more medication may be required with more severe disease. Pregnant women should be discouraged from sleeping for too long a period at above 3000 metres. Overall, data concerning contraindications for travel to higher altitudes do tend to be sparse and it is advisable that those with respiratory and cardiovascular problems avoid altitudes greater than 2500 metres and avoid those more than 5000 metres in pregnancy.

Acclimatisation to high altitude

People who travel to high altitudes will experience a degree of hypoxia that is apparent by reduced exercise tolerance and shortness of breath. The explanation is simply that as the altitude increases so the partial pressure of oxygen (Pao_2) in the atmosphere decreases e.g. at about 2000 metres there is a reduction by around 30% compared to sea level. There is an adaptive ventilatory mechanism that the body employs to counteract this fall in Pao_2:

- The respiratory centre in the CNS is able to respond to hypoxia by an increase in respiratory rate.
- Increased respiratory rate is accompanied by a degree of alkalosis, which in turn will tend to reduce the respiratory rate and so prevent a further rise.
- Excess bicarbonate is excreted by the kidney after a few days to reduce the alkalosis, although a slightly raised pH remains. The respiratory centre thus becomes set to increase respiration at a given altitude that is

maximal after about 5 days, having to readapt progressively as altitude is again increased.

Other adaptive processes occur, but may present some physiological problems. They include:

- There is increased production of erythropoietin resulting in a rise in red blood cell mass (polycythaemia).
- Diuresis and a hyperosmolarity tend to occur, giving rise to a reduced plasma volume and haemoconcentration. This is related to a peripheral venoconstriction, resulting in a rise in central blood volume which will then inhibit the release of aldosterone and suppress antidiuretic hormone, resulting in the increased diuresis.
- A fall in alveolar Pao_2 tends to cause pulmonary vasoconstriction and pulmonary hypertension. This is a normal adaptive response to lung damage where oxygen supply is diverted to healthy lung tissue, so aiding in an improvement of gas exchange. However, the mechanism is of no advantage at high altitude and may worsen pre-existing conditions such as heart failure.
- There is increased blood flow to the brain that, although delivering more oxygen, will also raise intracranial pressure.

It is a common observation that some individuals are better at adapting than others. This may be a reflection of genetically determined factors such as differences in the ventilatory response to hypoxia.

Overall adaptation will restore submaximal exercise tolerance, but has less effect on maximal exercise ability. In other words, the highest level of exercise that an individual finds achievable at sea level will not be achieved at altitude.

Pathophysiology of AMS

Box 8.1 summarises the range of symptoms associated with AMS. The condition most commonly manifests itself as mild or benign AMS, where the symptoms are troublesome but not life threatening. Headache is the most prominent feature, which is worse on bending over. The victim will feel tired and irritable and symptoms may resemble those of alcohol hangover or a viral infection. As the condition worsens the headache may be more severe, accompanied by nausea and vomiting, and there may be extreme lassitude.

Although AMS is a well-recognised condition, the causes remain controversial. Symptoms are related to a range of physiological effects on the body, which are caused by a reduction in atmospheric pressure

---

Box 8.1 Signs and symptoms of acute mountain sickness

Mild (benign)
- Headache
- Loss of appetite
- Nausea and vomiting
- Insomnia
- Tight sensation in the chest
- Poor performance
- Dizziness

High-altitude pulmonary oedema
- Dyspnoea
- Cough
- White sputum
- Cyanosis

High-altitude cerebral oedema
- Headache
- Drowsiness
- Loss of balance
- Abnormal behaviour
- Loss of consciousness or coma
- Nightmares

---

and hence the lower PaO_2. Other factors, such as cold and physical exertion, also contribute. However, there is little evidence that physical fitness confers any protection.[10] Table 8.2 lists some of the physiological effects that may have a bearing on developing AMS. Fluid retention and oedema seem to play a central role in the aetiology of symptoms experienced. In particular, vascular leakage within the CNS and the consequent rise in intracranial pressure is an important and well-documented pathophysiological observation. It is not known if cerebral oedema contributes to the CNS effects of AMS (e.g. dizziness and headaches), but this would be a reasonable explanation.

Hackett and Murdoch[11] have described a possible approach to the pathophysiology of AMS that places increased sympathetic activity as a central unifying component in the development of AMS. In this model it is proposed that the increased blood flow to the brain induced by hypoxia, as previously described, causes vascular leakage and changes

Table 8.2 Some physiological factors which can contribute to acute mountain sickness

Observation	Possible explanation
High alveolar CO_2	Poor respiratory response to hypoxia in some individuals
Development of pulmonary oedema	Changes in pulmonary perfusion and pulmonary vasoconstriction Increased capillary permeability
Central nervous system dysfunction	Cerebral swelling Increased capillary permeability or oedema Formation of blood clots due to nitrogen bubbles Central nervous system hypoxia
Fluid retention	Hormonal changes – possible role of atrial natriuretic peptide

in brain function that result in stimulation of the sympathetic nervous system. In the lungs such increased sympathetic activity worsens the pulmonary hypertension that may have occurred in response to alveolar hypoxia and also the release of atrial natriuretic peptide that has an effect of increasing vascular permeability. Increased sympathetic tone will tend to stimulate the renin–angiotensin system, worsening overall fluid retention. Fluid retention may also be worsened by an increased output of antidiuretic hormone, again due to the cerebral oedema/ vascular leakage. However, the precise mechanism by which cerebral oedema develops is not known.

A suggested explanation of why some individuals seem to develop symptoms of AMS more readily than others is that their tolerance to any minor brain swelling at high altitudes may be determined by their craniospinal anatomy.[12]

High-altitude cerebral oedema and high-altitude pulmonary oedema

It is possible for the benign form of AMS to result in more serious complications, affecting either the lungs (high-altitude pulmonary oedema: HAPE) or the CNS (high-altitude cerebral oedema: HACE), although both can exist together. More rarely, HAPE and HACE can occur with little warning. There is a 4% risk of AMS sufferers experiencing such complications,[4] and up to 8% was estimated for those climbing at around 4000 metres in Nepal.[5] Increased capillary permeability, caused by chemical mediator release in response to hypoxia, probably contributes to HAPE and HACE.

HACE can really be viewed as the most severe form of AMS, from which it can sometimes progress, and is characterised by severe neurological disturbances, eventually leading to coma and death. Headache may be absent and the subject will initially appear disoriented and confused. It is treated by descent, the administration of oxygen and the use of dexamethasone.

HAPE can be fatal but rapid descent and the administration of oxygen can just as quickly reverse the condition. It most commonly strikes on the second night at a particular altitude and rarely occurs after 4 nights. The symptoms are as would be expected with any form of pulmonary oedema: severe dyspnoea, reduced exercise tolerance and dry cough. Fever may also be present, which can confuse the diagnosis. The victim will become increasingly cyanosed and hypoxic, eventually leading to loss of consciousness. It seems likely that the condition is related to pulmonary hypertension, as described above, which may lead to damage of the microcirculation and capillary leakage. There may be a number of factors that are responsible for the pathophysiology of HAPE and the susceptibility of individuals, but this is still a matter of debate and further research.[13] Those with a previous history of HAPE should take extra care regarding acclimatisation.

Prevention of AMS

Whatever the true cause of AMS, ways of preventing the problem are well recognised. A slow rate of ascent is important. For instance, experienced mountaineers who carefully plan their climbs are less susceptible to AMS than casual trekkers. It is suggested that for every 1000 metres climbed over 3000 metres, 2 nights' acclimatisation should be allowed. Another maxim is to 'climb high but sleep low', indicating that AMS can be avoided if one always returns to lower ground when resting during the night. The altitude at which the climber sleeps can be quite a good predictor of developing AMS, sleeping below 2800 metres being a good strategy if practical. This is probably an important reason why AMS is less common among alpine skiers: night-time lodgings in the Alps tend to be on lower ground. It is always worthwhile advising travellers who are flying direct to the high Andes, for example, to take things easy for a few days. Other factors that may impair good acclimatisation to high altitudes include the use of respiratory depressants such as alcohol, hypnotics and narcotic analgesics. A low-salt diet may help to reduce fluid retention and there is some evidence that a high-carbohydrate diet may be helpful. Maintaining good hydration, but not overhydrating, is generally advisable in the cold dry climate at high altitudes, particularly during the physical exertions of climbing, and about 3 litres of fluid intake a day has been advised.[8]

One of the best predictors of problems from AMS is a previous history of the condition since it does tend to recur in susceptible individuals.[4]

Drug management of AMS

Immediate treatment of AMS is simple: go down to a lower altitude. Climbers developing the initial symptoms of benign AMS should be advised to rest and climb no further until the symptoms resolve. In the case of pulmonary or cerebral symptoms, a rapid descent can be life-saving. Oxygen will greatly improve symptoms, but this is not usually available. Climbers have reported that special inflatable hyperbaric bags (Gamow) are of use. These have been criticised for providing only short-term relief and potentially delaying descent.[14] They are useful in buying time while descent can be arranged. Ibuprofen is a safe and effective remedy for AMS-induced headache[15] and three doses of 325 mg aspirin taken prophylactically every 4 hours have been shown in one trial to reduce the incidence.[16]

A range of drugs have been used for both the prevention and treatment of AMS (Table 8.3). However, their exact mechanism of action in this situation is not well understood.

Acetazolamide

Acetazolamide is used to treat and prevent benign AMS (unlicensed indication), although its true place in therapy is somewhat contentious. It must be remembered that, in itself, this form of AMS is not fatal and there is not a great deal of evidence that acetazolamide prevents progression to a more serious form. Therefore, the benefits of taking acetazolamide should be weighed against the risk of adverse effects. A positive indication for such prophylaxis would be a past history of AMS or travelling from sea level to a sleeping altitude of 3000 metres in the same day.[13]

Acetazolamide is a carbonic anhydrase inhibitor and induces mild metabolic acidosis which tends to increase respiration. Its mode of action in AMS might therefore be through stimulation of respiratory drive, hence compensating for the low Pa_{O_2}. Being a diuretic it also helps to resolve the fluid retention associated with AMS. The most common adverse effect at the recommended dosage (Table 8.3) is paraesthesia in the fingers and toes. It may also cause a loss of taste of carbonated drinks and should be avoided by those with an allergy to sulphonamides.

A few trials have shown that acetazolamide can be used as prophylaxis, but it is unclear what the most effective regimen might be, whether it should be taken in advance of travel and how long before ascent. Some experts argue against it being used routinely in this way, except in cases where AMS is known to be particularly troublesome, or the rate of ascent is relatively fast. Others suggest a strategy of continuing for just 2 days on reaching altitude, but then restarting if symptoms become troublesome.[11] For most tourist treks in Nepal gradual ascent is practical and such prophylaxis is not required.

A recent review of published data concerning the prophylactic use of pharmacological agents for preventing AMS concluded that a daily dose of acetazolamide 750 mg was more efficacious than the widely used 500 mg daily dose. In addition prophylaxis was not thought to be worthwhile if the rate of ascent was less than 500 metres/day.[17] However, this particular analysis was criticised[18] for not including the results of important trials, for comparing two doses which considered different rates of ascent and for having too strict an endpoint regarding the presence of AMS.

Table 8.3 Drug management of acute mountain sickness

Name	Regimen	Principal use
Acetazolamide	Prophylaxis: 500 mg slow-release at night or 250 mg twice daily commencing the day before reaching 3000 metres (but see text) Treatment: 250 mg stat	Prophylaxis and management of mild symptoms
Dexamethasone	8 mg stat then 4 mg every 4 hours	Management of cerebral symptoms
Nifedipine	10 mg stat sublingual then 20 mg modified-release 6-hourly while at altitude. Repeat sublingual dose every 15 minutes if blood pressure does not drop more than 10 mmHg within 10 minutes	Management of pulmonary symptoms

Acetazolamide has also been used to resolve symptoms associated with benign AMS. The issue here might be one of safety, since it is theoretically possible that, on gaining symptomatic relief, a subject might be tempted to continue the ascent, which could in turn precipitate a more serious form of the condition. There are however no reported case studies where this seems to have been a problem. If acetazolamide is to be taken in this way, it is still wise to take time to rest and to have a slower rate of ascent. The evidence base for acetazolamide's use in the treatment of AMS is not as strong as that for prophylaxis.[4] A small study has indicated that a single dose of 250 mg could relieve symptoms in those with established AMS.[19] A dose of 125 mg has been claimed to be effective in relieving the sleep disturbances associated with high altitude.[11]

Dexamethasone

The principal use for dexamethasone is in the relief of HACE or more severe AMS[20] and for the latter it may have a quicker onset of action than acetazolamide. It is important not to rely on this agent alone for a cure and, again, descent to a lower altitude is essential. Unlike acetazolamide, it does not actually aid in acclimatisation, so further ascent whilst taking dexamethasone may be unwise. Its principal effect is probably a reduction of cerebral oedema, which it does by reducing vascular permeability. It may also be effective prophylactically, but acetazolamide is usually used in preference.

Nifedipine

Nifedipine's use in relieving HAPE in an emergency situation (unlicensed indication) has been demonstrated by studies.[21] However, to date, there is little evidence supporting its usefulness and the recommended regimen is largely empirical. Its mechanism of action is probably via pulmonary vasodilation. This relieves pulmonary hypertension, a physiological response to alveolar hypoxia known be present in HAPE.[22] Concomitant therapy for HAPE includes using oxygen, where available, and this combined with rapid descent, will give a better outcome than the use of nifedipine alone. For the treatment of oedema associated with HAPE and HACE, furosemide (frusemide) can also be used.

β-Agonists

A potential useful option in preventing HAPE in susceptible individuals is the use of β-agonists. This was demonstrated by a recent trial in which the incidence of HAPE was reduced by 50% in such individuals by the use of prophylactic salmeterol inhalers.[23]

Local and herbal remedies

In the high Andes, travellers are likely to come across a number of local remedies for the prevention of AMS; the condition is known locally as soroche. Chief among these is an infusion of tea made from coca leaves. There is probably little cocaine in this infusion, but, anecdotally, travellers have claimed some symptomatic relief from mild AMS from drinking it. The use of a paste of coca leaves, held in the mouth, could well help as a respiratory stimulant to relieve the symptoms of AMS, although such practice is not to be advised to travellers. Even more worrying, I have come across instances where respiratory stimulants, such as nikethamide, are freely sold to travellers. On the other hand there does seem to be some evidence supporting the use of ginkgo biloba prophylactically to reduce the incidence of AMS.

Marine hazards

The principal hazards at sea are due to accidents from swimming or watersports and the danger from marine animals; this last factor is discussed in Chapter 11.

Travellers going on diving holidays should be aware of the physiological dangers associated with scuba diving, e.g. decompression sickness. This would not usually be an area where most health professionals would be called on to give specific advice. However, all those who attempt this sport should be strongly advised to take a recognised diving course, either in the UK or at their destination. Travellers should be warned only to attend diving courses overseas that are certified by the Professional Association of Diving Instructors (PADI) or the National Association of Underwater Instructors (NAUI). The hazards of diving and their management will not be discussed further in this book; useful summaries can be found in Dawood's *Traveller's Health* and Dupont and Steffen's *Textbook of Travel Medicine*.

Certain medical problems, ranging from sinus to cardiac conditions, may make a person unfit for diving. A particularly important piece of advice to all divers is to avoid flying for a day or so after a dive to avoid decompression illness.

Very common problems associated with swimming in both the sea and swimming pools are middle-ear infections, discussed in Chapter 11.

Equipment and clothing

The importance of adequate planning for the particular environment at the destination has been emphasised throughout this chapter. One important aspect that is within the control of the traveller is the clothing and equipment carried during the trip. There are limits to the range and quantity that can be carried by an individual and in this section it will be assumed that the traveller is a backpacker where all equipment must be carried personally.

Clothing and equipment for hot climates

Clothing

In the tropics the principle is that the body should be able to sweat freely, allowing evaporation and so cooling of the skin. Cotton has traditionally been the material advocated for this purpose. In more recent years clothing made of polycotton and polyamides has been produced specifically for hot and wet tropical climates; these fabrics allow clothing to dry out more quickly and do not require ironing (Fig. 8.1). It is also claimed that the material allows sweat to wick away from close contact with the skin and thus provides more comfort. Whether to choose either of these materials is to some extent a matter of personal choice. In extremely wet tropical conditions it is likely that both cottons and synthetic types of material will become equally saturated. Some do not like the slightly slimy feel to the synthetic materials; others value their tendency to become less creased. Ripstop materials have specially woven cross-fibres that minimise tearing of material and will prolong the life of clothing when walking through heavy undergrowth.

Both long-sleeved shirts and trousers should be worn, particularly at night, to maximise protection from insect bites; ideally clothing should be treated with insecticide, as described in Chapter 6. At least two sets of such clothing should be carried and, for those who might like to wear shorts during the day if there are few biting insects, trousers with bottoms that can be removed are useful. Depending upon the time of year something warm to wear at night such as a light-weight fleece may also be advisable even in the tropics. For the rainforest, or if trekking in other wet/rainy conditions, some form of waterproof clothing will be required. It is usually more convenient not to wear waterproofs during the day in a hot climate, but on making camp and before

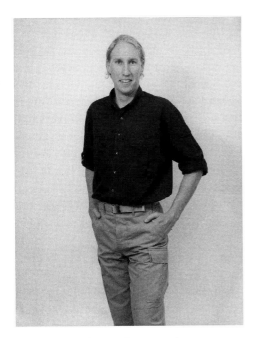

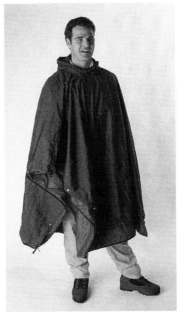

Figure 8.1 Shirt and trousers for tropics. Courtesy of Nomad.

Figure 8.2 Poncho with quilt lining. Courtesy of Nomad.

retiring it is important for comfort to try to stay dry. One of the most versatile coverings for trekkers and walkers is the army poncho (Fig. 8.2), as it allows good circulation of air and can also cover both the body and the rucksack. The poncho can also be used as a ground sheet or even an improvised shelter.

Headgear should not be too heavy in the tropics. It should both protect from the direct rays of the sun and also allow some evaporation of sweat. A bandana is a very useful item for a head covering, sweat rag or scarf. Where more sun protection is required, then a light wide-brimmed bush hat is advised. It may be tempting to purchase army-style khaki-green or camouflage tropical clothing, but this should be avoided when travelling to destinations of civil unrest as it is possible to be identified as hostile by local security forces.

In the desert white-coloured clothing will reflect radiated heat from the sun. Arab style cloth headwear is very useful both for protection of the head and for wrapping around the face to protect against sand storms.

Footwear

For jungle trekking, boots should have a higher ankle to protect against snake bites, jigger fleas or entry of other animals. The boots should be sturdy enough for walking, yet relatively light-weight and easy to dry off after a day's trekking in a wet environment. Jungle boots meeting these specifications can be purchased and have small ventilation holes near the bottom of the boot allowing water to circulate freely (Fig. 8.3). They can be purchased quite cheaply but do not have the high-tech features for comfort of modern walking boots. On the other hand, the rigours of jungle trekking are quite likely to ruin more expensive footwear. Socks should also be easy to dry out and wool or waterproof socks specifically designed for the jungle are suitable. Correctly fitting boots for any type of walking are extremely important and skin damage can lead to a chronic wound that is difficult to heal or even cellulitis (Plate 9). A further pair of shoes may be needed at the end of the day's trekking. Open-toed sandals may be best avoided if camping out in the jungle undergrowth where parasitic insects may be a problem.

Boots used specifically for the desert tend to be lighter in construction with rubber soles and a suede or canvas upper, and may not be suitable for rough hard terrains.

If heavy exposure to leeches is anticipated then it is worth considering canvas leech socks through which they are unable to penetrate (Fig. 8.4).

Equipment and sleeping

One priority piece of equipment for a hot climate is a suitable water bottle, and these bottles come in many shapes and sizes. If never too far from a reliable water supply, the type of bottle is not too critical. Those on expeditions and treks should choose with care. One very useful style of bottle is a bladder that will minimise the weight carried (Fig. 8.5). This is encased in an outer stronger material which can be kept moist with water, thus helping to cool the contents of the bladder by evaporation.

A tent is not always practical to be carried during long treks in the tropics, and in any case it is often more comfortable to sleep out-of-doors in hot climates. A light-weight hammock can be a useful piece of equipment in such circumstances, being strung up between trees and keeping the individual well above the ground. An insecticide-treated

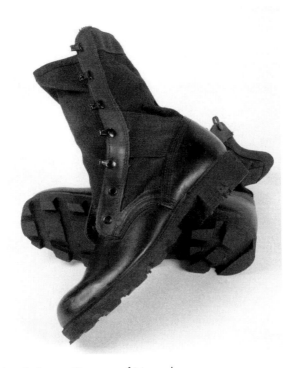

Figure 8.3 Jungle boots. Courtesy of Nomad.

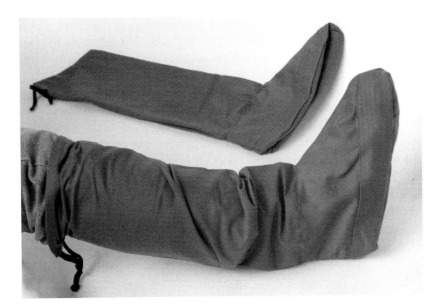

Figure 8.4 Leech socks. Courtesy of Nomad.

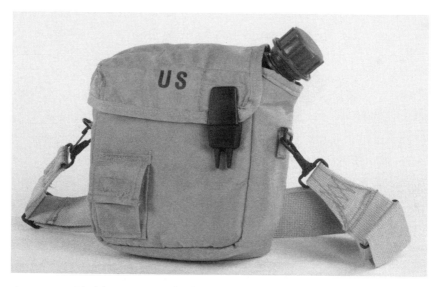

Figure 8.5   Bladder-type water bottle. Courtesy of Nomad.

mosquito net should additionally be hung over the hammock. A Basha sheet (or poncho) can also be hung over the hammock to protect from rain during the night.

Sleeping bags can be purchased for a variety of climates but may be too warm for the tropics, and a simple sleeping bag lining sheet may be all that is required. A more versatile alternative is to use a poncho liner or tropical quilt which is made of insulated light-weight synthetic fabric. This will provide warmth at night or during the day if required, and can provide comfort when spread on the ground.

Keeping things dry can be a continual problem for trekkers and hikers. It is particularly important to try and keep clothes worn on retiring as dry as possible. Waterproof stuff bags are very useful for this purpose, and using a number of them helps to organise a crowded rucksack. The rucksack itself should be carefully chosen if it is to be worn for long periods of time as inappropriate fitting can lead to back strain and rubbing straps to infected chronic wounds. It is a good idea to consult a specialist travel/camping supplier and try a number of rucksacks for comfort.

Walkers and trekkers in all climates must be aware of the need for basic survival equipment. A map and compass, and the ability to use them, may be life-saving in certain situations. A whistle is useful to attract attention in an emergency. Global positioning system (GPS) is becoming almost obligatory when undertaking any form of expedition away from civilisation. A torch, matches and emergency food rations – a chocolate bar will suffice – will also form part of the essential preparation for many outward-bound trips.

Cold climates

The principle in this situation is to wear multiple layers of clothes in order to trap air and thus aid insulation. The layer closest to the skin should be the thinnest and the outermost layer ideally completely waterproof, being made of strong modern synthetic fibres. It is however important that sweat evaporates from the skin during physical exertion and closed cloth material is best avoided. One means of ventilation is to use outer clothing that has small 'breathing holes' underneath armpits and allows ventilation around the neck and wrists. The poncho described above will also allow good circulation of air but windproof clothing may need to be worn underneath. Breathable semipermeable materials such as Goretex are very useful for outer garments.

In general, for subzero temperatures the principle is to leave little if any skin exposed to the environment. Hats enclosing the ears should be worn and the chin and neck covered with a scarf or balaclava. Mittens are said to be better than gloves and there should be no gap of exposed skin between glove and jackets.

An appropriate tent will be essential if camping out in cold or wet and windy conditions. General survival equipment is much the same as described above for hot climates.

Main points

In hot climates

- Expect to take a week to become acclimatised before undertaking a high level of physical activity.
- Always drink past the point of quenching thirst.
- Be aware of the first signs of heat exhaustion and take steps to cool down.
- If undergoing prolonged physical activity in hot climates, increase dietary salt.

In cold climates

- It is not possible to acclimatise so the correct clothing and equipment are important.

- Be aware of the signs of potentially developing frostbite or hypothermia.
- If frostbite does occur, then make sure that there is no danger of refreezing before thawing out the limb. For hypothermia, keeping warm and dry while seeking medical help is the principal objective.

At high altitude

- If at all possible, take time to acclimatise for each 1000 metres ascent over 3000 metres.
- Beware of the symptoms of AMS, HAPE and HACE. It may be up to others in a group to recognise the symptoms and help the victim to descend.
- If AMS is troublesome, acetazolamide can be taken. At onset of symptoms do not climb any higher and if they do not resolve or become worse then descend.
- For HAPE and HACE, always descend. Dexamethasone is useful for HACE, nifedipine for HAPE. For HAPE in particular oxygen should be given, and if not available a portable hypobaric chamber.

Frequently asked questions

What are the positive indications for taking acetazolamide if travelling to a high altitude?
There are probably three situations where acetazolamide is definitely worth considering:

1. those who have previously had a bad experience of AMS
2. if travelling directly from sea level by plane or train to the altitudes indicated in the text
3. potentially in situations where a fast ascent may be required

Those travelling to high altitudes may be recommended the medication by group organisers and there seem to be few contraindications to prescribing to otherwise healthy individuals. It is sometimes advocated to try a dose or two at sea level to test tolerability.

How is it best to take acetazolamide – prophylactically or as required?
Most of the research has examined the prophylactic use but there is a general consensus that it is effective at resolving symptoms of AMS. One approach might be to use as prophylaxis if there is a previous history of AMS or a very rapid ascent is anticipated, and to use as required in other situations.

Always warn to climb no higher despite taking acetazolamide until symptoms improve. If symptoms worsen or do not improve, then descend.

Are there any problems for children at high altitude?
Children are no more susceptible to altitude problems than older people, but it may be more difficult to identify problems in younger children who are unable to describe their symptoms. Parents may not wish to travel to high altitudes with very young children owing to the suggestion that high altitude may be associated with an increased risk of sudden infant death syndrome. There is another syndrome that can present a small risk to young children living above 3000 metres called subacute infantile mountain sickness.[24]

If people flying in an airplane are at risk of deep-vein thrombosis (DVT), might this also apply to those at altitude? If taking an oral contraceptive, could this increase the risk of DVT at altitude?
The principal factor for developing a DVT in an airplane is immobility (see Chapter 10). This could be a risk factor for mountaineers if prolonged periods are spent in a small tent. There are other risk factors at high altitude for DVT such as the tendency towards polycythaemia and dehydration. Oral contraceptives are not known to be an extra risk factor in this context.

Is coca tea or chewing coca leaves, as is the custom in some South American countries, useful for preventing AMS?
Certainly very little of the active alkaloids would be extracted from the tea in the normal process of infusion, so from that point of view it is thought to be a harmless placebo. Travellers should be cautioned that the tea is classed as a controlled drug and could present problems if they attempt to bring it through customs.

For chewing, the leaves must be mixed in a paste with other calcium-containing plants to release the cocaine. This will raise catecholamine levels sufficiently to increase respiration. However, adverse effects would be expected in novice users and travellers should be discouraged from this practice.

If someone is potentially allergic to acetazolamide, can dexamethasone be used?
Dexamethasone is considered as second-line treatment for AMS as it does not actually aid in acclimatisation, but is a reasonable alternative.

Is it useful to take electrolyte solutions regularly if trekking in a hot climate?
As described in the section on Heat stroke and heat exhaustion, above, the increased output of sweat can lead to salt depletion in hot climates, contributing to developing forms of heat exhaustion. Using electrolyte solutions, some of which are relatively low in salt (see Chapter 3) is not a very efficient way to make up the deficit and instead increased salt in the diet is recommended. Neither, again for reasons explained above, are they

particularly useful for treating heat exhaustion where a large fluid intake is the priority. Anecdotally some do report consumption of isotonic glucose/electrolyte solutions to improve well-being after extended treks in humid tropical conditions. This may be related to a more efficient water absorption from such solutions.

How much should a person in a hot climate aim to drink in a day?
The advice is always to drink beyond the point of thirst. As a benchmark, adults carrying out fairly heavy physical activity in humid hot conditions may need to consume around 10 litres of fluid per day. Maintain a pale-coloured urine: if a dark and/or low-output urine is seen, then insufficient is being drunk.

Are salt tablets useful for those travelling to hot climates?
As described in the text, these should be generally discouraged.

References

1. Johnson C. Effects of climatic extremes. In: Dawood R, ed. *Travellers' Health: How to Stay Healthy Abroad,* 4th edn. Oxford: Oxford University Press, 2002: 326–349.
2. Weiss E L. Medical risks of temperature extremes. In: DuPont H L, Steffen R, eds. *Textbook of Travel Medicine and Health,* 2nd edn. Hamilton, Canada: BC Decker, 2000: 113–119.
3. Hett H A, Brechtelsbauer D A. Heat related illness. *Postgrad Med* 1998; 103: 107–120.
4. Beeley J M, Smith D J, Oakley E H N. Environmental hazards and health. *Br Med Bull* 1993; 49: 305–326.
5. Helal B, Philipp E. Skiing. In: Dawood R, ed. *Travellers' Health: How to Stay Healthy Abroad,* 4th edn. Oxford: Oxford University Press, 2002: 381–392.
6. Hackett P H, Rennie D, Levine H D. The incidence, importance and prophylaxis of acute mountain sickness. *Lancet* 1976; ii: 1149–1154.
7. Honigman B, Thies M K, Koziol-McLain J *et al.* Acute mountain sickness in a general tourist population at moderate altitudes. *Ann Intern Med* 1993; 118: 587–592.
8. Basnyat B. Altitude illness. In: Dawood R, ed. *Travellers' Health: How to Stay Healthy Abroad,* 4th edn. Oxford: Oxford University Press, 2002: 224–231.
9. Murdoch D R. Altitude illness among tourists flying to 3740 meters elevation in the Nepal Himalaya. *J Travel Med* 1995; 2: 255–256.
10. Milledge J S, Beeley J M, Broome J *et al.* Acute mountain sickness susceptibility, fitness and hypoxic ventilatory response. *Eur Resp J* 1991; 4: 1000–1003.
11. Hackett P H, Murdoch D R. Medical problems of high altitude. In: DuPont H L, Steffen R, eds. *Textbook of Travel Medicine and Health,* 2nd edn. Hamilton, Canada: BC Decker, 2000: 80–92.

12. Hackett P H. The cerebral etiology of high-altitude cerebral edema and acute mountain sickness. *Wilderness Environ Med* 1999; 10: 97–109.

13. Hackett P H, Roach R C. High altitude illness. *N Engl J Med* 2001; 345: 107–114.

14. Pollard A J. Treatment of acute mountain sickness. *BMJ* 1995; 311: 629.

15. Broome J R, Stoneham M D, Beeley J M et al. High altitude headache: treatment with ibuprofen. *Aviation Space Environ Med* 1994; 65: 19–20.

16. Burtscher M, Likar R, Nachbauer W, Philadelphy M. Aspirin for prophylaxis against headache at high altitudes: randomised, double blind, placebo controlled trial. *BMJ* 1998; 316: 1057–1058.

17. Dumont L, Mardirosoff C, Tramer M R. Efficacy and harm of pharmacological prevention of acute mountain sickness: quantitative systematic review. *BMJ* 2000; 321: 267–272.

18. Hackett P. Pharmacological prevention of acute mountain sickness. *BMJ* 2001; 322: 48.

19. Grissom C K, Roach R C, Sarnquist F H, Hackett P H. Acetazolamide in the treatment of acute mountain sickness: clinical efficacy and effect on gas exchange. *Ann Intern Med* 1992; 116: 461–465.

20. Keller H R, Maggiorini M, Bärtsch P, Oelz O. Simulated descent v dexamethasone in treatment of acute mountain sickness: a randomised trial. *BMJ* 1995; 310: 1232–1235.

21. Oelz O, Maggiorini M, Ritter M et al. Prevention and treatment of high altitude pulmonary oedema by calcium channel blocker. *Int J Sports Med* 1992; 13 (suppl. 1): S65–S68.

22. Oelz O, Maggiorini M, Ritter M et al. Nifedipine for high altitude pulmonary oedema. *Lancet* 1989; ii: 1241–1244.

23. Sartori C, Allemann Y, Duplain H et al. Salmeterol for the prevention of high-altitude pulmonary edema. *N Engl J Med* 2002; 346: 1631–1636.

24. Murdoch D R, Pollard A J, Gibbs J S. Altitude and expedition medicine. In: Zuckerman J, ed. *Principles and Practice of Travel Medicine*. Chichester, UK: Wiley, 2001: 247–260.

9

Skin conditions associated with the sun and heat

This chapter covers the effects of ultraviolet radiation from the sun on the skin and the preventive measures that can be taken to avoid skin damage. The main message for the public is that sunscreens are an aid to protection and should not be used as a way of increasing exposure to the sun.

Overexposure to ultraviolet (UV) radiation from the sun is not a problem solely confined to travel abroad and much of the advice given below applies equally in the UK on sunny summer days.

There are a number of factors which can put travellers to certain destinations at short- or long-term risk from the harmful effects of the sun, particularly from certain skin cancers. Not least is the desire to obtain a tan and to sunbathe for longer periods than when at home. In addition, the amount of UV radiation increases nearer the equator, an important consideration if travelling to the tropics. Similarly, there is an increased risk of sunburn for those undertaking skiing holidays, where reflected UV from the snow can intensify exposure.

Much of this chapter will, therefore, consider the effects of UV radiation on the skin and the various preventive measures that can be taken to avoid skin damage. Particular emphasis will be placed on sunscreens, although they are only one part of the preventive strategies that can be used. Other, rarer conditions associated with exposure to the sun (photodermatosis) will be briefly discussed, along with prickly heat. The latter is a common complaint that, although not directly caused by overexposure to the sun, is a condition for which the public seek advice. Health professionals should also be aware of the potential of some drugs to cause photosensitivity reactions.

Effect of UV light on skin

There are three bandwidths of UV radiation that can have harmful effects on the skin: UVA (320–400 nm), UVB (290–320 nm) and UVC

(200–290 nm). UVA has been further subdivided into short-wave (UVAII, 320–340 nm) and long-wave (UVAI, 340–400 nm).[1] About 80% of the UV reaching the earth's surface is in the UVA range and 20% within the UVB range. Most UVC is filtered out by the ozone layer.

UVB is mainly responsible for sunburn. Both UVA and UVB are involved with the process of tanning, the development of certain skin cancers (photocarcinogenesis) and photoageing, as will be described below. The exact UV wavelengths responsible for chronic effects on the skin and the mechanism by which the changes take place are not well understood.[2] Factors concerning the intensity of the sun are summarised in Table 9.1.

Sunburn

Sunburn represents an acute problem which, if it involves a large enough surface area of the body, can be life-threatening. Sunburn is an inflammatory response to damage caused by radiation and thus the classic signs of acute inflammation will be observed: hot, red and swollen skin with associated pain and discomfort. There are two phases to the reaction. Immediately after overexposure to the sun, the skin will develop a pink coloration that disappears quickly. About 6 hours later, there is a more intense redness of the skin that becomes hot, slightly swollen and sore.[3] There may also be systemic symptoms, such as shivering, fever and nausea. These reactions result from an inflammatory response whereby chemical mediators cause vasodilation and increased capillary permeability. In more severe cases, blistering of the skin occurs. Peeling of the skin usually begins after 2–3 days. Mild sunburn is managed by the use of cooling lotions, such as calamine lotion, although a calamine cream may be a better option, because it will help to hydrate the skin. Analgesics, such as paracetamol and ibuprofen, can be taken to aid pain relief.

Non-steroidal anti-inflammatory agents, such as indometacin, can reduce UV-induced erythema,[4] but evidence for their usefulness in resolving symptoms and aiding healing is lacking.[5] More severe sunburn may require admission to hospital.

Suntan

The suntanning process is an adaptive mechanism by which the skin can become protected from UV radiation. There are two phases to the tanning process. The immediate phase involves oxidation of melanin that

Table 9.1   Factors affecting ultraviolet (UV) radiation exposure from the sun

Factor	Precaution
The higher the angle of the sun over the horizon, the smaller the distance radiation must travel through the atmosphere and so less radiation is absorbed by the atmosphere. At noon at midsummer the sun is directly overhead	Avoid the sun at least 2 hours either side of midday. The risks are much lower after 4.30 p.m.
UV is most intense at the equator	Take extra care in the tropics
Each 300 metre rise in altitude results in a 4% rise in the burning effect from UV	Take extra care at high altitudes at all times of the year
UV is scattered but not necessarily absorbed on a cloudy day	Take care, even if the temperature feels cool
Radiation is reflected from snow, ice and light-coloured sand	Take care, because sufficient protection may not be gained, even if shaded from the direct rays of the sun. There is some reflection from water, but no more than that reflected from grass
UV penetrates water and some wet clothing	Wearing a white T-shirt when swimming may not offer sufficient protection (about SPF 7). Wear dark, closely woven materials
Some items of clothing are penetrated by UV radiation to a greater extent than others	Choose clothing carefully if high exposure is expected
Wind can contribute to the skin damage caused by the sun	Skiers and sailors, in particular, should use protection

SPF, sun protection factor.

is already present in the skin, rendering it a brown colour. This phase is mediated by UVA radiation and lasts less than an hour. A true tan is obtained following more prolonged exposure to UVB radiation, which affects the epidermal basal cell layer of the skin. The melanocytes residing in this area are stimulated by UVB to produce more melanin, which is deposited on the outer layers of the skin. This type of tanning, in which UVA radiation plays little part, begins after 1–2 days of exposure. A further effect of UVB exposure is skin thickening, caused by epidermal hyperplasia that offers considerable protection to the skin. It is important to note that a suntan induced by UVA sunbeds will not induce such thickening and people should be discouraged from preparing themselves for sunbathing by developing such tans.

It is a common observation that some individuals will tan more readily and burn less than others. Although it is useful for people to be aware of their skin type (Box 9.1), it should not necessarily guide the choice of sun protection screen factors (as has previously been recommended), mainly because it is now advised that people should be discouraged from developing a tan at all. The argument is that, in developing a tan, considerable exposure to UV radiation occurs, resulting in the development of the chronic skin problems described below. Thus, although it is true that tanning will protect from sunburn, other problems remain.

Box 9.1   Skin types and characteristics

- Type 1: Always burns, never tans
- Type 2: Always burns, sometimes tans
- Type 3: Sometimes burns, sometimes tans
- Type 4: Never burns, always tans
- Type 5: Brown skin
- Type 6: Black skin

For those who insist on developing a tan it should be explained that this has only cosmetic rather than any perceived medical benefits. The potential problems concerning photoageing and skin cancers should be emphasised. Artificial tanning products, but not tan accelerators or enhancers, can be safely recommended.

Despite the accumulating evidence of harm to the skin, many holiday-makers are still intent on developing a tan. In a survey of Irish holiday-makers it was found that 90% intended to develop a tan and estimated that 40% would be likely to burn.[6] If the individual is still keen to develop a tan then the advice is that this should be done gradually. The suggested method[7] is that fair-skinned people initially only expose their skin to the sun when it is most intense for about 10–20 minutes, applying a sunscreen of factor of around 10. Exposure time can be gradually increased and factor reduced over a few days as a tan develops.

Skin cancers

The association between exposure to the sun and the development of certain skin cancers has initiated much of the interest in sun protection. The incidence of these cancers is greater in white-skinned people living near the equator, so it is not surprising that Australia has been at the fore in research into skin cancer. There are three types of skin cancer associated with sun exposure (Plate 10):

- Basal cell carcinoma (BCC) has been linked to intermittent, intense sunburn and in people with skin types 1 and 2.[8] It tends to occur on the face and is a slow-growing tumour that rarely metastasises, although it can invade deeply and cause considerable morbidity[9]
- Squamous cell carcinoma (SCC) appears to be associated with the lifetime cumulative dose of UV radiation. It therefore occurs on areas of the body most frequently exposed to the sun, e.g. face, scalp or backs of hands. An early lesion caused by such exposure is called actinic keratosis, a precancerous skin lesion comprising thickened scaly skin, but this converts to SCC in only one in 1000 people.[10] It is the second most common skin cancer in Caucasians and can metastasise.
- Malignant melanoma (MM) is the most serious of skin cancers and has the highest mortality of all skin conditions. It appears to be associated with exposure to the sun in childhood and subsequent episodes of burning.[11] MM results from an abnormality in melanocytes and presents as a characteristic mole (Table 9.2). MM usually occurs on the legs of women and the backs of men, often appearing in middle age. It is twice as common in women as it is in men.

There is much work to be done in determining the exact role of UV light in the development of skin cancers. Studies have been hampered by a lack of animal models that can confidently predict changes in human skin.[12] Current research is concentrating on the following areas:

- The effect of UVA and UVB on gene mutations. It is known that UV-induced mutations to the tumour suppressor gene p53 are found in over 90% of SCC cases and in 50% of BCCs.[1] Other mechanisms associated with DNA damage have been identified, particularly associated with dipyridamine dimers.
- The effect of UV exposure on immunosuppression. UV exposure is known to cause immunosuppression, resulting in a lowering of immune surveillance and tumour growth. About one-third of individuals seem to be prone to UV-induced immunosuppression and it has been observed in 90% of individuals with skin cancer.[1] The immunosuppression has largely been shown to be caused by UVA exposure.[12]

Table 9.2 The melanoma checklist[53]

Checkpoint	Comment
Is the mole increasing in size?	Could be an existing mole becoming larger or a new mole
Is it a centimetre or more in diameter?	A non-malignant mole will usually be smaller than the blunt end of a pencil
Is the mole's border irregular or jagged?	Ordinary moles have a regular, smooth shape
Does the mole have varying shades of black or brown within it?	Ordinary moles have even shading
Does the mole look inflamed?	Malignant moles may have a reddish edge
Is the mole bleeding, oozing or crusting?	Not usually seen in an ordinary mole
Is the mole itchy?	Ordinary moles are not associated with pain or itchiness

- The role of UVA exposure in MM and BCC. Both UVA and UVB have been shown to cause SCC, but the exact spectrum of UVA involved in MM and BCC development is not fully understood. A rare form of melanoma, lentigo melanoma, appears to have a strong association with UV exposure. Direct evidence of such a link with other forms of skin cancer is conflicting.[10]
- The type of melanin present in the skin. There is some evidence that developing a tan does not in itself prevent cancer in fair-skinned people. A possible explanation is the presence of a less protective form of melanin (pheomelanin) and reduced skin repair capacity compared with people with darker skin.[12]

On balance, it appears that exposure to UV radiation contributes greatly to SCC. Although the role played by UV exposure in MM and BCC is less well defined, it seems prudent to regard UV exposure as a possible risk factor. Certainly protection from the sun from an early age is a key strategy in reducing the incidence of such cancers.[13]

Skin ageing and damage

A variety of problems are seen in people who expose themselves to the sun and who tan frequently. These are caused by damage to the connective tissue in the dermis; photoaged skin is yellowed, coarse and wrinkled in appearance. These effects have been particularly associated with UVA exposure. It has been suggested that antioxidants and retinoic acid can help control such skin ageing.[1]

Eye problems

Over exposure to UV light can cause an acute eye problem commonly referred to as 'snow blindness'. This is most likely to be experienced when exposed to very bright and reflected sunlight, usually from snow and more frequently at higher altitudes. The UV may damage the surface of the eye, resulting in pain and inflammation. Vision will become blurred and the eyes very sensitive to light, with a resulting spasm of the eyelids. Milder forms can be relieved by the use of artificial tears such as hypromellose BP. In more severe cases a lubricating eye ointment such as Simple eye ointment may need to be applied underneath an eye dressing or pad.[14] Prevention is by adequate use of UV filter glasses for mountaineers; skier's goggles are to be recommended as they have the additional effect of protecting from the wind, which can result in watery eyes.

Chronic overexposure to UV sunlight can result in permanent retinal degeneration. This is of greatest risk in fair-skinned and blue-eyed individuals. Also potentially at risk are those who have had cataract surgery, as even implants with UV filters may not sufficiently protect the retina. Anyone with a family history of such problems or a history of retinal degeneration, more common in older people, should take special care in sunlight. Good-quality glasses with UV filters should be worn by all such individuals.

Polymorphic light eruptions

Ten per cent of the population are prone to a true hypersensitivity reaction to sunlight called polymorphic light eruption.[10] It is less common in those with a darker skin and more likely to be seen in younger women. The reaction most commonly presents as an intensely itchy, spotty (papular/papulovesicular) eczematous eruption. This is sometimes confused with heat rash or prickly heat. The reaction can occur within hours to days of exposure to the sun, sometimes appearing under clothing that allows some penetration of UV light. Such people need to screen themselves as much as possible, particularly from UVA, because it is mainly this wavelength that is responsible for the reaction.

There are some other chronic conditions associated with reactions to UV light that demand extra caution, such as lupus erythematosus and certain porphyrias. A cold sore (herpes simplex) can also be triggered by sunlight.

Drug-induced photosensitivity reactions

Health professionals should be familiar with drugs that have the potential to induce photosensitivity. There are drugs which are known to sensitise the skin to UV light, enhancing its potential to cause acute damage, i.e. sunburn, sometimes referred to as a phototoxic reaction. The more potent photosensitisers, such as the psoralens, have application in treating psoriasis where they are given, either topically or orally, to enhance the effects of UVA treatment. Obviously people treated with these agents should take great care against exposure to the sun until the psoralen has been eliminated from the body. The psoralens are found naturally in certain plants (e.g. bergamot) and contact with these may also cause photosensitivity. A photosensitivity due to contact with plant material is sometimes referred to as a phytophotodermatitis. The reaction may be caused by a number of common citrus fruits (limes and lemons), vegetables (e.g. celery or carrots) and herbs such as fennel and dill. There is also the potential for cosmetics and perfumes to induce a photosensitivity reaction.

There are a number of commonly used medications that will quite reliably cause phototoxic reactions. An example is amiodarone, where the incidence has been reported at 30–50%,[15] and patients on a hospital ward treated with this drug have shown a phototoxic reaction if simply sitting near a window on a sunny day. The reaction to amiodarone can persist for many months after discontinuing therapy. This type of reaction tends to occur a few hours after exposure to the sun; the inflammatory reaction appears as an exaggerated sunburn in well-demarcated areas of the skin that have not been protected from the sun. Continuous exposure can lead to chronic inflammatory changes and skin damage. Those drugs that absorb light in the UV range are potential photosensitisers, and in particular those that have a chlorine substitution within the molecule, e.g. chlorpromazine.[16] Of the medication carried by travellers, antibacterials of various classes are the most likely to cause phototoxicity, including the tetracyclines (e.g. doxycycline), a fluoroquinolone (e.g. ciprofloxacin) or a sulphonamide-containing drug such as pyrimethamine-sulfadoxine (Fansidar). Some non-steroidal anti-inflammatory agents may cause phototoxicity and these are frequently used by travellers as analgesics. Quinine has more rarely been associated with such reactions.

A different and less common form of photosensitivity is a photo-allergic drug reaction. In this form UV light is able to cause structural changes in a drug that has distributed systemically or been applied topically to the skin. A drug so affected, called a hapten, will combine with proteins conferring antigenic properties and initiating an immune response, leading to inflammation of the skin. The rash so formed is very similar to that seen in chronic eczema except that the distribution is confined again to parts of the skin unprotected from light, but perhaps less well demarcated than for phototoxic reactions.

General measures to avoid harm from the sun

Current guidelines are directed not only towards avoiding sunburn but also against developing a tan, although many individuals planning a holiday to sunny climates will take an active decision not to heed such advice. General recommendations regarding avoiding exposure to the sun are summarised in Table 9.3 and Box 9.2, where topically applied sunscreens form just part of the strategy. There is evidence that these guidelines are generally not well adhered to by the public, who view

Table 9.3 Measures to avoid harm from the sun

Advice	Comment
Avoid the sun when at its strongest	Around 3 or 4 hours either side of midday
Avoid direct exposure to the sun by sitting in the shade	Be aware of reflected sunlight
Wear appropriate clothing	Ensure the clothing has a sufficiently close weave
Wear a hat with a brim	Hats protect areas of the face, ears and back of neck
Apply high-factor sunscreen to exposed skin regularly before going out into the sun	Sunscreen should not be the only measure and should not be used to increase overall exposure to the sun. Pay particular attention to sensitive areas such as the soles of feet, backs of knees and nipples
Take particular care if there is a history of skin cancer	Particularly for people with skin types 1 and 2. Extra care is also required for those with precancerous lesions

---

Box 9.2 Health promotion messages

The mnemonic SHADE is Health Promotion England's campaign for safety in the sun. The key messages are to cover up, seek shade, apply sunscreens generously and protect children.

- **S**eek the shade – Especially at midday when the sun is strongest
- **H**ats on! – Protect yourself by wearing a wide-brimmed hat and tightly woven clothing
- **A**pply SPF 15 –Use plenty of high-protection sunscreen
- **D**o not burn – Burning will not protect you and it will not improve your tan
- **E**xercise care – Always protect babies and young children

SPF, sun protection factor.

---

sunscreens as the principal mode of protection against the sun and even these are probably not applied appropriately, as discussed in the section on sunscreens, below. For instance, a study in Switzerland[17] identified that clothing and other methods to shield from the sun were not much used by the public, and although sunscreens were used as the first line of defence they tended to be applied when out-of-doors, e.g. before swimming rather than before exposure to the sun. In a survey of data obtained from 1858 British adults, 35–40% of respondents were intending to develop a tan during the year of the study and about the same proportion reported sunburning in the previous 12 months, with a good correlation found between the observations.[18]

Wearing the correct type of clothing is important (Table 9.1). In Australia, a sun protection factor (SPF) rating for types of clothing has been introduced. Sunglasses that block UV should be used, particularly in situations where there is reflected sunlight, e.g. on ski slopes.

The use of fake or artificial self-tanning products can be recommended as a good cosmetic alternative to a natural tan. These self-tanning creams contain dihydroxyacetone, a chemical that reacts with proteins in the stratum corneum to produce brown coloration similar to a natural tan.[19] As the stratum corneum is shed, so the tan will tend to fade. These products do not offer much protection from the sun (SPF 3–4) and there is a risk that people will assume that they will not get burned with such tans. In one survey there was a tendency for fake tan users to cover up less when in the sun and suffer more sunburn than those who did not use these tanning products, although it was found that they were generally higher users of sunscreen.[20] Inclusion of a sunscreen into these products may give a further false sense of security, as the protection will wear off long before the artificial tan.[21]

A further useful strategy to help minimise skin damage after exposure to the sun is the use of moisturising creams and lotions, applied liberally to exposed skin. The formulation and type are according to personal preference and most would prefer less greasy products if applying to a wide area. It has been suggested that products containing antioxidants, e.g vitamin E and derivatives, will further help with skin repair and minimise damage, perhaps having a photoprotective effect if applied before exposure.[22]

Sunscreens

The first documented use of sunscreens were lotions and ointments of quinine used in the nineteenth century.[23] In the early twentieth century products based on an extract of chestnut were popular. From the 1940s onward, when para-aminobenzoic acid (PABA) was introduced, the range of agents and available formulations mushroomed. With greater affordability of travel overseas since the 1960s, there has been a tendency for holiday-makers to choose destinations of high sun exposure to develop a tan. At this time sunscreens were seen simply as a means of developing a tan gradually without burning, a position that is now thought to be disadvantageous, as discussed. More recently sunscreens of increasingly higher SPF factors have been produced. This concept is often misinterpreted by the public as a 'sunblock effect' that allows unlimited exposure throughout the day and the health professional should advise on their appropriate use by explaining such misunderstandings.

In recent years, there have been a number of controversies regarding the use of sunscreens. These include suggestions that they increase rather than reduce the risk of cancers, reduce vitamin D synthesis in the skin and lose potency when exposed to sunlight.

It is important, therefore, for health professionals to have a good understanding of the scientific principles concerning the use of sunscreens and the evidence for their effectiveness. In the USA, sunscreens are regulated as over-the-counter medicines, and the permitted type and concentration of active ingredients, labelling and definitions of protection are clearly defined.

The active ingredients contained in sunscreen preparations fall into two groups:

1. Absorbent sunscreens, also called organic sunscreens, are chemical agents that absorb UV energy at a molecular level (Fig. 9.1). They contain free electrons that are capable of delocalisation by UV radiation.[2] Energy is then released in the form of heat when the molecule returns to the ground state. Examples include PABA (less commonly used these days), esters of PABA, cinnamates and benzophenones (oxybenzone and mexenone), and dibenzoylmethanes (avobenzone). With the exception of avobenzone, absorbent sunscreens tend to be more effective in the UVB range. PABA and its esters are able to penetrate the outer horny layer of the skin in about 30 minutes to 2 hours so are less easily washed off than the other types.

2. Reflectant or inorganic sunscreens form a reflective barrier to both UVA and UVB radiation. It has also been suggested that they absorb UV radiation through a semiconductor effect.[2] Titanium dioxide is the most widely used compound. It leaves a white, silvery film on the skin, although this is reduced by micronisation. Products may also contain micronised zinc oxide. Thick zinc oxide paste, available as brightly coloured sticks, is a complete sunblock and can be applied to sensitive areas, such as the bridge of the nose. One study has indicated that microfine zinc oxide gives better protection against UVA and causes less whitening on the skin than an equivalent concentration of microfine titanium dioxide.[24]

There has been concern that certain organic sunscreens are not photostable, i.e. they are degraded by sunlight. This has been demonstrated specifically for avobenzone.[25] In spite of such degradation, it is likely that sufficient activity is maintained in periods between reapplication. Photostability can also be improved by formulating the sunscreen with stabilising agents.[1] The active ingredients of sunscreens currently prescribable on the National Health Service are listed in Table 9.4.

SPF and star systems

To allow selection of an appropriate sunscreen, a system of measuring efficacy at screening against UVB has been devised, called the sun protection factor (SPF) rating. The SPF is the difference in the time taken to burn between protected and unprotected skin. For this test, a standard 2 mg/cm^2 dose of sunscreen is applied to skin, which is then exposed to measured doses of UVB radiation until slight erythema appears. The process is repeated on untreated skin. The SPF is the amount of UVB required to produce erythema on treated skin divided by that for untreated skin.

The disadvantage of the SPF system is that it can encourage people to expose their skin to longer periods of sunlight, perhaps contributing to the link between sunscreen use and an increased risk of MM (discussed later). It is also a common observation that some people burn despite the use of high-protection sunscreens. Diffey[26] has attempted to explain these apparent contradictions and has suggested that SPF numbers be dropped in favour of classifying sunscreens as having low to very high protection. He points out that even in tropical conditions, most people are unlikely to receive more than 35 standard erythema doses (a measure of erythemal radiation) of UV in a day. Since two to three doses are required to start burning, an SPF that reduces this by about 15 times (i.e. SPF 15) is all that is required by skin types 2 and 3. However, it has been found that many people only apply sunscreen at a thickness of 0.5–1.3 mg/cm^2, so it is not surprising that most require SPFs of 30 or more to avoid burning. In addition, it has been shown that people often do not cover exposed skin evenly and fail to reapply sunscreen at appropriate intervals. As a result of this observation, suggestions have been made that could enable users to identify the correct amount of product to be applied.[27] In this method the body is divided into 11 areas and two strips of sunscreen, as measured out on the index and middle finger from the middle of the palm, are applied to each area. This will result in an application rate of around 2 mg/cm^2. It is recognised that few people will be willing to apply such copious amounts, so applying just one fingerlength will result in half the SPF stated on a bottle – to achieve an SPF of 15 therefore an SPF 30 cream would need to be used. Furthermore, the rule does not apply to the very popular sunscreen lotions or spray formulations.

There is no agreement on the best method of defining protection from UVA. Because of the long exposure time required before UVA-induced erythema becomes apparent, *in vitro* models have to be used. These models measure the absorbance of UVA light passing through specially prepared tape treated with sunscreen.[28]

Boots the Chemists Ltd was one of the first UK companies to adopt a star system on its sunscreen products in addition to an SPF number. An important factor in any test of UVA screening is the bandwidth of UVA filtered, which should cover both UVAI and UVAII. Table 9.4 lists the UVA/UVB range and maximal absorbance of some common agents. From the table, it can be seen that a blend of sunscreens is required to achieve coverage of all spectra. In particular it is important to check for the presence of avobenzone or micronised zinc oxide in products for adequate protection against UVAI.

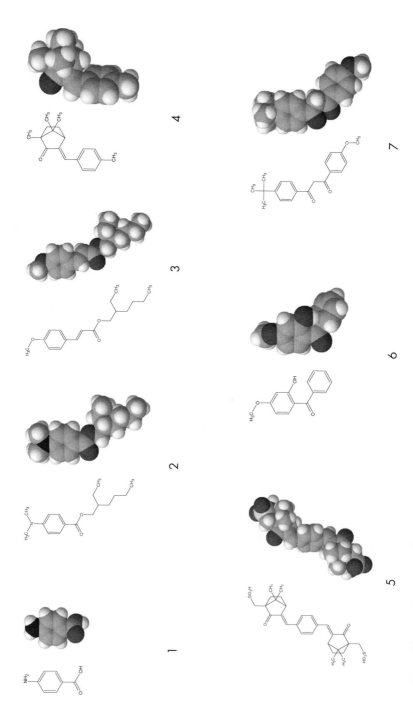

Figure 9.1 Chemical structure of some organic sunscreens.

Table 9.4 The properties of some commonly used sunscreens

Class	Chemical name	Other names	UV absorbance	UV protection
Para-Aminobenzoic acid and derivatives	p-Aminobenzoic acid (1)	PABA	283	UVB
	2-Ethylhexyl p-dimethylamino benzoate (2)	Padimate O; Octyl dimethyl PABA	311	UVB
Cinnamates	2-Ethylhexyl p-methoxycinnamate (3)	Octyl methoxycinnamate; Octinoxate	311	UVB
Camphor derivatives	3-(4-Methylbenzylidene) bornan-2-one (4)	3-(4-Methylbenzylidene)camphor; Enzacomene	300	UVB
	3,3'-(1,4-Phenylene-dimethylidyne)-bis-(7,7-dimethyl-2-oxobicyclo-[2.2.1]) heptane-1-methane-sulfonic acid (5)	Terephthalylidene dicamphor sulfonic acid; Ecamsule	345	UVB, UVAII
Benzophenones	2-Hydroxy-4-methoxy-benzophenone (6)	Oxybenzone Benzophenone-3	288, 325	UVB, UVAII
Dibenzoyl methane derivatives	1-(4-tert-Butylphenyl)-3-(p-methoxyphenyl)-1,3-propanedione (7)	Avobenzone Butylmethoxydibenzoylmethane	358	UVAI
Titanium dioxide			(Range of protection 250–240)	UVB, UVAII
Zinc oxide			(Range of protection 250–380)	

UV, ultraviolet

Some experts have the view that the SPF system does not really reflect protection achieved against the long-term effects of the sun. It has been suggested that products should be classified according to their ability to screen against known markers of skin damage. For instance, it is possible to assess the protection against damage to DNA dipyridamines, mutations to the p53 gene and suppression of immunity.[29] SPF still remains an internationally recognised standard for protection against sunburn.

Choice and application of sunscreen

Until recently, it was common practice to select a sunscreen appropriate to a person's skin type, i.e. those with skin type 1 were advised to use the highest factors. Charts were produced that recommended progressing to lower-factor sunscreens as a tan developed. However, although this approach prevents burning, it does not help prevent longer-term complications.

The philosophy best adopted is that 'no tan is a safe tan' and that sunscreens should be used to prevent tanning. It is now recommended that, rather than selecting specific sunscreens for skin types, those products of SPF 15 or above should be used by all Caucasians. This will simplify choosing a sunscreen and emphasise that the desired outcome is not to develop a tan. Those insisting on a tan may wish to step down the factor used, although anything below SPF 8 is not worthwhile. It is of interest to note that SPFs have been capped at 30 in the USA. In addition, US sunscreens have a standardised measure of UVB, but not UVA protection.[30] A few important points regarding the application of sunscreens are listed below:

- Most people fail to apply sufficient sunscreen. Some groups of users have been identified as particularly poor users of sunscreens. Men in general are less likely than women to use a sunscreen or apply it correctly.[31] Amongst 18–24-year-old European students the median thickness applied was only 0.39 mg/cm^2.[32] It has been estimated that 100 ml will only cover the entire body three times.[33]

- Sunscreen should be applied 30 minutes before exposure to the sun and should be reapplied every 2 hours. There is little evidence to support this suggested reapplication rate, although it would seem reasonable to allow for removal by sweating or abrasion. It has also been pointed out that the normal rate at which the stratum corneum is shed would result in the loss of efficacy in any product after a few hours.[34] However, a study examining efficacy of sunscreens in children found that a single application within a 6-hour period provided the same level of protection as four applications.[35] Applying sunscreen before exposure is more important for PABA-containing products, and is especially important for people with a tendency to burn. Most products become effective 5–10 minutes after application.[2]

- Sunscreens should not be used as a method of increasing the total time of exposure to the sun. Rather they are a convenient way of protecting exposed skin that is not covered by clothing in warm climates.
- Water-resistant sunscreens are claimed to be effective after the body has been immersed in water. In the USA, a 'water-resistant' label is allowed if the SPF level is maintained after 40 minutes of immersion and 'water-proof' after 80 minutes. A recent comparative study found that there was a gradual reduction in protection to between 60 and 90% after four 20-minute immersions in water with a variety of products labelled as either waterproof or water-resistant.[36] This may be particularly important for children playing around water for long periods, where regular reapplication would be prudent.
- The effectiveness of sunscreens can be reduced by storage conditions, e.g. exposure to heat on a beach. For this reason, a fresh supply of sunscreen should be purchased each year.

The correct application of sunscreens will prevent burning. Evidence also indicates that the use of broad-spectrum sunscreens helps to prevent photoageing[34] and is essential for those with photodermatosis. However, as will be described in the next section, there is much debate over the role of these products in preventing skin cancers.

Cancer prevention

There is conflicting evidence that sunscreens protect against MM and not all experts agree on the aetiological link between exposure to UV radiation and certain skin cancers.[37] Some studies have demonstrated protection against MM[38] but others have shown either no protection[11] or an increased risk in those using sunscreens.[39,40] Such research is the subject of much media interest. Health professionals should be aware of the factors that may contribute to these findings:[41]

- Studies often involve questionnaires given to the public. These might be poorly controlled or contain recall bias.
- High-protection sunscreens may not have been available some years ago, and certainly would have given poor protection against UVA, which could have an influence on the development of MM now. Products with good protection against UVAI have only become available relatively recently.

- People developing MM could have been using sunscreens inappropriately to allow increased exposure to the sun, combined with an insufficient rate of reapplication. This former point seems to be borne out by a study conducted on Swiss and French tourists who were randomly assigned to use either an SPF 10 or SPF 30 sunscreen; the group with the higher factor spent a significantly longer time sunbathing.[42]
- There is no good evidence that sunscreens possess carcinogenic properties or that they directly damage the skin.
- Reviews and meta-analysis of the various trials that have examined the relationship between MM and sunscreen use do not appear to indicate any association.[43]

There is more evidence that sunscreens offer good protection against the development of non-melanoma skin cancers. Two trials demonstrated that actinic keratosis is reduced by the application of high-factor sunscreens.[44,45] This correlates with the finding that sunscreens can reduce mutations to p53 tumour suppressor gene.

Adverse effects

Local reactions to sunscreens are often reported and can be associated with the cream formulation and/or active ingredients. Allergic reactions to the active ingredients in sunscreens appear to be uncommon.[46] In one study, despite a reaction rate of 19%, there was no difference between the reaction rate in active and placebo-treated individuals, indicating that the vehicle rather than the active ingredients was responsible for the reaction. Fewer than 10% of these reactions were found to be allergic in nature.[47] Photoallergic reactions to sunscreens are also only very rarely encountered. In a retrospective analysis of photopatch testing on 2715 patients, 52 exhibited photosensitivity to chemicals used in sunscreens, the most common being oxybenzone, accounting for 14 reactions.[48] Physical sunscreens containing only titanium dioxide may be expected to produce fewer adverse events than the organic types, but this has not been proved in practice.

It has also been claimed that overuse of sunscreens can lead to a lack of vitamin D production in the skin, although no clinically relevant effects from this lack have been found and there is no evidence that they increase a tendency for developing osteoporosis.[49]

There appear to have been no well-documented reports of adverse effects due to absorption of sunscreens. It is known that benzophenones are absorbed through the skin and that absorption will be greater for alcohol-based formulations,[50] but there is little in the way of data concerning other individual or combinations of sunscreens.

Prickly heat

Prickly heat, or heat rash, is a common complaint among holiday-makers going to hot, and especially humid, climates.

Despite popular belief, it is not related to exposure to the sun. The correct term for this condition is miliaria rubra and it is caused by a blockage of the sweat glands. The rash is caused by leakage of sweat out of the blocked ducts into the surrounding epidermal tissue, causing an inflammatory reaction.[51] Blockage occurs as a result of prolonged exposure of the skin to sweat (e.g. under occlusive clothing), which forms a keratin plug. It is possibly associated with the presence of certain bacteria.

Common sites for miliaria are the skin folds in areas where clothing may be rubbing. It can also be found in other areas, such as the neck, face and groin, in infants. The red papules give an uncomfortable prickling sensation, rather than itching, and an attack can last several weeks while the blockage clears.

Prickly heat is prevented by ensuring that susceptible areas are kept clean and dry. Wearing loose-fitting, light clothing, showering each night and drying the skin thoroughly can also help to prevent it. The best method of prevention is to stay in a cool or air-conditioned environment.

Calamine lotion or cream will provide some relief, as will hydrocortisone 1% for more severe cases. One small study indicated that symptoms were improved by taking 1 g ascorbic acid daily for 1 week.[52]

Main points

1.   There are three broad problems associated with overexposure to the sun: acute sunburn, chronic skin damage and skin cancers.
2.   Sunburn can be avoided by either taking steps to avoid exposure to the sun or developing a tan. The latter course of action is not advised as developing a tan in Caucasians is known to be associated with skin damage. The relationship between tanning and skin cancers has not been established.
3.   MM is a potentially life-threatening skin cancer related to overexposure to the sun, possibly due to episodes of sunburn. SCC has a stronger link to sun exposure.
4.   There are other conditions called photodermatosis that are activated by sunlight and a number of drugs are known to be associated with

photosensitivity. Prickly heat is not related to sun exposure, but to the plugging of sweat glands.

5.   There are a variety of measures that can be taken to reduce exposure to the sun apart from applying sunscreens, which should be used as part of an overall strategy.

6.   The SPF in sunscreens gives an indication of protection against UVB, measured as the length of time the individual may expose the skin to the sun before burning. Reapplying sunscreen after that time will not give further protection.

7.   There is no universally recognised standard for assessing protection against UVA. Ideally the sunscreen should contain ingredients known to protect against UVB, UVAI and UVAII.

8.   Sunscreens need to be applied quite generously and evenly to achieve the stated SPF and then reapplied during the day. There may be some merit in using factors higher than SPF 15 to allow for lower application rates.

Frequently asked questions

Will a tan protect from developing skin cancer?
Developing a tan will certainly damage skin. Also as a person with a tan will be likely to increase overall exposure to the sun, there will be an increased risk of certain skin cancers.

It has been said that sunscreens actually increase the risk of skin cancer. Is this true?
There is no evidence that the sunscreens themselves are carcinogenic. Studies that seem to show a relationship between sunscreen use and skin cancer are not particularly robust. Some data relate to the use of older sunscreens that did not protect against UVA. It is also possible that the association is due to people using sunscreens to develop a tan gradually, thus increasing overall exposure to the sun.

How do I choose the best sunscreen for my skin type?
If planning to develop a tan then factors lower than SPF 15 can be used depending on destination, fairness of skin and tendency to burn. However, this course of action is not recommended and travellers should be counselled against tanning if possible, and should generally use higher factors.

What is the best way to treat or avoid prickly heat?
This is a very common question and there is a lack of data concerning the best treatments. Photodermatosis or other allergy should be ruled out. Otherwise treatment is empirically based upon that used for any

inflammatory skin reaction, i.e. emollients, oral antihistamines and mild corticosteroids. Keeping the skin dry and clean is advised as a preventive measure.

Can a sunbed prepare for exposure to the sun?
Although modern sunbeds emit more UVB than older types and thus may give some protection, overall this may be insufficient to protect against sunburning and a sunscreen should still be used. Tanning in this way could still predispose to photoageing and cancer, so no more than two courses a year are recommended.

Is an artificial tan safe and will it protect against the sun?
Yes, modern artificial tans have a good safety profile – some older types contained bergamot that should be avoided. They will not offer protection against the sun's rays.

If PABA and its derivatives actually penetrate the skin and therefore need less reapplication, is this an ideal product if swimming?
PABA does not protect against UVA. Therefore in a broad-spectrum screen containing PABA the UVA screen will not penetrate the skin and therefore will more easily be washed off. Also it is important to remind people that, even if PABA is used, it should not encourage overall greater sun exposure.

Is it a good idea always to use cosmetics containing sunscreens? Should sunscreens be used throughout the year in temperate climates to protect against photoageing?
It is unlikely that enough of the product will be used to achieve the stated SPF and other measures should be used to protect the face. In the UK there is little to be gained by applying sunscreens during the winter months (October–March).[54]

References

1. De Buy H, Lev S, Murry J *et al*. Modern approaches to photoprotection. *Dermatol Clin* 2000; 18: 577–590.
2. Rosen C F. Photoprotection. *Semin Cutan Med Surg* 1999; 18: 307–314.
3. Purvis J, Barker D. Sun and the skin. *Pharm J* 1989; 243: 225–227.
4. Hughes G S, Francom S F, Means L K *et al*. Synergistic effects of nonsteroidal and topical corticosteroids in the therapy of sunburn in humans. *Dermatology* 1992; 184: 54–58.
5. Driscol M S, Wagner R F. Clinical management of the acute sunburn reaction. *Cutis* 2000; 66: 53–58.

6. Manning D L, Quigley P. Sunbathing intentions in Irish people travelling to Mediterranean summer holiday destinations. *Eur J Cancer Prev* 2002. 11: 159–163.

7. Hawk J. Sun and the traveller. In: Dawood R, ed. *Travellers' Health: How to Stay Healthy Abroad*, 4th edn. Oxford: Oxford University Press, 2002: 350–354.

8. Kricker A, Armstrong B K, English D R, Heenan P D. Does intermittent sun exposure cause basal cell carcinoma? A case-control study in Western Australia. *Int J Cancer* 1995; 60: 489–494.

9. Dicesare D, Herbert A. Diseases and disorders caused by the sun. In: DuPont H L, Steffen R, eds. *Textbook of Travel Medicine and Health*, 2nd edn. Hamilton, Canada: BC Decker, 2001: 119–130.

10. Taylor C R, Sober A J. Sun exposure and skin disease. *Annu Rev Med* 1996; 47: 181–191.

11. Osterlind A, Tucker M A, Stone B J, Jensen O M. The Danish case-control study of cutaneous melanoma. II The importance of UV-light exposure. *Int J Cancer* 1988; 42: 319–324.

12. Gasparro F P. Sunscreens, skin photobiology, and skin cancer: the need for UVA protection and evaluation of efficacy. *Environ Health Perspect* 2000; 108: 71–78.

13. Armstrong B K, Kricker A. The epidemiology of UV induced skin cancer. *J Photochem Photobiol* 2001; 63: 8–18.

14. Ffytche T. Eye problems. In: Dawood R, ed. *Travellers' Health: How to Stay Healthy Abroad*, 4th edn. Oxford: Oxford University Press, 2002: 427–435.

15. Lee A, Thompson J. Drug-induced skin reactions. In: Lee A, ed. *Adverse Drug Reactions*. London: Pharmaceutical Press, 2001: 19–43.

16. Moore D E. Drug-induced cutaneous photosensitivity: incidence, mechanism, prevention and management. *Drug Safety* 2002; 25: 345–372.

17. Berret J, Liardet S, Scaletta C *et al.* Use of sunscreens in families living in Switzerland. *Dermatology* 2002; 204: 202–208.

18. Stott M A. Tanning and sunburn: knowledge, attitudes and behaviour of people in Great Britain. *J Public Health Med* 1999; 21: 377–384.

19. Draelos Z D. Self-tanning lotions: are they a healthy way to achieve a tan? *Am J Clin Dermatol* 2002; 3: 317–318.

20. Beckmann K R, Kirke B A, McCaul K A, Roder D M. Use of fake tanning lotions in the South Australian population. *Med J Aust* 2001; 174: 75–78.

21. Levy S B. Tanning preparations. *Dermatol Clin* 2000; 18: 591–596.

22. Dreher F, Maibach H. Protective effects of topical antioxidants in humans. *Curr Probl Dermatol* 2001; 29: 157–164.

23. Urbach F. The historical aspects of sunscreens. *J Photochem Photobiol* 2001; 64: 99–104.

24. Pinnell S R, Fairhurst D, Gillies R *et al.* Microfine zinc oxide is a superior sunscreen ingredient to microfine titanium dioxide. *Dermatol Surg* 2000; 26: 309–314.

25. Sayre R M, Dowdy J C. Photostability testing of avobenzone. *Cosmetics Toiletries* 1999; 114: 85–91.

26. Diffey B. Has the sun protection factor had its day? *BMJ* 2000; 320: 176–177.

27. Taylor S, Diffey B. Simple dosage guide for suncreams will help users. *BMJ* 2002; 324: 1526.

28. Diffey B L, Robson J. A new substrate to measure sunscreen protection factors throughout the ultraviolet spectrum. *J Soc Cosmetic Chem* 1989; 40: 127–133.

29. Gil E M, Kim T H. UV-induced immune suppression and sunscreen. *Photodermatol Photoimmunol Photomed* 2000; 16: 101–110.

30. Draelos Z D. A dermatologist's perspective on the final skin monograph. *J Am Acad Dermatol* 2001;44: 109–113.

31. Wright M W, Wright S T, Wagner R F. Mechanisms of sunscreen failure. *J Am Acad Dermatol* 2001; 44: 781–784.

32. Autier P, Boniol M, Severi G, Dore J F. Quantity of sunscreen used by European students. *Br J Dermatol* 2001; 144: 288–291.

33. Morton O. Sunscreens today. *Chemist Druggist* 1997; 247: 22–23.

34. Schaefer H, Moyal D, Fourtainer A. State of the art sunscreens in the prevention of photodermatoses. *J Dermatol Sci* 2000; 23 (suppl.): S62–S67.

35. McLean D, Gallagher R. Sunscreens: use and misuse. *Dermatol Clin* 1998; 16: 219–226.

36. Stokes R P, Diffey B L. The water resistance of sunscreens in day-care products. *Br J Dermatol* 1999; 140: 259–263.

37. Karnauchow P N. Melanoma and sun exposure. *Lancet* 1995; 346: 915.

38. Holly E A, Aston D, Cress R D et al. Cutaneous melanoma in women. 1. Exposure to sunlight, ability to tan and other risk factors to ultraviolet light. *Am J Epidemiol* 1995; 141: 923–933.

39. Westerdahl J, Olsson H, Masback A et al. Is the use of sunscreens a risk factor for malignant melanoma? *Melanoma Res* 1995; 5: 59–65.

40. Autier P, Dore J F, Scifflers E et al. Melanoma and use of sunscreens: an EORTC case-control study in Germany, Belgium and France. *Int J Cancer* 1995; 61: 749–755.

41. Do sunscreens prevent cancer? *Drug Ther Bull* 1998; 36: 49–51.

42. Autier P, Dore J F, Negrier S et al. Sunscreen use and duration of sun exposure: a double-blind, randomized trial. *J Natl Cancer Inst* 1999; 91: 1304–1309.

43. Huncharek M, Kupelnick B. Use of topical sunscreens and the risk of malignant melanoma: a meta-analysis of 9067 patients from 11 case-control studies. *Am J Public Health* 2002; 92: 1173–1177.

44. Thompson S C, Jolley D, Marks R. Reduction of solar keratoses by regular sunscreen use. *N Engl J Med* 1993; 329: 1147–1151.

45. Naylor M F, Boyd A, Smith D W et al. High sun protection factor suncreens in the suppression of actinic neoplasia. *Arch Dermatol* 1995; 131: 170–175.

46. Scauder S, Ippen H. Contact and photocontact sensitivity to sunscreens: a review of a 15-year experience of the literature. *Contact Dermatitis* 1997; 37: 221–232.

47. Foley P, Nixon R, Marks R et al. The frequency of reactions to sunscreens: results of a longitudinal population-based study on the regular use of sunscreens in Australia. *Br J Dermatol* 1993; 128: 512–518.

48. Darvay A, White I R, Rycroft R J et al. Photoallergic contact dermatitis is uncommon. *Br J Dermatol* 2001; 145: 597–601.

49. Farrerons J, Barnadas M, Lopez-Navidad A et al. Sunscreen and risk of osteoporosis in the elderly: a two-year follow-up. *Dermatology* 2001; 202: 27–30.

50. Benson H A. Assessment and clinical implications of absorption of sunscreens across skin. *Am J Clin Dermatol* 2000; 1 :217–224.

51. Feng E, Janniger C. Miliaria. *Cutis* 1995; 55: 213–216.
52. Shamim S M. Treatment of miliaria rubra with ascorbic acid: an open pilot study. *J Pakistan Assoc Dermatol* 2000; 10: 41–43.
53. Grant N. Sun protection and the pharmacist. *Pharm J* 1992; 248: 689–690.
54. Diffey B L. Is daily use of sunscreens of benefit in the UK? *Br J Dermatol* 2002; 146: 659–662.

10

Health problems associated with air and sea transport

This chapter looks at some of the problems encountered when travelling by air or sea. The general area of flight hygiene will also be discussed, together with measures that can be taken to avoid discomfort during the flight. Finally, fitness for flying, an important consideration for those with certain medical conditions, will be discussed.

There are several health problems associated with travelling. Motion sickness is a problem common to any mode of transport via land, sea or air for which pharmacists and other health professionals are often called on to give advice about prevention. For air travel there has been intense media interest in the dangers of 'economy class syndrome', with pharmacists being asked to supply appropriate support stockings to prevent deep-vein thrombosis (DVT) and to offer advice on the necessity of low-dose aspirin. Jet lag is a perennial problem which can be minimised by certain measures in-flight and for which some complementary therapies are claimed to be of help. A further common in-flight problem is associated with barotrauma, particularly concerning the middle ear, and here over-the-counter (OTC) decongestant remedies may be useful.

Motion sickness

Any form of transport, from automobiles to spaceships, can cause motion sickness in animals as well as humans. The exact physiological processes are still not fully understood, despite descriptions of the problem being recorded from ancient times. Undeniably, it is a result of the brain responding inappropriately to certain types of 'unnatural' forms of motion. The implication is that the human brain is designed to register and respond to a regular motion on a two-dimensional plane associated with human self-propelled motion, i.e. walking or running. Evolution has not yet adapted humans to other artificial methods of transport. Motion sickness can also be experienced in other circumstances where the senses are subjected to unusual forms of motion, real or apparent, for instance in flight simulators or in computer-generated virtual environments.

Cause of motion sickness

A popular theory[1] is that of neuronal mismatch, where the brain has developed a particular internal model for controlling posture and balance against normal locomotor activity. When the signals from the senses do not match this internal model over a period of time due to some atypical sustained movement, then the symptoms of motion sickness are experienced. This certainly explains why most will eventually adapt to the form of transport by an updating of the internal model after a few days, but it is not understood how the mismatch gives rise to the specific symptoms. It has been suggested that the vomiting centre in the brainstem region, possibly the nucleus tractus solitarius, controlling orientation is also responsible for detecting the presence of certain poisons.[2] Therefore, the sensory mismatch initiates a physiological response to poisoning, e.g. nausea and vomiting. This hypothesis may explain why smells and tastes can potentiate the sickness, i.e. a reaction to a potential poison. The vomiting centre in the brainstem is thought to receive a number of inputs, including those from the vestibular apparatus, chemoreceptor trigger zone and autonomic nervous system to cause emesis. Inputs from the higher centres may explain the relationship of a tendency to motion sickness and anxiety or certain personality types, although sickness from the anxiety of flying is unrelated to motion sickness.

The motion sickness response also involves activation of the autonomic nervous system, with parasympathetic stimulation causing stomach emptying and sympathetic stimulation causing other symptoms such as increased heart rate and cold sweats. A large part of the sensory input is connected to the vestibular sensory system that is mediated via the middle ear, and deaf mutes as well as dogs that have had the vestibular apparatus removed are known not to suffer from motion sickness. However, this is not the only important input and a visual mismatch as well as that contributed by mechanoreceptors in the skin and musculoskeletal system will all contribute.

A common observation is that not all individuals are equally susceptible to motion sickness. It has been estimated that, although everyone is susceptible to some form of motion sickness, about 5% will suffer very badly and a further 5% will only have minimal symptoms.[3] In any particular journey the incidence among passengers and crew will vary depending on the severity of stimulus, e.g. disturbance in motion due to the weather.

Table 10.1 summarises those characteristics that have been shown to predispose an individual to motion sickness. An increased susceptibility during pregnancy may be expected to occur, particularly during the early stages, compounding so-called morning sickness. General gastrointestinal upset and hormonal changes associated with menstruation might also be expected to worsen motion sickness. In particular, headache at the time of menstruation increases the incidence of motion sickness and those suffering from migraine are also more likely to be affected.[4] Motion sickness is uncommon in children under the age of 2 years and most common in those aged between 2 and 12 years. In air sickness, anxiety may play a large part in the syndrome, and being well rested can help, although general fitness is not protective. Chinese people seem more prone to the problem than those of European origin. Studies have also identified the types and frequencies of motion most likely to initiate motion sickness (Table 10.1). Surprisingly, those who are more fit tend to have a greater susceptibility. Being well rested may lessen symptoms, but sleep loss through a prolonged period of motion sickness may set up a vicious cycle of sleep deprivation. Many will experience worsening symptoms when exposed to strong smells or foods, as described above.

Table 10.1 Predisposing factors to motion sickness

Factor	Comment
Gender	More common in women than in men (1:1.7). Also greater around menstruation and during pregnancy
Age	< 2 years rare 2–12 years common, maximal at 12 years 12–21 years, declining incidence > 21 years significant decline with advancing age
Mental state	Fatigue, sleep deprivation, anxiety
Race	Chinese
Physical fitness	Aerobic fitness increases
Secondary provocative agents	Unpleasant smells, smell or sight of food, sound of others vomiting
Primary provocative agents	Ships – vertical oscillations at 0.2 Hz Cars/airplanes – linear acceleration and cornering/banking

Symptoms and strategies to avoid motion sickness

The symptoms of motion sickness can vary from mild fatigue and drowsiness to a life-threatening dehydration due to excessive vomiting. Most will experience varying degrees of nausea and vomiting accompanied by malaise, abdominal discomfort and cold sweats. There is often an 'avalanche' of symptoms, beginning with slight abdominal discomfort followed by pallor, sweating, light-headedness and depression which progress to nausea and vomiting. Drowsiness and lethargy may persist for some hours after vomiting has resolved. As described, the phenomenon is associated with autonomic nervous activity and a number of common symptoms reflect the stimulation of the parasympathetic system such as increased salivation, flatulence and the sympathetic system, e.g. cold sweats and pallor. Drowsiness seems particularly pronounced in children.

There are a number of common strategies that can be employed to alleviate the symptoms, although none is usually completely successful. The principle here is to attempt to minimise the sensory input of the abnormal plane of movement:

- For those on board a ship it is often recommended to try to stay on the deck and fix the eyes on the horizon. This will provide a fixed point of reference for the senses. If below deck, the centre of the ship will provide the least movement at the frequencies causing motion sickness. If it is not possible to stay on deck, the recommendation is therefore to lie down with eyes closed towards the centre of the ship. One trial has indicated that position on the ship makes no significant difference to motion sickness.[5] Generally, lying down produces less nausea then upright positions.
- In an airplane less turbulence is felt by those sitting over the wings.
- Car sickness is a particularly common problem for children, who for safety reasons are usually sitting in the back seats. It is acknowledged that sitting in the front is associated with less sickness. The driver also does not usually suffer from the motion sickness and can help the passenger by taking bends slowly and avoiding powerful acceleration. Reading as a passenger also seems to promote sickness and therefore looking out of the window should be encouraged. The advantage of good forward vision was demonstrated in a study of coach passengers.[6]

After a few days most individuals will adapt to the new type of motion, popularly referred to as 'getting your sea legs', which could be explained as a resetting of the neuronal mismatch. On return to land after a long sea journey the new internal model will have to readapt to the more stable conditions and after a few months the adaptation will be lost.

This process can initially manifest as 'mal de débarquement' where the individual who has adapted to motion sickness then develops symptoms of disorientation and nausea on return, for instance, on reaching land after a long sea journey. The symptoms from this syndrome are much milder than those of motion sickness, and probably represent a far easier adaptation to the internal model (i.e. correction of neuronal mismatch), suggesting that the model of normal motion is 'remembered' by the individual and therefore quickly replaces that used to adapt to the abnormal motion.

As most individuals will adapt to the new motion at sea after a few days, this probably represents the best form of treatment. Alcohol is best avoided due to the effect on the vestibular apparatus and the effects of the disturbance on balance can last for several hours after consuming even minimal amounts of alcohol.[7] In particular, it is a common experience that consuming too much alcohol results in 'room spinning' when lying down, so obviously such an effect would be extremely undesirable if suffering from motion sickness.

Airsickness is less common except in extremes of air turbulence. A further strategy in all types of travel is to try to restrict head movements, for instance, by pressing the head firmly against a seat.

Medication used to prevent and treat motion sickness

The pharmacist will become most closely involved when asked to recommend prophylactic OTC medicines for motion sickness. The two most widely used classes of medication are the antihistamine and anticholinergic groups. The mechanisms of action of drugs that prevent motion sickness are obscure and they have been identified as having a beneficial effect from the vast number of substances used over the past century. It is probable that they inhibit the inputs from the vestibular nuclei to the vomiting centre, i.e. the cholinergic activity responsible for initiating vomiting. It is likely that the anticholinergic central nervous system (CNS) properties of the antihistamines used in the management of motion sickness account for most of their activity, and the newer non-sedating antihistamines are not known to be effective. The principal side-effects of such medications are well known: drowsiness in the case of antihistamines, and dry mouth and eyes for anticholinergic agents. Anticholinergic agents can also cause drowsiness and there are some contraindications to their use, such as glaucoma and urinary retention.

Table 10.2 summarises the OTC products available for motion sickness. All must be taken in advance of travel and are of little use once

Table 10.2 Over-the-counter drugs for motion sickness

Drugs	Brand name	Minimum licensed age	Time for onset of maximum effect	Duration of action
Hyoscine hydrobromide	Kwells Joy-rides	4 years	30 minutes	4 hours
Cinnarizine	Stugeron	5 years	4 hours	8 hours
Promethazine teoclate	Avomine	5 years	2 hours	24 hours
Promethazine hydrochloride	Phenergan	2 years	2 hours	18 hours
Meclozine hydrochloride	Sea-legs	2 years	1 hour	12 hours

symptoms have begun. Hyoscine takes the shortest time for onset of action but also has the shortest duration; it is the preferred choice for relatively short journeys. Of the antihistamines, promethazine has the most potent CNS anticholinergic properties and would tend to induce a high degree of drowsiness, sometimes being the preferred medication for young children during a night-time journey. Cinnarizine is believed by many to be the drug of choice if longer protection is desired and of all the antihistamines has the least tendency to cause drowsiness. Onset of action for cinnarizine has been claimed to be improved if the tablets are allowed to dissolve in the mouth.[8] Part of the action of cinnarizine may be related to its calcium antagonist properties, although no conclusive evidence regarding the usefulness of calcium antagonists such as nifedipine in the management of motion sickness has been demonstrated.[7]

Use of hyoscine in the form of transdermal patches (prescription-only medicine) will increase the duration of action. The usual side-effects may be present and sometimes persist long after the patches are removed, owing to accumulation in the skin.[9] They may also actually delay the adaptation process.[10] Very young children should not take hyoscine and it is best avoided in the elderly. If one drug does not work in an individual it is worth trying another, ideally of a different class.

Dopamine antagonists, such as metoclopramide, are generally ineffective in motion sickness. One study did report a synergistic effect in the combined use of cinnarizine and domperidone.[11]

Phenytoin has been shown to be one of the most effective agents in preventing motion sickness.[12] In cases of severe motion sickness, 25–50 mg of intramuscular promethazine is the usual treatment. A further effective regimen is the combination of dexamfetamine 5–10 mg with hyoscine,[3] but as the former is a controlled drug it would not normally be prescribed for this indication.

Other measures of preventing motion sickness

There have been a number of suggestions regarding treatments and methods of preventing motion sickness which do not have any strong evidence base. These include:

- Wrist bands that apply pressure to the acupuncture point called P6; laboratory trials indicate that they are ineffective.[13] One trial using a device designed to simulate abnormal motion demonstrated that subjects experienced less nausea and gastric activity on the days the band was worn compared to other days when it was not applied.[14] However, the trial did not include a control group of any type for comparison. There does appear to be some evidence that small devices worn on the wrist that electrically stimulate P6 may provide some relief of motion sickness.[15]
- Ginger tablets or powder were identified in an early study as possibly being superior to some antihistamines[16] but this was not confirmed by a later study, which found it to be ineffective.[17] Ginger has been shown to be equally as effective as seven other commonly used compounds, including cinnarizine and hyoscine, in a more recent trial conducted on seafarers in quite extreme weather conditions.[18]
- Conductive metal strips fitted to the rear of cars.
- Dietary strategies.
- A small piece of cotton in the external ear canal (left ear if right-handed, opposite if left-handed).
- It has been observed that children wearing prism glasses for reading problems did not suffer car sickness.[4]

Jet lag

Jet lag is a distinctly modern problem associated with flights across multiple time zones. It is essentially due to a disruption of the circadian rhythm. The body's physiological processes are timed to a day-and-night cycle, and the timing of these cycles is taken from certain environmental cues or 'zeitgebers', of which light and temperature are the strongest contributors. Other cues may include the timing of meals and social factors, such as work or home environments. The effect of light on the retina will suppress melatonin release from the pineal gland and there has been much interest in the role of this hormone in modulating circadian rhythm and the effects of jet lag. A further consideration, beyond disturbance to circadian rhythm, is that air travel at night may well disturb the usual cycle of rest and contribute to the symptoms experienced.

The typical symptoms consist of daytime fatigue and sleeplessness at night after arrival at the destination. This will make it difficult for the individual to concentrate and carry out complex tasks. The affected person may be irritable, exhibit poor motivation and suffer from headaches. The symptoms can persist for up to a week after arrival. There is a variation among individuals to susceptibility and the type of trip undertaken has also been shown to influence severity (Table 10.3).

Recovery after eastern flight takes longer than western flight and is related to the fact that the body clock is set to a cycle of around 25 hours, so that adaptation to an extended day after westward flight does become easier. This is central to understanding the adaptive processes that can be used in altering the sleep/activity cycle to help resolve jet lag. As an example, assume that an individual travels from New York to London and leaves at 10 a.m., which is 3 p.m. in London. Assuming an 8-hour flight, the local time of arrival will be 11 p.m. but the internal body clock (still on New York time) will believe it to be just 6 p.m. Therefore the body clock is required to shift forward by 5 hours (phase advance), in other words the individual must try to get to sleep at a time when the body clock is saying it is early evening. However, if the same situation takes place travelling westward then leaving at 10 a.m. with an arrival at 1 p.m. local time will be equivalent to an internal clock set at 6 p.m. This means the individual needs to move back the body clock (phase delay), i.e. will have to stay awake longer but will find it easier to get to sleep (equivalent to going to bed late). In general the body does resynchronise more easily to a longer day, as described. A further factor

Table 10.3 Factors that influence severity of jet lag

Factor	Comment
Direction	Westward flight is better tolerated than eastward flight. It is easier to adapt to the new time by a phase delay
Age	Worse in older people
Zones crossed	The more time zones that are crossed, the more sleep and activity cycles become out of phase with other circadian rhythms
Napping	Unplanned napping on arrival reinforces zeitgebers from departure time zone

is that eastern flights are often scheduled in the early evening, so that leaving New York at 6 p.m., the plane will arrive at 7 a.m. local time, with the internal clock set at 2 a.m. and unless the subject has slept in flight, a potentially great deal of sleep has been lost and there are many hours until bedtime at the destination. Problems will particularly arise, therefore, if a phase delay is attempted after an eastward flight – in the first example the individual progressively goes to bed later in local time, and the required phase shift is 17 hours. On the other hand, for an eastward trip over 10 times zones a phase delay would be more practical.[1]

Managing and preventing jet lag provoke a great deal of interest and many strategies have been suggested ranging from proven, useful measures to outright quackery. Box 10.1 describes a variety of countermeasures that have been selected. Essentially these fall into three categories: planning of the journey and sleep adaptation strategies, attempting to improve awareness/wakefulness on arrival and adjusting the circadian rhythm. Ultimately experienced long-haul travellers will discover a combination of strategies that works the best for them.

Advanced planning and sleep adaptation

An important measure is to be well-rested before departure by ensuring a few nights of good, uninterrupted sleep. Anticipating some jet lag in the itinerary on arrival is also useful so that any activities requiring a high level of alertness can be avoided. The most consistently proven strategy is that of adaptation to the local sleep/activity periods. This will involve phase shifting to attempt to sleep at times outside the home-set circadian rhythms.

Sleep should be attempted at the local time on arrival even if not feeling tired and the usual 'sleep hygiene' measures may prove useful: avoiding caffeine, sleeping in a quiet, darkened room, warm baths, not going to bed too soon after eating a large meal and taking milky drinks. It is generally better to get up rather than lying in bed for long periods of time unable to sleep. Alcohol should be avoided to induce sleep, as quality of sleep is poor and early wakening is likely to occur. Often the traveller will have little problem sleeping on the first night of arrival owing to the rigours of the flight and lack of sleep, so problems are more likely to be experienced on subsequent nights. Hypnotics may have a use here, particularly in the second night after arrival when sleep can be fragmented. In this case, a low dose of a short-acting hypnotic such as zopiclone could be prescribed to be taken on no more than 3 consecutive nights. It may be worth considering trying the medicine to

---

Box 10.1 Prevention and management of jet lag

Advance planning
- Sleep well for a few nights before departure
- Avoid undertaking critical tasks immediately on arrival
- Adapt to local time – consider hypnotics (moderate evidence of usefulness[47])
- Keep to original local time if visit is less than 72 hours
- During flight, sleep and eat at destination times – consider hypnotics
- Take 'power naps' if tired during the daytime on arrival

Increase alertness
- Caffeine
- Aromatherapy
- High-protein meals

Reset circadian rhythms
- Exposure to bright light at appropriate times (moderate evidence of usefulness[47])
- Melatonin
- Exercise

---

identify adverse or hangover effects before departure. Zopiclone has been demonstrated in one study to have a beneficial effect on sleep fragmentation and daytime activity, although this was only examined after westward flights.[19] A trial on a similar hypnotic called zolpidem found it to be somewhat superior to melatonin when taken during the flight and for 4 days thereafter.[20] In general it is best to aim for the same amount of sleep taken within a 24-hour period as the individual normally has at home.

The adaptive process should really begin while in flight by setting watches to the destination times, then taking meals and sleeping according to those times. Sleep will be aided by good 'flight hygiene', as summarised in Box 10.2. Otherwise a short hypnotic could be considered to aid sleep in anticipation of the destination times, but the warnings below regarding DVT should be noted.

If the stay is less than 72 hours it may be advisable to avoid adapting to the new time zone as this will cause less disruption on return. Whether attempting to adapt or not, there will be times during the day when fatigue will necessitate a nap. In these circumstances 'power naps' of around 40 minutes have been suggested as the best approach. It has

---

Box 10.2 General recommendations for healthy flying

- Avoid large meals at unusual times
- Avoid excessive caffeine and alcohol
- Drink plenty of water or soft drinks
- Wear loose-fitting clothing
- Try to move around as much as possible and perform leg exercises

---

been observed that a nap of between 40 and 120 minutes can result in sleep inertia such that the subject feels more fatigued on awakening. If attempting adaptation then such naps should coincide with afternoon or night at home time.[21]

Improving alertness

Caffeine as a stimulant is recommended in a number of sources when wakefulness is critical. Other strategies, such as aromatherapy and high-protein diets, are lacking in good evidence to support their usefulness.

Synchronisation of circadian rhythm

The area of circadian rhythm synchronisation has been of interest, particularly since the use of melatonin was suggested in the early 1990s. It has been well demonstrated that light is important in setting the circadian rhythm and it has been shown in some studies that exposure to bright sunlight will improve adaptation. There have been further suggestions that phase shifting is enhanced by careful exposure to light at certain times of the day. Therefore, bright light in the morning (5–11 a.m.) has been claimed to advance the body clock and bright light in the evening (10 p.m.–4 a.m.) to delay the clock. This will result in avoiding morning light and seeking evening light after an eastward flight and the opposite after westward flights. Tables have been produced which describe the ideal times of day to seek or avoid bright light depending on the direction of travel and the number of time zones crossed.[22] A useful programme produced on the Medical Advisory Service for Travellers Abroad (MASTA) website allows entry of the flight itinerary and then produces a list of suggested light exposure times (see Chapter 1). Unfortunately, bright sunlight cannot always be found at the stated times of day and artificial light has not been demonstrated to have the same benefits. It is probably more practical to advise daytime exposure generally at the destination after westward flights and perhaps to avoid morning light after eastward flights crossing 8–10 time zones.

Linked to the findings that light can alter circadian rhythm is the contentious issue of the role of melatonin. This substance is secreted at night by the pineal gland. Production is suppressed by daylight. It is thought to play an important role in setting the circadian rhythm:[23] if taken in the morning it delays the circadian rhythm and if taken at night it will induce an advance.[24] The theory is that oral melatonin can act as a chronobiotic if taken at destination night-time.

Anecdotally many travellers have claimed benefit from taking melatonin tablets, currently unlicensed for this indication in the UK. The mode of action is uncertain, because as well as potentially altering circadian rhythm it also has a mild sedative affect in its own right, thus aiding sleep. It has been suggested that the hormone is best taken in the early evening at the new time zone if being used for its potential as a hypnotic. In terms of use as a chronobiotic then timing of dosing may be more critical. For eastward flights it has been suggested that melatonin should be taken before flight at the time of the destination's early evening and then at bedtime for 4 days after the flight. However, melatonin should not be taken during during the day prior to a flight due to its sedative properties. For westward flights it can be taken after about 11 p.m. for 4 days following the flight.[25] A dose of 5 mg of a non-sustained-release tablet may be optimal.[26] More precise tables for timing melatonin dosage have been devised, describing optimal timing of melatonin following flight across different time zones.[27]

The evidence concerning the effectiveness of melatonin does remain controversial. A number of small trials[28] have indicated that melatonin may reduce the severity and duration of jet lag, although the results do not show a consistent benefit in all situations. For instance, one study on westward flight in passengers showed little benefit on arrival, whereas some benefit was seen after the return journey. These studies tend to use subjective methods to assess benefit, such as visual analogue scores. Laboratory studies examining sleep quality and sleep/wake cycle changes have yielded inconsistent results.[29] A larger study involving 586 travellers[29] did note a 50% reduction in jet lag scores compared with placebo. The major side-effect of sleepiness occurred in 8.3% of the melatonin group. This side-effect will contraindicate its use by airline pilots. A review of nine trials by the Cochrane database concluded that there is sufficient evidence to support the use of short-acting preparations of melatonin in relieving jet lag if taken before bedtime at the destination country, particularly after an eastward flight.[30] They found little evidence regarding adverse effects, other than drowsiness if taken at inappropriate times. It was also noted that melatonin should be avoided by epileptics and those on warfarin therapy.

Melatonin is not currently licensed in the UK, although it is available as a dietary supplement in the USA. As the usual strict manufacturing guidelines regarding pharmaceutical preparation are not applicable to such preparations, large variations in quality and bioavailability have been found,[31] perhaps accounting by the interindividual variations in response sometimes reported.

Deep-vein thrombosis

There has been much controversy in recent years over the claim that those flying long-haul are more prone to developing DVTs, potentially leading to the life-threatening complication of pulmonary embolism. The most important factor in this problem is believed to be the cramped conditions and long periods of immobility encountered, particularly in standard-fare cabins, giving rise to the term 'economy class syndrome'. In fact, a similar problem may occur if a traveller using other forms of transport, e.g. coaches, is immobile for many hours. There is some evidence that the lower partial pressure of oxygen during flight compared with that at ground level, as discussed later, may also have an influence on blood-clotting mechanisms.[32] Consuming large amounts of alcohol during flight could contribute to dehydration and a sluggish circulation.

DVTs developing in the leg may be symptomless and can lead to embolism without warning. Otherwise pain, worse if the foot is flexed upward, and tenderness may indicate the presence of a clot.

Proving that DVTs are an increased risk overall to those who undertake long-haul flights poses a number of methodological problems:

- There is general agreement that the risks of developing DVTs during flight or shortly after is low taking into account the number of people travelling by air. Also the incidence of DVTs in the general population is of a low order. Therefore large studies may be needed to demonstrate the increased risk for travel.
- Many who develop DVTs have no symptoms and only a very small number will progress to life-threatening pulmonary embolism. Others may experience local damage and some morbidity.
- The risk factors known to be associated with DVTs have been derived from studies on postsurgical patients (about 10% of postsurgical patients

developing a DVT suffer from a pulmonary embolism) and may not relate precisely to those most at risk due to flight.

- There is a known subgroup of the population who have an inherent disposition to developing DVT but it is not possible to identify such individuals easily.

Until recently there were just three case-control studies which gave somewhat conflicting results regarding an association between DVT and flying.[33] In two of these studies, which did record an increased risk of thromboembolism, there was no differentiation in the results between transport via land and air, and possible potential for referral bias. A third study found no association, but the number of subjects involved with air travel was small.[34] A randomised trial examining the protential benefits of compression hosiery[35] found that 10% of airline passengers not wearing below-knee stockings developed signs of clotting when assessed by ultrasonography, whereas none was found in those using such stockings. Unlike the case-control studies, those with a previous history of thromboembolism were excluded and flight duration was much longer. There was some possibility of bias in the ultrasonography used to assess the subjects. In the LONFLIT2 study of similar design,[36] 4–5% of high-risk subjects developed DVT, which was significantly reduced in those wearing below-knee stockings. In the LONFLIT1 study comparing high- and low-risk groups, no DVTs were observed in the low-risk subjects compared with 4.9% in the high-risk subjects. Recently, a study examining the incidence of pulmonary embolism in a large number of passengers arriving at Charles de Gaulle airport in Paris[37] did find a strong association between distance travelled and incidence: 0.01 cases per million in journeys under 5000 km, 1.5 cases per million over 5000 km and 4.8 cases per million over 10 000 km. Because of the design of the study, the actual incidence is likely to be an underestimate.

There now seems to be general agreement that the conditions posed by long-haul flight represent an increased risk that is as yet not fully quantified. Furthermore, it seems reasonable to assume that those individuals (Table 10.4) known to be at increased risk generally of DVT would also be prone to developing flight-related DVT. Other possible risk factors may include smoking and varicose veins, although it has been claimed that physiological changes in smokers who are not allowed to smoke during flight may contribute to a risk. Obesity may be a risk if it contributes to poor mobility. Also those who are tall may encounter problems with posture.

Table 10.4 Recommendations for the prevention of travel-related deep-vein thrombosis (DVT)

Class	Recommendation
All passengers	• Move around as much as possible and exercise calf muscles half-hourly by flexing and rotating ankles for a few minutes • Avoid excessive alcohol and caffeine. Drink plenty of other fluids
Extra precautions for those at minor risk One or more of: • 40 years • Very tall/short • Previous leg swelling • Recent minor leg injury or minor surgery • Extensive varicose veins	• Avoid caffeine, alcohol or tranquillisers • Take only short naps unless in a normal sleeping position • Avoid leg discomfort and crossing legs • Consider support stockings
Extra precautions for those at moderate risk One or more of: • Recent heart disease • Pregnant or hormonal medication • Recent major leg injury or surgery • Family history of DVT	As for moderate risk plus: • Seek professional medical advice concerning potential risks, need for support stockings and prophylactic aspirin
Extra precautions for those at substantial risk • One or more of: • Previous or current DVT • Known clotting tendency • Recent major surgery or stroke • Current malignant disease or chemotherapy • Paralysed lower limb	• Consider postponing flight and take medical advice • Use all of above recommendations and low-molecular-weight heparin instead of aspirin

Essentially any factors, including posture when asleep and tight clothing, that restrict movement and hence circulation may increase risk. It has been suggested that taking hypnotics may present a danger in the overlong maintenance of a poor posture when asleep. Similarly, somnolence due to alcohol may contribute to the overall reduced mobility.[38]

The reduced oxygen pressure may lead to abdominal distension further impeding circulation (discussed later). Low cabin humidity combined with a tendency to drink coffee and alcohol could lead to a reduced circulating volume. Undoubtedly it is the sum of a combination of factors which would most contribute to the development of DVTs.

The UK House of Lords expert committee has recently made recommendations[39] concerning the approach to be taken regarding prevention of DVTs in air travellers and these are summarised in Table 10.4. It follows that if immobility is the prime causative factor for these problems then moving around the cabin as much as possible would help minimise the risks. This is not very practical in a full airplane, where there are great restrictions in space. It is commonly advised that passengers attempt regular leg exercise from the seated position as an alternative. Unfortunately such strategies do not appear to improve circulation greatly.[40] It has been suggested that in order to attain such improvements then exercising the legs against some resistance is required, and portable inflatable paddle devices are now available for this purpose. It may be tempting to believe that the greater space available in higher-class seating would allow greater movement and hence less incidence of DVT. There does not seem to be any direct evidence that this is the case, presumably because such passengers still spend a large proportion of the flight relatively immobile.

Maintaining hydration is a useful general measure by consuming soft drinks and avoiding alcohol or coffee, which has a diuretic effect. The other main strategies involve improving venous return by compression stockings and the use of anticoagulant strategies. Those at highest risk may require prophylactic injections of heparin.

Pharmacists may be particularly involved regarding a decision to take aspirin and the choice of appropriate compression hosiery. Those falling into minor risk groups may wish to take aspirin even though not specifically recommended for such individuals by the expert committee. The use of low-dose aspirin has been suggested for the prevention of thrombosis, although the evidence base for use in this context is not strong. Most of the evidence is derived from studies in prevention of DVT in postsurgical patients, but even here heparinisation is still the prophylactic of choice. Furthermore, the suggested regimen has been derived purely empirically and there is no consensus. Taking just one 150 mg dose 2 hours before travel has been suggested.[41] In addition this is as yet an unlicensed indication for any aspirin products currently marketed, so it remains a professional judgement to be made by pharmacists when supplying aspirin for this use.

Also the subject of some debate is the ideal compression hosiery to be used. It has been suggested that class 1 stockings (14–17 mmHg compression) be used because class 2 (18–24 mmHg) may be difficult for people to fit during flight, although this view is not shared by all experts.[42] Of the ready-made stockings marketed for travellers, Mediven are rated at 18–21 mmHg, Scholl and Activa at 14–17 mmHg.

A further consequence of immobility is the commonly experienced swelling of the legs during a long-haul flight. It is best to avoid tight-fitting shoes when flying for this reason.

Other problems of air travel

When flying in a pressurised aircraft the partial pressure of oxygen is not equalised to that at sea level, but is the same as that at about 6000 feet in altitude. Expansion of gas in body cavities can lead to potential problems and the low oxygen partial pressure poses a danger for those with various medical conditions.

Barotrauma

A common problem is pain in the ears when there is a rapid change in altitude, particularly when descending. This is known as otic baro-trauma and is due to a failure in equalisation in pressure between the area behind the eardrum (the middle ear or tympanic cavity) and the outside environment. As the outside pressure rises, so the air in the middle ear shrinks, creating a negative pressure that must be equalised by air entering the middle ear, otherwise the inward pressure on the tympanic membrane could be painful and potentially damaging. Such equalisation is made via the Eustachian tube that connects the ear to the nasopharynx. On rapid descent the negative pressure tends to close the tube and physical manoeuvres may be needed to force it open. In particular any middle-ear inflammation or congestion would tend to impede the opening of the tube. Thus it is advisable to avoid flying if suffering conditions such as acute otitis media or sinusitis.

To relieve the symptoms there are two manoeuvres described which can aid in the opening of the Eustachian tubes:[43]

- Toynbee manoeuvre. Swallowing with the nose held shut is effective on the ground and is used in diagnosis when examining the ear.

- Valsalva manoeuvre. Attempting forcible expiration with the lips closed and nostrils squeezed together is probably the most popular method.

A useful variation on the Valsalva manoeuvre, called the Frenzel manoeuvre, involves also swallowing at the same time as the forcible expiration with closed lips and nostrils. The sinus must also vent into the back of the nose through small holes called ostia and this may be impeded by sinusitis. Sinus barotrauma is uncommon but unpleasant.

The pain will often continue on landing as the tissues behind the eardrum are damaged and inflamed (otitis). Fluid from inflamed tissue will tend to accumulate, being felt moving when the head is shaken, further increasing pressure and pain. Complications of barotrauma can include rupture of the tympanic membrane and secondary ear infections. However, the small perforations that may result will heal spontaneously after about a week. Treatment involves the use of decongestants such as pseudoephedrine, oral antibiotics when indicated and attempting to open the Eustachian tubes using the manoeuvres described above. Similarly, a sinus barotrauma may result in an infection and sinusitis requiring antibiotic treatment, e.g. a broad-spectrum antibiotic such as amoxicillin.

Decongestants are often recommended prophylactically for those who have a cold, sinus congestion or a history of middle-ear infections. It has been suggested that oral pseudoephedrine be taken an hour or so before descent. It can be combined with a topical nasal decongestant such as xylometazoline. There have been few studies to quantify the usefulness of such decongestants, and commercial airline pilots are not permitted to take such oral medicines. One study did examine the effects of a high-dose pseudoephedrine preparation (120 mg) compared with xylometazoline in those with a history of barotrauma. Although pseudoephedrine was of some benefit, xylometazoline was found to be no different from placebo.[44]

One potential minor problem is that any gas held in the gastrointestinal tract tends to expand and stretch the abdomen at altitude. This is a common experience on airplanes, where passengers may feel bloated and clothing around the waist feels tight. It is advisable to avoid eating foods such as Brussels sprouts and beans, which are known to produce excessive gas.

A further complication of barotrauma is experienced as a toothache during flight, known as aerodontalgia. In this condition air becomes trapped under a filled tooth cavity, so that as gas expands at altitude the resulting pressure beneath the tooth gives rise to the discomfort experienced. Replacement with a new filling will often solve the problem. Sometimes the problem is due to a decaying tooth that releases gas which then becomes trapped in a cavity.

Fitness to travel

Fitness for air travel is a frequent reason for consultation with a medical practitioner before flight. This should be done well in advance of travel, to allow completion of a International Air Transport's standard Medical Information form (MEDIF) detailing the general fitness to travel and any special medical requirements during flight.

The fact that some individuals have a chronic condition that may be exacerbated by lower oxygen partial pressure, for instance, those with a severe chronic obstructive airways disease or heart failure, is an important consideration. In some circumstances flight would not be advised unless extra oxygen is available, and this can usually be arranged in advance. The range of conditions that require special consideration is summarised in Table 10.5 and all patients in these categories should consult their general practitioner before flying.[45,46] Also note the problems of decompression sickness mentioned in Chapter 8, and that deep-sea divers should leave an adequate time between last dive and flight.

Recent myocardial infarction, unstable angina or unstable heart failure can all potentially be contraindications to flying. If an individual is able to walk 100 metres without experiencing symptoms of angina or dyspnoea then it is generally considered that he or she will be fit to fly without an additional oxygen supply provided the condition is stable. As a rule of thumb this is roughly the distance that may be walked from departure gate to aircraft. People with severe chronic obstructive airways disease may not be able to fly; others with less severe disease may require supplemental oxygen.

Because of potential gas expansion in body cavities, flying may be contraindicated after some forms of recent surgery, when air could become potentially trapped within a body cavity. This would include recent abdominal and thoracic surgery and a pneumothorax. Gas gangrene would also present a danger and malodorous wounds may be offensive to other passengers.

People with diabetes need to be well prepared for travel. They must carry all necessary medication, blood-testing equipment and glucose in case of hypoglycaemia. Those with type 1 diabetes may be at risk of loss of control of diabetes when crossing a number of time zones

Table 10.5 Fitness for travel – considerations for some common conditions (consult other texts for precise advice)

Problem	Advice
Cardiovascular	
Myocardial infarction	Do not fly within 7 days. Avoid flight for 3 weeks, if uncomplicated; 6 weeks if complicated
Unstable angina	Flight contraindicated until stabilised
Uncontrolled heart failure	Flight contraindicated until stabilised
Respiratory	
Chronic obstructive airways disease	Assess respiratory function
Asthma	Carry medicines
Pneumothorax	Not unless fully inflated for at least 2 weeks
Central nervous system	
Stroke	Not within 3 days
Epilepsy	Not within 24 hours of a fit
Diabetes	Take care with appropriate alteration of insulin regimen
Surgery	Avoid flying for 2–3 weeks after certain types of surgery, including thoracic, abdominal, brain and intracranial surgery and surgery of the middle ear. Fractures in a plaster within the last 48 hours are also often prohibited, unless splint has a bivalve
Blood disorders	Do not fly if Hb < 7.5 g/dL or within 10 days of sickling crisis

thus interfering with the timing of their usual insulin regimens. Eastward travel will tend to shorten the day length and reduce insulin requirements; westward travel has the opposite effect. There are algorithms available to calculate appropriate changes to insulin regimens. The suggested alterations in insulin dose/timing may be quite difficult to follow under the rigours of air travel and frequent self-monitoring of blood glucose is usually strongly advised.

Women in the later stages of pregnancy require special consideration in order to avoid labour in flight. Airlines would not generally allow travel over 36–40 weeks' pregnancy and it is best to check individual airlines for their precise limits. Other potential complications, such as a history of premature labour, may also contraindicate flight earlier in pregnancy. A further factor is the potential increase in exposure to ionising radiation at altitude that may contribute to fetal damage. This would not be significant if undertaking a few long-haul flights during pregnancy, but should be limited to no more then a total of 200 hours. For other individuals more than 2000 hours a year would need to be flown before there was significant risk. This is dependent on the actual routes taken, as radiation tends to be less at the poles than the equator and the figures quoted reflect hours of flight in those areas of highest cosmic radiation exposure.

An unresolved issue is the safety of flying for young babies following reports of a potential link to sudden infant death syndrome (SIDS). Flight during the first 2 weeks of life is probably best not undertaken unless unavoidable, but evidence concerning a direct link to SIDS is not conclusive.

Any passenger with a potentially infectious disease would be excluded from air travel. One of the most common problems is the child with chickenpox skin lesions who may well be prevented from boarding an aircraft. Flight would not then be permitted until the lesions had healed over some 5–7 days later after medical assessment. Of course the 5-day period when the child could transmit infection before the rash develops would probably go unnoticed.

Mental health problems are another potential area that may require some advanced planning, particularly where behavioural problems may distress fellow passengers. Also within this category may be included a fear of flying, which can present very real problems to fellow passengers and crew. In these cases sedation may sometimes be required.

Cabin air quality

Concern is sometimes expressed regarding the quality of air on-board aircraft and the possibility of contracting contagious diseases from other travellers. Airlines claim that the air is filtered efficiently and there is little chance of pathogenic organisms being circulated around the cabin. Air is recirculated around the cabin area, but not through the toilets and galley, every few minutes by passing over filters that are small enough to remove most bacteria and viruses. The result is that air is carrying fewer microorganisms than might be present in most air-conditioned buildings. However, owing to the fact the people can be in close proximity for long periods there would be an increased risk of contracting an infection from a passenger seated nearby. For this reason the airlines must be notified of passengers who are suffering from tuberculosis.

It is true that there is a low air humidity in aircraft cabins, and economy class is greatly more affected due to the higher passenger density. Normal thirst mechanisms do compensate so that individuals do not generally experience any degree of dehydration, although note the warnings above concerning alcohol consumption. Dry eyes may be experienced and contact lens wearers may be better advised to use spectacles during long flights. Dry throats can be relieved by sucking lozenges but a sore nose can be more difficult to treat. Skin may also feel dry and itchy and regular application of an emollient cream is recommended. Dry air in the aircraft could exacerbate asthma, so it is important that inhalers are ready to hand.

Main points

1. Motion sickness is believed to be due to a mismatch between the sensory inputs of motion and the CNS model of normal motion, the best cure being to allow adaptation to the abnormal stimuli. Either antihistamine or anticholinergic agents are of use in preventing motion sickness, but must be taken in advance of travel. Other measures can be taken to minimise the sensory disturbance caused by the abnormal motion.

2. Jet lag is caused by upsetting the circadian rhythm with respect to the usual sleep/wake cycle and is corrected once the cycle has been re-established at the new time zone. Symptoms are often more severe after eastward journeys. Preparation before travel may help if the traveller is well rested. During flight it may be desirable to sleep, avoiding heavy meals and alcohol. Sleep at destination night-time only will help with adaptation as well as exposure to daylight at the appropriate hours. There is some evidence supporting the use of melatonin and short-acting hypnotic agents.

3. 'Economy class syndrome' is probably a misnomer and represents the increased risk of DVT when individuals experience long hours of immobility with limited leg movement. General measures for all include maintaining fluid intake, avoiding alcohol and regular effective leg exercising. Risk groups require additional measures which may include wearing graduated compression hosiery, prophylactic aspirin and anticoagulation.

4. Expansion of gas in body cavities at altitude can cause a number of problems, referred to as barotraumas. The most common is otic barotrauma due to expansion of gas behind the eardrum. This may be relieved by special manoeuvres that open the Eustachian tube. Inflammation from an inner-ear or sinus infection can exacerbate the problem and oral and/or topical decongestants are indicated.

5. Fitness for flight must be considered well in advance of travel. In particular those with any recent surgery, cardiovascular, circulatory, blood or respiratory problems should consult their medical practitioner. There are a number of other medical conditions, e.g. insulin-dependent diabetes, that may require special consideration.

Frequently asked questions

Is it safe from the point of view of potential SIDS to take babies on long-haul flights?
As indicated in the text, there appears to be some evidence of physiological changes when babies are exposed to periods of a lowered atmospheric pressure as in an aircraft. It has not been proven that this is related to SIDS. Parents should be advised of this and must decide upon the advisability of travelling with very young children. As the risk of SIDS declines with increasing age, then for children over 2 years of age there would be less concern. Parents might be most cautious during the first 3 months of life. The risk of postpartum complications and DVT may be a consideration for the mother wishing to travel in the first few weeks after delivery.

Should aspirin be taken routinely by those over 40 years of age as prophylaxis against DVT during long-haul flights?
The evidence supporting the use of aspirin in this situation is not very strong. It would be preferable to focus on the use of compression hosiery and other in-flight strategies to reduce DVT. Ideally those seeking such prophylaxis should be referred to a medical practitioner.

Is there an increased risk of DVT during long-haul flights in pregnancy?
There is a general increased risk of DVT in pregnancy, especially for the older woman, but it is not known if this also increases the risk of such problems as a result of flying. Compression stockings and other in-flight measures are advised, together with heparin for those with a previous history of DVT and other particular indications.

Is it useful to suck sweets to prevent otic barotraumas in-flight?
There is no evidence that this provides any particular protection or relief of symptoms. The manoeuvres described in the text should be used.

What is the best medication for preventing motion sickness in children?
For young children who are being cared for by parents the sedative properties of promethazine syrup may offer some advantage during travel. This must be started well in advance of travel.

References

1. Nicholson A N, Pascoe P A, Spencer M B, Benson A J. Jet lag and motion sickness. *Br Med Bull* 1993; 49: 285–304.
2. Treisman M. Motion sickness: an evolutionary hypothesis. *Science* 1977; 197: 493–495.
3. Oosterveld W, Landolt J P. Motion sickness. In: DuPont H L, Steffen R, eds. *Textbook of Travel Medicine and Health,* 2nd edn. Hamilton, Canada: BC Decker, 2000: 396–402.
4. Bles W, Bos J E; Kruit H. Motion sickness. *Curr Opin Neurol* 2000; 13: 19–25.
5. Gahlinger P M. Cabin location and the likelihood of motion sickness in cruise ship passengers. *J Travel Med* 2000; 7: 120–124.
5. Turner M, Griffin M J. Motion sickness in public road transport: the relative importance of motion, vision and individual differences. *Br J Psychol* 1999; 90: 519–539.
7. Bagshaw M. Aviation medicine. In: Zuckerman J, ed. *Principles and Practice of Travel Medicine.* Chichester, UK: Wiley, 2001: 220–245.
8. Morley A, Blenkinsopp J, Nicholls J, Nicholls J. Travel sickness. *Pharm J* 1987; 239: 71–72.
9. Scopoderm: transdermal hyoscine for motion sickness. *Drug Ther Bull* 1989; 27: 91–92.
10. Van Marion W F, Bongaerts M C M, Christiaanse J C *et al.* Influence of transdermal scopolamine on motion sickness during seven days' exposure to heavy seas. *Clin Pharmacol Ther* 1985; 38: 301–305.
11. Van-Driessche R. Combination of cinnarizine and domperidone for the prevention of motion sickness: double blind comparative study versus cinnarizine against seasickness. *Curr Ther Res* 1985; 38: 61–67.
12. Stern R M, Utydehage S H, Muth E R, Koch L H. Effects of phenytoin on motion-induced motion sickness and gastric myoelectrical activity. *Aviation Space Environ Med* 1994; 65: 518–521.
13. Bruce D G, Golding J F, Hockenhull N, Pethybridge R J. Acupressure and motion sickness. *Aviation Space Environ Med* 1990; 61: 361–365.
14. Stern R M, Jokerst M D, Muth E R, Hollis C. Acupressure relieves the symptoms of motion sickness and reduces abnormal gastric activity. *Altern Ther Health Med* 2001; 7: 91–94.
15. Sherman C R. Motion sickness: review of causes and preventative strategies. *J Travel Med* 2002; 9: 251–256.
16. Mowrey D B, Clayson D E. Motion sickness, ginger and psychophysics. *Lancet* 1982; i: 655–657.
17. Wood C D, Manno J E, Wood M J *et al.* Comparison of efficacy of ginger with various antimotion sickness drugs. *Clin Res Pract Drug Regul Affairs* 1988; 6: 129–136.
18. Schmid R, Schick T, Steffen R *et al.* Comparison of seven commonly used agents for prophylaxis of seasickness. *J Travel Med* 1994; 1: 203–206.
19. Daurat A, Benoit O, Buguet A. Effects of zopiclone on the rest/activity rhythm after a westward flight across five time zones. *Psychopharmacology* 2000; 149: 241–245.

20. Suhner A, Schlagenhauf P, Hofer I *et al*. Effectiveness and tolerability of melatonin and zolpidem for the alleviation of jet lag. *Aviation Space Environ Med* 2001; 72: 638–646.
21. Dawson A G. Medical aspects of air travel. In: DuPont H L, Steffen R, eds. *Textbook of Travel Medicine and Health*, 2nd edn. Hamilton, Canada: BC Decker, 2000: 390–397.
22. Waterhouse J, Reilly T, Atkison G. Jet-lag. *Lancet* 1997; 350: 1609–1614.
23. Brsezinski A. Melatonin in humans. *N Engl J Med* 1997; 336: 186–195.
24. Lewy A J, Ahmed S, Jackson J M, Sack R L. Melatonin shifts human circadian rhythms according to a phase–response curve. *Chronobiol Int* 1992; 9: 380–392.
25. Arendt J. Jet lag (letter). *Lancet* 1998; 351: 293–294.
26. Suhner A, Schlagenhauf P, Johnson R *et al*. Comparative study to determine the optimal melatonin dosage form for the alleviation of jet-lag. *Chronobiol Int* 1998; 15: 655–666.
27. Melatonin for jet lag? *Drug Ther Bull* 1998; 36: 15–16.
28. Samel A. Melatonin and jet-lag. *Eur J Med Res* 1999; 4: 385–388.
29. Arendt J, Deacon S. Treatment of circadian rhythm disorders – melatonin. *Chronobiol Int* 1997; 14: 185–204.
30. Herxheimer A, Petrie K J. Melatonin for the prevention and treatment of jet lag. Update of Cochrane Database System Review 2001;(1):CD001520; 11279722.
31. Di W L, Kadva A, Johnston A, Silmann R. Variable bioavailability of oral melatonin. *N Engl J Med* 1997; 336: 1028–1029.
32. Geroulakos G. The risk of venous thromboembolism from air travel: the evidence is only circumstantial. *BMJ* 2001; 322: 188.
33. Hissh J, O'Donell M J. Venous thromboembolism after long flights: are airlines to blame? *Lancet* 2001; 357: 1461–1462.
34. Kraaijenhagen R A, Haverkamp D, Koopman M M *et al*. Travel and risk of venous thrombosis. *Lancet* 2000; 356: 1429–1493.
35. Scurr J H, Machin S J, Bailey-King S *et al*. Frequency and prevention of symptomless deep-vein thrombosis in long haul flights: a randomised trial. *Lancet* 2001; 357: 1485–1489.
36. Belcaro G, Geroulakos G, Nicolaides A N *et al*. Venous thromboembolism from air travel: the LONFLIT study. *Angiology* 2001; 52: 369–374.
37. Lapostolle F, Surget V, Borron S *et al*. Severe pulmonary embolism associated with air travel. *N Engl J Med* 2001; 345: 779–829.
38. Malone P C. Air travel and the risk of venous thromboembolism. *BMJ* 2001; 322: 1183.
39. House of Lords Science and Technology – fifth report: Air Travel and Health. November 2000. Available at http://www.parliament.the-stationery-office.co. uk.
40. Landgraf H, Vanselow B, Schulte-Huerman D *et al*. Economy class syndrome: rheology, fluid balance, and lower leg oedema during a simulated 12 hour long distance flight. *Aviation Space Environ Med* 1994; 65: 930–935.
41. Bellingham C. Giving advice on traveller's thrombosis. *Pharm J* 2001; 266: 116–117.
42. Anonymous. Confusion over compression level for prevention of DVT in travellers. *Pharm J* 2001; 267: 181–186.

43. King P F. The eustachian tube and its significance in flight. *J Laryngol Otol* 1979; 93: 659–678.

44. Jones J S, Sheffield W, While L J, Bloom M A. A double blind comparison between oral pseudoephedrine and topical xylometazoline in the prevention of barotrauma during air travel. *Am J Emerg Med* 1998; 16: 262–264.

45. Shand D. The assessment of fitness to travel. *Occup Med* 2000; 50: 566–571.

46. Bettes T N, McKenas D. Medical advice for commercial airline travellers. *Am Family Phys* 1999; 60: 801–810.

47. Paulson E. Travel statement on jet lag. *Can Med Assoc J* 1996; 155: 61–66.

11

Medical kits and the self-management of first aid and minor medical conditions for travellers

Key to the self-management of medical problems for travellers, particularly where medical facilities are poor, is an appropriate first-aid/medical kit and the knowledge of how the items are used. Supply of an appropriate medical kit to travellers is an important role for pharmacists. Most holiday-makers should be advised to carry a basic first-aid kit and a small selection of over-the-counter (OTC) medicines. When travel to more exotic destinations is to be undertaken, a wider range of medical supplies might have to be considered. This chapter describes the factors that should be taken into consideration when advising holiday-makers and travellers in what items to purchase and serves as a summary on the management of various ailments, e.g. travellers' diarrhoea, discussed elsewhere in this book. In particular the management of bites and stings is discussed as a general first-aid consideration for the traveller.

There is little information to be found about the design of medical kits for travellers – only a few reviews that discuss the subject in any depth are available.[1-3] This chapter will focus on the general principles that should be followed when designing a medical kit for a variety of travellers (Fig. 11.1).

For many travellers, particularly backpackers, luggage space is limited and only those items most likely to be needed or those of greatest importance can be carried. The traveller's itinerary should be considered when giving advice, and certain activities can carry a greater need for specific or more extensive first-aid items. In addition, pharmacists should always ask about any long-term medicines being taken, in order to arrange sufficient supplies. Sometimes customers can overlook medicines that are required only occasionally (e.g. for mild asthma or hayfever) and lack of supplies can then become a problem overseas.

Any medical kit should be packed appropriately for travel – most packaging is designed for the bathroom cabinet rather than the rigours

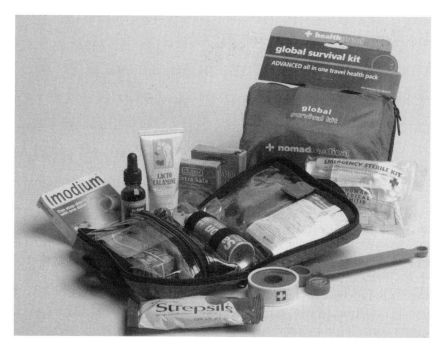

Figure 11.1 A comprehensive personal medical and first-aid kit. Courtesy of Nomad.

of the open road. Finally, health care professionals should ensure that the traveller understands what to do with the items in the kit and that appropriate instructions have been included.

Purchase of medicines overseas

Travellers can often be tempted to obtain supplies of drugs when they reach their destination rather than in the UK. This may be for financial reasons, because some medicines can be purchased more cheaply abroad. Some travellers may not wish to carry items that might never be used and that take up luggage space.

There are a number of important considerations that travellers should be advised to take into account when purchasing medicines overseas.

Communication

Travellers can have difficulty explaining their requirements in a foreign language. Equally, pharmacists or doctors overseas may not be able to give sufficient information, even in written form, about medicines that they have supplied or prescribed.

Identifying the medication

Names for generic medicines may not be the same in different countries, e.g. paracetamol in the UK is called acetaminophen in the USA. In addition medicines with the same proprietary names but from different countries may contain different or additional ingredients to the product available in the UK.

Availability of medicines

In some developing countries or remote areas, a good range of medical supplies may not be available or a specific medicine required to treat a chronic condition may not be marketed.

Quality of medicines

In certain developing countries, counterfeit medicines or medicines of poor quality may be supplied. Some studies have investigated the quality of medicines in certain parts of the world. The most common problem seems to be one of quality control. In one study,[4] a range of antibiotics and antimalarial drugs obtained from 35 pharmacies in Nigeria was analysed for the content of active ingredients. A total of 48% of samples were found to be outside pharmacopoeia limits. In some cases, this could have lead to treatment failure. Another interesting finding was that the medicines were substandard whether they were locally produced or had been imported. The authors hypothesised that the packaging and stated origin of some of these products could have been counterfeit (forgeries of marketed medicines).

Occasionally, such medicines can be formulated with dangerous ingredients and this can have catastrophic effects. A recent example occurred in India, where cough medicine was intentionally formulated with diethylene glycol instead of propylene glycol, resulting in the deaths of 33 children.[5] The prevalence of counterfeit medicines in which no active ingredient is present is a problem that is difficult to quantify, because reports of such medicines are often anecdotal.

For travellers who must purchase supplies of medicines overseas, a common-sense approach is to use reputable sources, rather than buy the cheapest medicines. An embassy or consulate can advise on reliable retailers.

Packaging

When taking medicines abroad, some thought should be given to appropriate packaging for travel.

If loose tablets are dispensed, there is the potential for them to become pulverised while being carried in a rucksack. It is, therefore, preferable to dispense tablets that are in blister packs wherever possible.

Many backpackers lose the outer cardboard containers and instructions that go with medicines. To reduce the likelihood of this, pharmacists should advise such travellers to place tablets, together with the outer box and patient information leaflet, into resealable plastic bags that will also protect against moisture. Items can also be stored in a sealable Tupperware-type box but this can be considerably more bulky and harder to pack than a plastic bag. Backpackers may wish to consider using one of a variety of specially designed fabric pouches that are available. Medicines are usually sold and dispensed with an accompanying patient information leaflet, but it is sometimes worth including a full data sheet for prescribed medicines in addition, because this may be useful to prescribers consulted overseas.

Packing medical and first-aid kits for large groups of individuals requires special consideration. The outer container should be strong and, in some circumstances, completely waterproof. Many items can be stored and organised in individual Tupperware-type boxes.

There has been no formal assessment of the stability of medicines carried by travellers to warm climates. The short holiday times involved probably do not result in significant degradation but it may be worth advising travellers to discard unused medicines after a longer trip to places of climatic extremes. Other problems, such as the integrity of suppositories or pessaries, can be anticipated because of their low melting point.

Legal and ethical issues

The legal status of medicines can vary between countries, which can cause problems for travellers. There have been relatively few reports of incidents involving travellers who have been carrying medicines, other than those that have occurred with controlled drugs. However, this does not mean that travellers will not encounter problems occasionally.

Medicines should be well packaged and labelled, as mentioned above, and it is advisable to carry a note from a doctor or a copy of a prescription for medicines for chronic conditions (particularly since further supplies may be needed in an emergency).

The variation in country regulations regarding carrying medicines for personal use across international boarders has been recognised by the United Nations International Narcotics Control Board, particularly with respect to narcotics and psychotropics.[6] A survey of these requirements for 57 countries was conducted by King's College London and the results are summarised in Table 11.1. An initial search for information on carrying medicines for personal use was conducted through the internet and e-mails were sent to relevant contacts if these could be identified. If insufficient information was obtained by this method or further clarification was required, the UK-based consul or embassy was contacted by telephone. Relevant internet sites were identified for 29 countries and for 23 an e-mail address for enquiries was provided. A total of 24 countries were telephoned, but only information of a general nature could often be obtained by this method. For nine countries no data could be obtained by any method.

Of the 48 countries where information was available, 50% recommended maximum amounts of medication to be carried, usually 3 months' supply, and that a letter/prescription should be carried; 13% only recommended letter/prescription and 17% only a maximum supply. Some countries also recommended a maximum supply of OTC medicines, usually no more than five packets. Nineteen countries described a variety of narcotics and psychotropics which were specifically prohibited; diamorphine was listed for 10 countries. Maximum periods of less than 3 months' supply for certain categories of medicines were described by 12 countries and for a further 10 countries special permission was required for medicines, usually narcotics or psychotropics.

Certain countries appeared to have anomalous regulations; Japan specifically bans even mild stimulants such as pseudoephedrine and Vicks inhalers, whilst Moroccan regulations stipulated that a general practitioner letter endorsed by the Moroccan embassy should be carried for all medicines. Some countries like Mexico were more notorious for random enforcement of regulation, particularly narcotic and psychotropic drugs, and the US state department had issued specific warnings to travellers.

Table 11.1 Study of 57 countries regarding recommendations and restrictions for travellers carrying medicines for personal use across international borders (does not reflect the actual legal requirements: only information available by internet, e-mail or telephone is included)

Country	Prohibited items	Restricted	Maximum quantities of restricted items without permit and comments
Argentina[a]	Morphine		
Australia[a,b]	Diamorphine	Any injectable except insulin, growth hormones, anabolic steroids, kava, ma huang, khat	
Austria[a,b]	–		Non-EU residents require permits for all medicines
Bahamas[a,b]	–		
Bahrain[a,b]	–		
Belgium[a,b]	Methadone, melatonin	Narcotics, Viagra	Max. $430 Viagra
Belize[a]			
Brazil			Unidentified
Canada		Narcotics, traditional medicines	Narcotic 2–3 weeks, traditional medicines max. 3 months' supply
China[a,b]			Doctor's prescription also required
Cyprus[a,b]			
Czech Republic			No data
Denmark[a]	Khat, diamorphine	Narcotics, psychotropics	2 weeks' supply
Egypt[a,b]			
Estonia		Narcotics, psychotropics, hormones, blood preparations, vaccines	Only with special permit

Table 11.1   continued

Country	Prohibited items	Restricted	Maximum quantities of restricted items without permit and comments
Fiji[a,b]			
Finland		Narcotics	Permit for max. 14 days' supply narcotics. Other medicines from EU countries 1 year's supply; non-EU, 3 months' supply
France[b]	Diamorphine		
Germany	Diamorphine	Narcotics	Narcotics max. 30 days
Greece[a,b]		Narcotics	Narcotics max. 30 days
Hong Kong		Narcotics, pharmaceutical products and medicines	Permission required
Iceland[b]		Narcotics, psychotropics	Some max. of 10 days, others max. of 1 month. Other medicines max. 100 days' supply
India[a,b]		Narcotics	Permit required
Indonesia			No data
Israel[a,b]			
Italy[a,b]	Morphine, methadone		
Jamaica			No data
Japan	Amfetamines, diamorphine, some stimulant sinus medicines, e.g. Vicks inhalers, pseudoephedrine	Narcotics, psychotropics, sex hormones, natural products, vitamins	Narcotic and psychotropics, sex hormones permission required; vitamins max. quantities 4 months, natural products 2 months

Table 11.1 continued

Country	Prohibited items	Restricted	Maximum quantities of restricted items without permit and comments
Malaysia[a]		Narcotics	Maximum 1 month
Malta[b]	Amfetamines, morphine, diamorphine, barbiturates		
Mauritius	Tranquillisers and hypnotics. Some analgesic preparations (e.g. co-proxamol)	Narcotics	
Mexico[a]		Narcotics, psychotropics, HIV medication	Possession can result in arrest. Caution is required when carrying any prescription medicine
Morocco[b]	Narcotics	All medicines	Approval needed unless accompanied by letter from general practitioner which must be certified by Moroccan consulate/embassy
Netherlands	All UK category controlled drugs		
New Zealand[b]		Methadone, morphine	Permit required
Norway[a,b]		Narcotics	Legal narcotics max. 1 month
Peru			No data
Philippines[a,b]		Narcotics	Permission required
Poland			No information
Russia			No information
Roumania			No information

Table 11.1 continued

Country	Prohibited items	Restricted	Maximum quantities of restricted items without permit and comments
Saudi Arabia[a]			
Singapore[b]	Morphine, diamorphine		
South Africa[a,b]	Diamorphine	Narcotics, prescribed medicines	Max. 1 month supply of any medicine
Spain[a,b]			
Switzerland[a]		Narcotics	Max. 1 month supply
Thailand[a,b]		Narcotics, psychotropics	Psychotropics max. 30 days. Narcotics permission required and max. 30 days
Tanzania			No information available
Trinidad[a,b]			
Turkey[a,b]	Methadone		
United Arab Emirates[b]		All prescribed medicines	For all medicines a certificate from Dubai embassy required
USA[a,b]	Diamorphine		
Uruguay[a]			
Zimbabwe[a]	Diamorphine	–	–

HIV, human immunodeficiency virus.
[a] Maximum of 3 months of prescription items for personal use allowed.
[b] Prescription and/or letter from a doctor should be carried.

From this study it can be seen that it may not be easy, or in some cases possible, for travellers to obtain specific advice before departure and a comprehensive website of information compiled by an international agency would be useful. Particular care should be taken regarding narcotic and psychotropic drugs, as discussed in the next section.

Controlled drugs

The position regarding controlled drugs is more problematic. Even the low doses of codeine present in OTC medicines available in the UK could, in theory, present problems if carried across some borders.

Pharmacists should advise travellers to check with the relevant authorities before travelling abroad if carrying Schedule 5 controlled drugs. Relevant authorities would be the Home Office for controlled drugs, the Medicines Control Agency (MCA) if export licences are required, and the embassies of the destination country and countries travelled through for all drugs. Although this may not always be practical, it is up to individuals to decide whether or not they make these checks and health professionals can only advise that it is recommended.

For controlled drugs in Schedule 2 (e.g. morphine), an export licence must be obtained from the UK Home Office before travel. Small quantities can be exempt from this but the Home Office should be contacted before travelling in all cases. This licence is relatively easy to arrange provided it is done in advance.

More problematic is that an import licence or authority may have to be sought from the country of destination, although, as the survey in Table 11.1 shows, most will allow quantities for personal use without special permission. Arranging such permission can be almost impossible if the medicine is not allowed to be used in a particular country (e.g. diamorphine in the USA).

Healthy travellers who need to carry stronger analgesics for emergency use should consult a doctor, who may agree to prescribe an alternative analgesic, such as tramadol. Travellers requiring Schedule 2 controlled drugs for chronic conditions should ensure that they obtain appropriate licences.

Group travel

The supply of medicines for expeditions or groups, where one kit is intended for use by a number of individuals, is an area for which there is poor provision in current UK legislation.

Prescription-only medicines (POMs) and pharmacy medicines (Ps) can be sold by wholesale supply to individuals allowed to purchase them in this way under the Medicines Act (e.g. a doctor who takes responsibility for and who administers medicines to members of a group). Such supply requires a wholesale dealer's licence, unless wholesaling is an inconsiderable portion of total pharmacy business. As a general rule, the requirement for a wholesale dealer's licence is over-looked by the Medicines Control Agency if wholesaling is less than 5% of turnover in licensed medicinal products. A disadvantage of wholesale supply of POMs is that repackaging and labelling cannot be undertaken without an assembly licence. In reality, groups and expeditions some-times repackage their own supplies after a doctor has made a requisi-tion, which is not ideal.

Another practice common among small groups is for one individ-ual to obtain a prescription from a doctor and subsequently share the medicine once it has been supplied. Health professionals should always discourage sharing of prescribed medicines and should recommend that travellers obtain individual medical supplies, appropriately packaged and labelled, for their particular circumstances, unless travelling in groups where a doctor is taking responsibility for the group's medicines. If a doctor has prescribed a prescription medicine for all members of the group, the group may choose to purchase only one supply for economic reasons.

A further ethical consideration is whether or not a POM should be given to travellers for use 'just in case'. This is particularly true of antibiotics, where some general practitioners believe that medical help should always be sought in the destination country. Balanced against this is the argument that medicines supplied abroad may be of poor quality or it may not be possible to obtain them at all.

A final consideration is that only 3 months' supply of medicines can be given on a National Health Service prescription for people leav-ing the UK. This is because after this time individuals cease to be regis-tered with their general practitioner.

Export

Pharmacists may sometimes be called upon to supply medicines to people already overseas, for instance, an expatriate worker.

There are two ways in which a pharmacist can supply POMs for export. The first is against a prescription written by a doctor, who must be registered with the General Medical Council in the UK. The second is sale by way of wholesale dealing. Sales by wholesale dealing can only be made to a person who, in the course of business, buys the product for selling, supplying or administering to another person. In terms of export, this definition includes hospitals, clinics, other wholesale busi-nesses, pharmacies and doctors resident abroad (provided the medicine is for supply to a patient rather than for the doctor's personal use).

Pharmacists must ensure that the order originates from a bona fide source before making this type of supply. Supply of controlled drugs by wholesale dealing can only take place when a licence from the Home Office has been obtained.

Before exporting any medicine, pharmacists should check with the MCA to see if any export certificates are needed, and with the embassy of the recipient country to see if any import certificates are required. It is possible to post medicines overseas, provided the necessary declaration of contents is made on the package and any special packaging requirements are met. Information about packaging can be obtained from HM Customs and Excise offices. Pharmacists should ensure that the medicine will reach the intended user and should consider whether sending medicines in this way will affect the safety, quality and efficacy of the product.

Designing first-aid and medical kits

There are three principal groups of products to consider when designing kits for travellers:

1. first-aid medicines
2. OTC medicines
3. POMs

The range of items in each category included in any kit will depend upon the type of traveller. Broadly these fall into:

- tourists on short holidays to developed countries who will require only basic first aid and a small range of OTC medicines
- tourists visiting developing countries and areas where malaria is endemic who will need a more extensive kit but for whom POMs, other than malaria prophylaxis or treatment for current chronic conditions, are rarely needed
- people travelling to developing countries and tropical areas for long periods who may require larger kits and some POMs
- expeditions far from medical help which will need comprehensive kits

Business travellers who leave the country frequently are a special case and may find a comprehensive range of supplies useful. Such a kit may be needed for trips arranged at short notice and could, perhaps, be held by occupational health departments in larger companies.[7]

An important consideration for most travellers is to make sure that those items most likely to be used are included in the medical kit. This will be very largely dependent on the factors described above. A further study conducted by King's College London gives some insight into the level of usage of medical and first-aid items used by travellers to a variety of destinations in largely developing countries. In this study travellers visiting a specialist pharmacy were surveyed to identify those items included in their medical kits, what was actually used whilst away and any items purchased whilst away. These were mainly young backpackers visiting a variety of destinations in developing countries and the results will be discussed by way of illustration in the following sections.

First-aid items

The priority when putting together first-aid items is to ask about the exact itinerary and activities to be undertaken. First-aid kits can become bulky and it is often best if the group identifies an individual to carry the kit instead of other equipment. However, each individual should carry at least some first-aid items, such as plasters, for personal use. The use of various first-aid items in the King's College study is shown in Table 11.2.

Table 11.2 First-aid items carried and used by a cohort of travellers to developing countries

Item	Number of kits where item carried (% of total kits; n = 127)	Number of kits where item used (% of kits where item carried)
Plasters	112 (88)	52 (46)
Non-adherent dressing	57 (45)	6 (11)
Surgical tape	67 (53)	18 (27)
Wound dressing	45 (35)	7 (16)
Antiseptic wipes	68 (54)	23 (34)
Steristrips	42 (33)	6 (14)
Gauze swabs	40 (31)	6 (15)
Cotton buds	54 (43)	22 (41)
Antiseptic	82 (65)	32 (39)
Crêpe bandage	56 (44)	3 (5)
Safety pins	52 (41)	12 (23)
Scissors	94 (74)	37 (39)
Tweezers	82 (65)	32 (39)
Blister dressing	33 (26)	10 (30)
Sterile AIDS/HEPB kit	55 (43)	3 (5)

AIDS, acquired immune deficiency syndrome; HEPB, hepatitis B.

It is important for all individuals to have an understanding of how to use the components of a kit and an appreciation of wound management. A first-aid course is invaluable for those on more adventurous trips.

All travellers should be prepared to deal with cuts and grazes and to have to hand the items listed in the first part of Box 11.1. All wounds should be washed before applying a dressing. Antiseptics are not greatly used by health professionals in wound management owing to potentially adverse effects on wound healing and for the cleaning of cuts and grazes soapy water would be sufficient. In the situation concerning wound management by the lay person, particularly in the field conditions of trekkers, wound cleaning may not be adequately performed so that use of antiseptics may offer some additional protection from infection. Antiseptic wipes can be useful if a convenient source of clean water is not readily available. It is best to avoid tubes of antiseptic cream when travelling, because organisms may be introduced into the tube with frequent use. An iodine-based preparation gives the broadest spectrum of activity, therefore, a dry-powder spray of povidone-iodine is ideal. Also of use to travellers are small bottles of povidone-iodine tincture, which contain a brush for application. Any organisms that contaminate the brush are killed when it is replaced in the solution.

Certain types of travellers should consider the items listed in the second part of Box 11.1. Backpackers who are travelling rough in tropical areas should be particularly vigilant with any minor injury. A minor wound, often resulting from vigorous scratching of an insect bite, can become contaminated and fail to heal. The resulting, exudating wound is often then covered with a dressing that is changed frequently because of leakage, resulting in removal of any granulation tissue that has formed. Over time a chronic wound can develop.

There have been no detailed studies regarding these 'tropical ulcers' in travellers generally, although they have been reported in visitors to the tropics.[8] It has been suggested that specific organisms requiring antibiotic treatment can play a part in the aetiology of such ulcers.[9] Whatever the origin of these wounds, it is essential that people living in tropical conditions treat even the most minor abrasion. Therefore, appropriate cleaning and application of an antiseptic, with a covering to prevent contamination, are essential.

It can be worthwhile for travellers to carry dressings for such purposes: a non-adherent dressing would be the best option. For emergencies where it is not convenient to wash the wound with clean, soapy water, Steripods (containing liquid antiseptic or saline) can be useful. It

---

Box 11.1 First-aid items

Most travellers
- Antiseptic
- Plasters

Tropical, long-term or special activities holidays
- Crêpe bandage
- Foot blister plaster
- Hydrocolloid dressings
- Iodine-based antiseptic
- Non-adherent dressing
- Sterile kit
- Steristrips
- Surgical tape

---

is best to clean wounds with sterile gauze rather than cotton wool, which can shed fibres.

If a wound heals poorly, a dressing that provides a good healing environment may be required. Anecdotally, travellers report that hydro-colloid dressings, such as Granuflex, produce good healing. Once applied, the dressing can be left *in situ* for up to 5 days. The strong, waterproof outer layer seems to allow integrity of the dressing to be maintained in tropical environments.

The requirements for other types of dressing should be considered carefully, and, as can be seen in Table 11.2, may well not be needed. A crêpe support bandage may be useful if a person is walking or trekking a lot and when sprains and strains are likely. However, it may not be worth carrying Tubigrip, because a range of sizes would be needed for different limbs. Other items, such as open-weave bandages, are rarely of use to travellers.

Field dressings are appropriate for those undertaking activities in which there is potential for serious injury (e.g. mountaineering). However, suturing equipment is unnecessary, unless there is someone in the travelling group who is trained in stitching. Steristrips are a use-ful alternative for deeper cuts and can be held in place more securely by applying tincture of benzoin (friar's balsam) to the edges of the strip. Users of these products should be reminded of the need to clean thoroughly and remove any debris from such wounds before closure.

Walkers and trekkers may find a specially designed hydrocolloid dressing such as Compeed useful for treating blisters on the feet.

Other items such as a pair of tweezers and scissors should be included. Many find the small sterile lancets used to obtain blood from a fingerprick test useful for removing splinters. They can also be used to prick a foot blister, which should always be done carefully and covered with a sterile dressing, leaving the skin over the blister in place.

In recent years, it has become common for travellers to carry kits containing sterile needles and syringes. The intention is that these would be used, if needed, in areas where such equipment is in short supply. In such areas, there is the danger that needles could be reused, thus potentially transmitting blood-borne diseases such as hepatitis B and human immunodeficiency virus (HIV). People on long trips to developing countries may wish to carry such kits, although they are unlikely to be needed. Problems are not usually encountered at Customs, provided the kit is well packaged and clearly labelled. It is worth reminding travellers that they should make sure they are aware of their blood group. Some groups of travellers should be encouraged to pack condoms in view of the worldwide problems relating to sexually transmitted diseases.

Over-the-counter medicines

A range of OTC medicines can be recommended to travellers (Box 11.2). For example, most people will need to carry a supply of analgesics/antipyretics, as shown by the results in Table 11.3. Travellers' diarrhoea can be a problem in a variety of destinations. Treatment has been discussed in Chapter 2 and the use of loperamide and oral rehydration solutions (ORS) appeared to be high in the King's College study. In particular, ORS appears more popular than loperamide and, as described in Chapter 2, perhaps loperamide could be more widely used in the context of travellers' diarrhoea without dysentery. Very similar results were obtained from a survey of users of travel health kits by corporate travellers produced by an occupational health department of the Coca-Cola company.[10] The items felt to be of most use were analgesics and those for the treatment of diarrhoea. However, water purification tablets were felt to be of little use by the corporate travellers, contrasting with around half of the travellers in the King's College study who carried water purification chemicals, using them whilst away.

Protection against the sun and the management of sunburn are covered in Chapter 9 and most in the King's College survey appear to have purchased and used suitable preparations. This contrasts with the

Box 11.2   Over-the-counter medicines

Most travellers
- Analgesics/antipyretics
- Loperamide
- Rehydration sachets
- Soothing/moisturising cream (e.g. calamine cream)

Other possible requirements
- Antacids
- Antifungal creams and powders
- Antihistamine tablets
- Hydrocortisone cream
- Laxatives
- Treatments for motion sickness

Coca-Cola study, where it was found to be of least use, possibly due a low level of outdoor activity. Travellers who suffer from motion sickness may wish to carry appropriate remedies, as described in Chapter 10.

In hot, humid climates, there can be an increased risk of fungal skin infections. Those with a history of recurrent tinea pedis (athlete's foot) who are planning walking trips may find the condition flares up.

Table 11.3   Medicines carried and used by a cohort of travellers to developing countries

Medicine	Number of kits where medicine carried (% of total kits; n = 127)	Number of kits where medicine used (% of kits where medicine was carried)
Analgesics	109 (86)	70 (64)
Antihistamine tablets	67 (53)	24 (36)
Antihistamine cream	33 (26)	25 (76)
Antifungal cream	41 (32)	12 (29)
Hydrocortisone cream	46 (36)	11 (24)
Rehydration sachets	80 (63)	40 (50)
Loperamide	84 (66)	29 (35)
Laxative	11 (9)	2 (18)
Vitamins	65 (51)	52 (80)
Antibiotics	34 (27)	12 (35)

A similar condition quite common in men is the so-called 'Dhobi itch', a tinea infection around the groin area. Such travellers should carry an antifungal imidazole powder or cream (e.g. miconazole, clotrimazole). Women with a history of vaginal candidiasis may find it useful to carry an oral remedy, such as fluconazole, or a vaginal cream, rather than pessaries.

Reactions to insect bites and stings can be troublesome. People known to react may wish to carry a corticosteroid preparation, such as hydrocortisone, and those who react badly may need to consider a more potent, prescribed preparation. Antihistamine tablets are also useful for allergic reactions. A sedating antihistamine (e.g. chlorphenamine) may be useful at night if insect bite reactions are disturbing sleep. The King's College survey seemed to indicate a high use of antihistamine creams, although, as discussed under Bites and stings, below, a corticosteroid cream may be the preferred agent.

A trip to hot climates can lead to constipation because of inadequate fluid intake and a change in diet. Potential sufferers should carry a mild laxative such as senna.

Unless away for more than a few months and eating quite a restricting diet, it is unlikely that vitamin preparations would be required in otherwise healthy young adults. Table 11.3 shows that half of travellers carried such preparations and in over 80% of cases they were taken, a greater compliance even than with insect repellents, where only 78% of those carrying repellents used them, despite visiting malaria-endemic areas.

Prescription-only medicines (POMs)

Apart from providing POMs for chronic conditions, it is also important to remember to provide medicines for conditions that present as occasional acute problems (Box 11.3). This might include inhalers for mild asthma, courses of antibiotics for recurrent cystitis or, sometimes, ciprofloxacin for self-treatment of travellers' diarrhoea. If such items are intended for self-treatment in emergency situations, it is important that the individual is well versed in their appropriate use and that full written instructions are provided. In many countries, antibiotics can be purchased OTC. In the King's College study, it was found that 23 individuals (18%) used antibiotics, but, in half of these cases, the antibiotics were obtained overseas.

Analgesics such as dihydrocodeine or tramadol tablets may sometimes be indicated for use by travellers who will be some hours away

Box 11.3 Prescription-only medicines (POMs)

- Adrenaline (epinephrine)
- Antibiotics
- Antibiotic creams or powders
- Antibiotic eye ointment
- Standby treatment for people who develop malaria
- Remedies for mountain sickness
- Strong analgesics
- Treatments for chronic or recurrent conditions

from medical help and for whom injury might be a possibility. This might include trekkers or mountaineers visiting remote regions.

For nausea and vomiting, an antiemetic might be useful in certain situations. Oral preparations may not be kept down long enough to be ingested and suppositories may melt in hot climates. A useful preparation is prochlorperazine buccal tablets (Buccastem) which dissolve in the mouth.

Topical antibiotics (e.g. fusidic acid) or powders (e.g. Cicatrin) can be useful for superficial skin infections. Anecdotally, travellers to the tropics claim that such preparations are of help in preventing and managing chronic wounds but there is no good evidence for this. Chloramphenicol eye ointment can be useful in the event of conjunctivitis.

Any individual known to suffer anaphylaxis arising from allergic reactions (e.g. to bee stings) should be advised to carry adrenaline (epinephrine) for self-administration, such as an EpiPen. Treatment of malaria and mountain sickness have been covered in previous chapters.

Some travellers do need to carry courses of antibiotics. These include people:

- travelling for longer than a few weeks to destinations where medical supplies are unreliable. However, medical advice should be sought before instituting a course of antibiotics in such cases
- visiting areas far from medical facilities where self-treatment may be necessary

Antibiotics that are most suitable for travellers to carry should:

- cover the most likely problems that might require antibiotic treatment. These include travellers' diarrhoea of bacterial or protozoal origin, or infection of the urinary tract, chest or wounds. It may also be desirable to use antibiotics that cover against community-acquired pneumonia and cellulitis

- have few side-effects. In addition, the individual should not be allergic to the antibiotic or class
- be a well established antibiotic, rather than a newly introduced one, with which clinical experience might be limited
- have a simple regimen
- be cheap

Table 11.4 lists those antibiotics that have been cited as suitable for certain travellers.[1,2,7] The aim should be to carry a course of a single antibiotic that covers all potential infections. However, no antibiotic is indicated for all possible contingencies. Ciprofloxacin has a less satisfactory Gram-positive spectrum than some antibiotics, making it unsuitable for treating community-acquired pneumonia or cellulitis. Levofloxacin is claimed to have an improved Gram-positive spectrum but clinical data are limited.

Co-amoxiclav seems a potentially useful candidate, provided the traveller is not allergic to penicillin. However, it has not been evaluated for use in travellers' diarrhoea and can sometimes cause diarrhoea.

Table 11.4 Antibiotics that may be suitable for inclusion in medical kits

Drug	Travellers' diarrhoea (bacterial)	Travellers' diarrhoea (protozoal)	Respiratory and community-acquired pneumonia	Urinary tract infection	Wounds and cellulitis
Ciprofloxacin	Indicated	Not indicated	Not indicated	Indicated	Limited use
Co-amoxiclav	Limited use	Not indicated	Indicated	Indicated	Indicated
Erythromycin	Limited use	Not indicated	Indicated	Not indicated	Limited use (use if penicillin allergic)
Doxycycline	Limited use	Not indicated	Limited use	Not indicated	Limited use
Cefalexin/cefadroxil	Not indicated	Not indicated	Limited use	Indicated	Limited use
Metronidazole	Not indicated	Indicated	Not indicated	Not indicated	Not indicated

Concerns also exist regarding its potential to cause cholestatic jaundice,[11] although this is rare and occurs mainly in older people. A similar spectrum of activity can be gained from a combination of amoxicillin and flucloxacillin.

Erythromycin might be suitable for people with penicillin allergy. However, it often causes nausea and vomiting and would not be indicated for urinary-tract infections. Of the other macrolides, azithromycin has been suggested as being useful for travellers' diarrhoea. Clarithromycin causes less nausea than erythromycin but is more expensive.

Doxycycline is not normally considered the antibiotic of choice for most of the infections listed in Table 11.4, nor is it used for cellulitis or pneumonia. The same argument would apply to cefalexin, even though it can be used for certain mild to moderate chest and skin infections. Metronidazole and tinidazole are useful for protozoal or anaerobic infections.

In practice, ciprofloxacin and metronidazole are commonly recommended for travellers. Popular choices to cover chest and skin problems are co-amoxiclav or a combination of amoxicillin and flucloxacillin.

Expeditions and groups

Requests for kits for large groups of individuals should be referred to specialist organisations. However, in addition to the group or expedition kit, each individual is usually expected to carry personal supplies of some items that can be obtained through most pharmacies. Such a kit can consist of many of the first-aid items and OTC medicines discussed earlier. There is usually little need for individuals to obtain POMs, because these will be available in the group kit.

Expeditions

In the case of an expedition, a medical officer or group members with appropriate medical training may be present, and will be expected to administer certain medicines in an emergency. Supplies for an expedition are usually arranged such that there is a comprehensive large base camp kit, and a mobile kit to be carried by parties away from camp. Each individual on an expedition should carry his or her own kit of mainly first-aid items. This might consist of plasters, non-adherent dressings with tape/fixative, large wound dressing, support dressings such as a crêpe and triangular bandage, antiseptic wipes, blood lancets for splinters or blisters and a small supply of paracetamol.

For the mobile expedition kit (Figure 11.2) to be carried by one or two members within the group, all the items listed in Boxes 11.1–11.4 as well as those in Box 11.5 should be considered, depending on the situation. For instance, those at altitude may wish to carry altitude sickness remedies, whereas in highly malaria-endemic areas a standby malaria treatment would be carried. The main criteria to consider are the size of group, the time to be spent abroad and the distance of the destination from medical help. The range of antibiotics, other POMs and first-aid items carried by an expedition is larger than normal to cover a variety of situations.[12] Additional first-aid items to the ones carried by individuals for this larger kit might include sterile gauze swabs, cotton buds, a selection of different wound dressings, including for the eyes, disposable gloves, Steristrips and a bottle of liquid antiseptic such as aqueous povidone-iodine. A thermometer should be carried, particularly to malaria-endemic areas, and a small selection of syringes and needles is useful. The OTC medicines for such a kit would include the following: mild analgesics such as ibuprofen and paracetamol, chlorphenamine and loperamide. For prescription medicines, oral antibiotics discussed previously and a stronger analgesic such as tramadol or dihydrocodeine would be required. A preparation for treating eye infections (conjunctival) such as chloramphenicol or fusidic acid eye ointments should be included. Single-dose Minims amethocaine (tetracaine) 1% are very useful for those experiencing painful eye trauma. Finally, a variety of instructions on the use of the items in the kit and a suitable medical textbook should be included – the *Where there is no Doctor*[13] series is particularly useful.

The base camp kit can be larger in size and range as it does not have to be carried by individuals and can usually be transported by road or air. This will contain all of the items described in the mobile kit, in larger quantities to replenish supplies for those in the field. The sorts of extra first-aid items that might be included are burn water gel dressing or paraffin tulles, hydrocolloid dressings and a range of sizes of Tubigrip. A fairly comprehensive range of sterile equipment might include syringes and needles, forceps, suturing equipment, scalpels, cannulae and giving sets. Splints can also be carried in a variety of sizes (the flexible aluminium SAMs splints are very popular), or alternatively an inflatable splint is quite easy to use but correct inflation is important so that fitting is not too tight or loose. Organisation of the kit is extremely important so that items can be found easily; the best option is to arrange the items into individual Tupperware boxes that are clearly labelled with the contents. The individual boxes should be placed in a strong metal or fibreglass container.

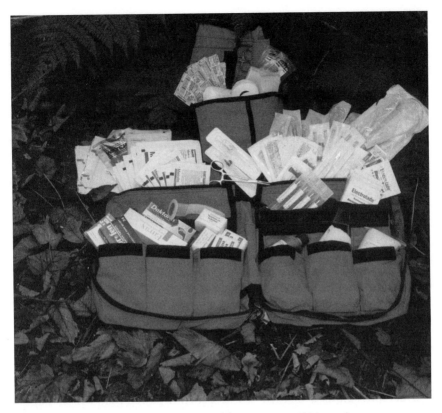

Figure 11.2 Mobile expedition medical kit. Courtesy of Nomad.

Box 11.4 Other products

- Contraceptives
- Insect repellents
- Other protection from bites (e.g. mosquito nets)
- Sunscreens
- Water purification tablets

For OTC medicines a greater range can also be included to cover a variety of minor ailments. This might include an antacid, throat lozenges, senna tablets, remedies for motion sickness, antifungal and hydrocortisone creams. Additional POM medicines that may be useful

---

Box 11.5   Extra supplies for expeditions and groups

- Antibiotic ear drops
- Antiemetics (e.g. buccal prochlorperazine)
- Inflatable or aluminium splints[a]
- Infusion fluids[a]
- Lidocaine (lignocaine) 1%
- Minims amethocaine (tetracaine)
- Over-the-counter items (e.g. throat lozenges, decongestants)
- Parenteral analgesics[a]
- Parenteral antibiotics[a]
- Prednisolone tablets
- Rectal diazepam
- Suturing equipment

[a] Usually expeditions only

---

include buccal prochlorperazine, prednisolone, diazepam and antibiotic ear drops. A greater range of antibiotics can also be included, such as co-amoxiclav and metronidazole.

A base camp kit will usually contain some parenteral preparations if a person qualified in their use is present. Adrenaline for managing anaphylaxis is one of the most useful preparations to include, usually in the form of pre-filled easy-to-use syringes such as an Epi-Pen. Parenteral cefotaxime is often the preferred antibiotic because of its broad spectrum of activity against both Gram-positive and Gram-negative organisms. Parenteral analgesics could include nalbuphine and diclofenac. Nalbuphine is not classed as a controlled drug despite its opioid properties, having a ceiling of analgesic effect above which additional doses do not increase analgesia. It is also claimed to cause less respiratory depression than other opiate drugs. Parenteral diclofenac gives adequate pain relief when an effect on the central nervous system is undesirable or pain is of an inflammatory nature. In an emergency, infusions may become necessary but space is a limiting factor. Dextrose/saline and a plasma expander (e.g. Haemaccel) would cover most situations.

Overland groups

For an overland group (an example of which would be a group of 10–20 individuals in trucks on a 6-month trans-African tour) or small groups of travellers, most POMs should only be used under medical advice if local supplies are unreliable. The truck kit for an overland group might be similar to that taken as a base camp kit by an expedition, although parenteral medicines, apart from adrenaline, might not be needed. In addition, individuals are usually requested to bring their own medical and first-aid supplies for use in the first instance, so all the OTC and first-aid items discussed under First-aid items and Over-the-counter medicines, above, should be considered.

Special environments

Cold environments

The kits described so far would be useful in most tropical or temperate environments. Cold environments, although sometimes requiring specialist survival equipment, do not call for many specific changes to the kits.

Diving

People on diving trips may be at risk of developing ear infections, particularly when diving in tropical waters. Otosporin ear drops are sometimes recommended but need to be stored at low temperatures. Alternatives to Otosporin include a combination of gentamicin and hydrocortisone. The risk of infection can be minimised by avoiding waterlogging of the ears, and some divers claim that aluminium acetate ear drops can help. However, aluminium acetate drops can be difficult to obtain, have a short shelf-life and are expensive. Spirit ear drops are used by some divers: a potential drawback is that they can remove protective ear wax. Acetic acid ear drops (Earcalm) may be a useful OTC preparation for the management of minor otitis externa infections.

Stings from jellyfish can be painful and, in some cases, dangerous. It is useful to have a dilute solution of acetic acid to hand to treat such stings for certain species (see below).

Bites and stings

Bites and stings from a variety of creatures are very common for travellers who may spend a longer time exposed to the outdoors than when at home. By far the most likely injury is from a biting insect such as a mosquito which does not in itself carry a poison or venom, but is seeking a blood meal. The second most common encounter would be stings from bees, wasps and ants where a venom is injected as part of the insect's defence mechanism. Stings from insects such as spiders and scorpions are less likely to be encountered, but the latter can cause serious problems. The next most common problem would probably be encountered with marine animals and these are generally associated with a more severe outcome than bee or wasp stings. Least likely for the traveller, but often most feared, are bites from venomous snakes.

Finally, bites from mammals should be treated with particular caution if in a rabies-endemic area, as described in Chapter 5.

Biting insects

The sheer numbers of mosquitoes in certain situations make a bite almost inevitable even if stringent bite avoidance measures are taken. The skin reaction experienced is an allergic-type reaction to the saliva of the mosquito, which contains a cocktail of potentially allergenic substances. There is frequently an immediate allergic reaction consisting of an extremely itchy red wheal that can last for a day or so. Some individuals experience a more delayed reaction that does not appear until several hours after the bite and can last for a few days. It is a common observation that there is a large interindividual variation in the severity of local response, with some developing very little reaction, whereas other experience quite severe blistering eruptions. There is also a possibility that tolerance develops with repeated exposure to a large number of bites. The most serious consequence of such bites is that a local infections leads to cellulitis or that scratching by the individual leads to the development of a chronic wound, as described under First-aid items, above. Travellers should be warned that a rapidly spreading red area around the bite, particularly if accompanied by fever, warrants immediate medical attention and treatment with the appropriate antibiotic, e.g co-amoxiclav.

With other biting insects, such as ticks and fleas, a similar type of allergic reaction is experienced. Certain insects are notorious for producing more severe reactions; these include certain blackflies and the tsetse fly.

As described under Over-the-counter medicines, above, the management of the allergic reaction to such bites would entail the use of a corticosteroid cream and oral antihistamines. Topically applied antihistamine creams are very popular, but theoretically considered inferior to a corticosteroid preparation. They must be applied very soon after the bite in order to inhibit the itching and would have less effect on any local swelling. They would therefore be expected to have little effect on the late reaction. They also have the potential to cause sensitisation of the skin and are sometimes discouraged for that reason. There appears to be very little evidence regarding efficacy but anecdotally many claim they are of benefit. In the UK hydrocortisone creams cannot be bought OTC for use on those under 12 years of age.

Also lacking in strong evidence regarding efficacy, but claimed by users to be of benefit, are certain other products designed to give relief from insect bites. Small devices that deliver an electric current when applied to the area of the bite are claimed to bring relief to a wide variety of bites and stings. A systematic survey of the literature found that there is little evidence supporting the efficacy of such devices.[14] Also popular are pens containing a roll-on preparation of ammonia (Afterbite) that must be applied as soon as the bite is experienced.

Stinging insects

Stings from hymenopterans such as wasps, bees and ants are not particularly a problem restricted to travel, but travellers may be required to deal with the consequences of a sting without resource to medical facilities. These insects may be more likely to sting if the individual is moving, hence the advice to keep still when they are threatening, and may be attracted by perfumes. There does not seem to be any strong evidence supporting the use of various bee repellents that are available.

The venom sack of a bee sting is left *in situ* after the sting, and there has been some debate regarding the best way of removing the sting. In theory, removal by pinching and pulling away the sting could squeeze out more venom into the skin, thus causing a more intense reaction. The usual advice is therefore to remove by scraping away the sting with an object such as a credit card. However, one study seemed to indicate that the most important factor was removing quickly, whether this was performed by pinching or scraping.[15]

The effects on the skin are not particularly related to toxicity from the venom, but to an allergic reaction to its components. Thus a local allergic reaction of pain, swelling and itching will be treatable by the use of local steroid and oral antihistamine preparations. If available, a cold pack can be applied immediately to the skin in order to limit the spread of the venom. There is quite a large variation in the population regarding severity of reaction, ranging from mild local reactions to life-threatening anaphylaxis. If the sting is on the throat or mouth than local swelling could compromise breathing and may require more aggressive treatment. Large numbers of stings can initiate toxicity to the venom, but this is a relatively rare problem. One author has claimed that the use of dilute solutions of meat tenderisers containing extract of papaya are very beneficial in removing the pain of a bee sting.[16]

Those who have experienced severe reaction in the past, including anaphylaxis, angioedema or more severe local reaction, might consider carrying a course of oral corticosteroids to be taken as soon as a sting is experienced. People who have previously experienced an anaphylactic reaction should be advised to carry adrenaline, for use after administration of oral corticosteroid at the first indication that such a reaction is occurring.

Sea animals

For sea bathers, encounters with the wide varieties of cnidarians (jellyfish, anemones and corals) are the most common source of problems. Reactions can vary from mild to life-threatening, with some species of jellyfish. Most species of jellyfish only cause local reactions, whereas a few, such as the box jellyfish and the Portuguese man of war, can induce systemic toxicity that can very rapidly result in death from cardiovascular or neurological complications. The advice is to avoid swimming where the jellyfish may be present. Some very dangerous species of box jellyfish are no bigger than a thumb and swimmers may be completely unaware of their presence: they can sometimes kill a victim within minutes. In Australia an antivenom against box jellyfish has been introduced. Cardiopulmonary resuscitation should be performed and maintained as long as possible until medical help can be sought, as recovery may take place when the relatively short-lived venom has been inactivated in the body.

The problem for travellers is that they may be unaware of the local danger of swimming from certain beaches at particular times of the year. The Australian authorities are quite thorough in posting warnings to avoid swimming and travellers should take heed of these. There have been cases of certain Indonesian beaches where no such warnings were placed, resulting in fatalities amongst tourists.

Vinegar has been shown to relieve the stings of box jellyfish by inactivating the nematocytes, which are minute threads released from specialised cells in the jellyfish that can contain venom. However, for other species, including the Portuguese man of war, this treatment is ineffective and may even stimulate the nematocytes.[17] A full-body wet suit would offer good protection and other special 'stinger' swimsuits are also available.

Venomous fish, e.g. stonefish or weaver fish, are most likely to be encountered when wading in shallow waters, resulting in a sting to the foot or leg. These can be excruciatingly painful, sometimes warranting a nerve block using local anaesthetic. Some also advocate bathing the affected limb in hot water, as hot as the patient can bear without causing tissue damage, as the toxins are heat-labile. There is an argument against this approach due to the potential for hot water to cause further damage to the skin. For most species there is rarely any systemic complication. Sea snake fangs are generally too small to penetrate the skin deeply and they will not bite unless mishandled. There are a few species whose venom is known to cause severe neuromuscular complications with quite a high mortality, so contact with sea snakes should always be avoided.

Encounters with echinoderms (sea urchins) can leave very painful spines buried in the foot. Again, the venom in these spines is heat-labile and the hot-water immersion method described above can be tried. Otherwise small spines may be left and eventually reabsorbed into the body. Larger sea urchin spines may need to be removed surgically.

Snakes, scorpions and spiders

These have been considered as a group largely because the venom causes a true toxicity, rather than allergic reaction, sometimes indicating the use of specific antivenoms.

Spiders are generally not a great risk to the traveller. There are only a few potentially dangerous species, such as the funnel web and black widow species, that carry a neurotoxic venom, and fatal envenomations are extremely rare. This is because there is often too little venom actually passed during the bite. In many cases the actual bite can go unnoticed, only being apparent when a local skin reaction has developed. These reactions from some species of spider can be quite long-lasting, resulting in necrosis and considerable pain. It is generally a wise precaution for campers to check sleeping bags and footwear for the presence of spiders.

Similarly, scorpion stings are rarely fatal in adults, although because of their smaller body mass, they are a greater danger in children. Unlike a spider bite, the immediate pain felt would certainly be noticed, and pain is the chief and most distressing feature of a scorpion bite. The systemic symptoms are due to a generalised autonomic nervous stimulation caused by the venom, leading eventually to respiratory and cardiac failure. The best approach to treatment of systemic effects is using drugs that will block or reverse the effects of catacholamines released by the venom, including α-adrenergic blockers such as hydralazine or prazosin and calcium antagonists. Again, checking footware, clothes and bedding is advisable if scorpions are known to be present in a particular locality. Always avoid walking barefoot.

Snakes are more likely to be encountered by those who are working on field projects rather than the casual traveller or trekker. It is useful though for travellers to be aware of the first-aid options in the management of snake bites. There are two potential dangers from envenomation by snakes: local reactions that can produce quite severe tissue necrosis and pain and systemic toxicity. The range of systemic reactions will depend upon the species of snake and can include neurotoxicity, cardiotoxicity, bleeding or coagulation, shock, myotoxicity and renal failure. There are some species of snake whose venom tends to produce systemic reactions, and other species where local necrotic reactions are more common. It is not possible for most lay people to be aware of the particular dangers of the various species of snake, and the following general first-aid points should be adopted:

- Immobilising the effected limb is one of the first and most useful strategies. This will slow the spread of the venom until medical help can be sought. In some cases it may be wise to splint the limb and carry the patient to seek help. Take care to maintain the airway at all times. Keeping the patient calm is important, remembering that at least half of snake bites do not result in a serious envenoming. Also remember that effects of the venom may not appear for 24–48 hours, so close observation of the victim for a few days is strongly advised.

- A tight arterial tourniquet should *not* be used as this will cause serious complications by impeding blood flow. Instead the use of a crêpe bandage applied to the whole limb should be considered. This may act by slowing the flow of venom through the lymphatic system, reducing spread and onset of systemic symptoms while seeking medical help.[16] A potential disadvantage is that the venom may be held at the puncture sight, so worsening the skin damage and swelling. For this reason some experts do not advocate the use of a tight crêpe bandage.[17]

- For pain control, paracetamol and not aspirin or other non-steroidal anti-inflammatory drugs should be used. This is because snake venom has anticoagulant properties, contraindicating the use of the drugs.

- The various suction and other devices sold in snake bite kits have no proven value and may worsen local tissue damage by holding higher concentrations of venom at the puncture site. In all cases seek medical help and if possible take along the snake if it has been killed.

The other major consideration for treating snake bites is the potential use of an antivenom. In general travellers should be dissuaded from carrying their own antivenom unless there is someone present who is proficient and experienced in its use. It must be administered intravenously, ideally where there are intensive care facilities, and usually stored below 4°C. Anaphylactic reactions are not uncommon and in some cases the danger from the antivenom may outweigh the risks from the bite, and premedication with adrenaline has been advocated in some situations. The main circumstance where supply of antivenom may be indicated is if an expedition or group is travelling to an area with a known snake problem, planning to be working for some weeks or months on rural projects where local supply may be poor, and suitably experienced practitioners are available. If supply of antivenom at the destination is known to be good and reasonable transportation is available from the base camp, there may be no need to carry supplies. In some situations supplies may not be available. Some research is needed to identify the correct type of antivenom to be taken as these may be species-specific and this falls to good expedition planning. Probably of most use in such circumstances are the polyspecific types prepared to treat a range of venoms from snakes in the area being visited. The monospecific types however tend to be less antigenic. The antivenoms are much more efficient at reversing coagulation problems than neurotoxicity, for which anticholinesterases are sometimes effective.

Avoiding encounters with snakes involve common-sense measures: wearing boots and relatively thick trousers, taking care when lifting objects such as stones and using a torch when out at night.

Main points

1. All travellers should consider the following when preparing a medical and first-aid kit:

    *   Obtain a prescription for supplies of long-term medicines or treatments for infrequent but recurrent conditions that could cause problems.
    *   Purchase medicines in the UK if possible.
    *   Consider travel itinerary and activities.
    *   Discuss with a doctor the need for POMs for emergency use.
    *   Understand how to use the components of the travel kit.
    *   Package medicines in a manner that is suitable for travel and that satisfies legal requirements. If necessary, carry a letter from the doctor or a photocopy of the prescription.

- Consider appropriate first-aid and OTC products and malaria prophylaxis, where appropriate.

2.   Those in groups or expeditions:

- Ensure that a comprehensive base camp or truck kit is available and what items are for use by individuals.
- The main kit should be comprehensive and suitable for the destination, e.g. containing malaria standby treatment for malaria-endemic areas.
- A field kit should be available for smaller groups when travelling away from a base camp.
- All individuals should carry their own personal medicines and first-aid items.

3.   For bites and stings:

- Bites and stings that elicit mild local skin reactions can be managed using topical corticosteroid creams and oral antihistamines.
- Snake bite envenoming is best treated by immobilising the patient and rapid transfer to seek medical help. Splinting of the limb and use of a crêpe bandage may be useful in slowing the spread of venom.

Frequently asked questions

Am I likely to get into trouble if carrying OTC products containing codeine into another country?
The research conducted at King's College, discussed in the text, identified that most countries allow OTC-type medicines provided that it is in quantities for personal use. There are certain countries, e.g Mexico, that are notoriously erratic in their application of legislation and others, like Japan, which appear very restrictive in what is allowed. Anecdotal experience is that travellers rarely encounter problems with these medicines providing they are appropriately packaged and labelled.

Is it worth carrying antibiotics in my medical kit?
From the study conducted in the text it may be worthwhile considering for those on longer trips, e.g. 1 month, and where medical supplies may be poor or unreliable. The general advice is that such antibiotics should be taken under medical guidance.

If I decide to take antibiotics in my kit, which ones are best?
A quinolone seems to offer the broadest spectrum against pathogens encountered in travel, although Gram-positive activity may not be optimal.

In addition co-amoxiclav, erythromycin or a cepahalosporin could be considered. For certain destinations metronidazole or tinidazole may be useful.

I am on a tight budget. What is the minimum to include in my medical kit?
For first aid, plasters and an antiseptic, some tape and non-adherent dressing would be useful. Carry an analgesic and treatment for travellers' diarrhoea. In malaria-endemic areas take prophylaxis and in all areas where there are mosquito-borne diseases carry repellent.

I am going away for my gap-year to work on a project organised by a charitable organisation. What medical supplies do I need?
A good organisation will provide a main kit to be used by a group of people and advise on the contents of personal kits, although don't forget any regular medicines that you use.

I am worried about snake bites. Should I carry antivenom or a snake bite treatment kit?
The answer to both questions to most travellers will be *no*. In particular the kits which contain equipment to 'suck out' the venom should always be discouraged. For expeditions where there may be a need for antivenom it is appropriate to refer to a specialist centre.

References

1. Goodman P H, Kurtz K J, Carmichael J. Medical recommendations for wilderness travel: medical supplies and drug regimens. *Postgrad Med* 1985; 78: 107–115.
2. Sakmar T P. The traveller's medical kit. *Infect Dis Clin North Am* 1992; 6: 355–370.
3. Goodyer L I, Dawood R. Medicines and medical supplies for travel. In: Dawood R, ed. *Travellers' Health*, 3rd edn. Oxford: Oxford University Press, 1992: 573–582.
4. Taylor R B, Shakoor O, Behrens R H *et al*. Pharmacopoeial quality of drugs supplied by Nigerian pharmacies. *Lancet* 2001; 357: 1933–1936.
5. Deadly medicines warning issued by the World Health Organization. *Pharm J* 2001; 266: 208.
6. International Narcotics Control Board. *Annual Report of the INCB for 2000.* New York: United Nations Publications, 2000.
7. Deacon S P, McCulloch W J. Medical kits for business travellers. *J Soc Occup Med* 1990; 40; 103–104.
8. Webb J, Murdoch D A. Tropical ulcers after sports injuries. *Lancet* 1992; 339: 129–130.
9. Anon. Tropical ulcers. *Lancet* 1987; ii: 835–836.

10. Harper L H, Bettinger J, Dismukes R, Kozarsky P. The evaluation of the Coca-Cola Company travel health kit. *J Travel Med* 2002; 9: 244–266.
11. Revised indications for co-amoxiclav. *Curr Probl Pharmacovig* 1997; 23: 8.
12. Warrell D, Anderson S, eds. *Expedition Medicine*. London: Profile Books, 1998.
13. *Where There is no Doctor Series*. Oxford: Macmillan Press, 2002.
14. Ben Welch E, Gales B J. Use of stun guns for venomous bites and stings: a review. *Wilderness Environ Med* 2001; 12: 111–1171
15. Visscher P K, Vetter R S, Camazine S. Removing bee stings. *Lancet* 1996; 348: 301–302.
16. Theakston D G, Lalloo D G. Venomous bites and stings. In: Zuckerman J, ed. *Principles and Practice of Travel Medicine*. Chichester, UK: Wiley, 2001: 321–340.
17. Bodia M, Junghanss T. Envenoming and poisonings caused by animals. In: DuPont H L, Steffen R, eds. *Textbook of Travel Medicine and Health*, 2nd edn. Hamilton, Canada: BC Decker, 2001: 376–390.

Index

Page numbers in **bold** refer to main discussions in text, those in *italics* refer to figures, tables and boxes. Plates are indicated by Plate number.